ACUPUNCTURE
FROM SYMBOL TO
CLINICAL PRACTICE

ACUPUNCTURE
From Symbol to Clinical Practice

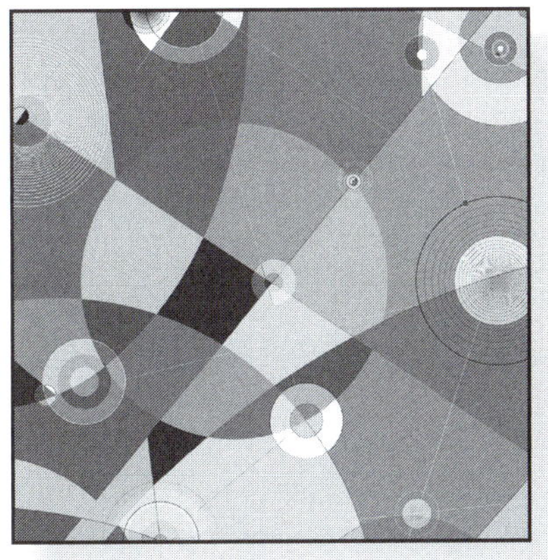

Jean-Marc Kespi

EASTLAND PRESS ▸ SEATTLE

Published by Eastland Press, Inc.
P.O. Box 99749
Seattle, WA 98139, USA
www.eastlandpress.com

Library of Congress Control Number: 2012954520
ISBN: 978-0-939616-79-4

2 4 6 8 10 9 7 5 3 1

Translation from the French by Dagmara Meijers-Troller and Sylviane Burner
Cover design by Gary Niemeier and Patricia O'Connor
Book design by Gary Niemeier

To Lisbeth, my close companion in life, who supported me throughout the writing process. She was my loyal interpreter during meetings with the editor and also a precious help in proofreading.

TABLE OF CONTENTS

FOREWORD

From 1974 through 1977 I shuttled back and forth between Berkeley and Paris, borrowing time from my day job in the emergency rooms and urgent care clinics of Berkeley and San Francisco to participate in the training offered by the French Medical Acupuncture Association. During the 1970s and 80s, Jean-Marc Kespi was president and the dominant of three driving personalities in the association. I had the good fortune to spend time attending his formal lectures and evening workshops, observing him in private practice, and watching him analyze patients and plan treatments at the monthly meetings of the dozen French acupuncture societies.

These were heady times for acupuncture in France. In the 1960s and early 70s, Albert Chamfrault and Nguyen Van Nghi's translations and teaching had generated a cadre of enthusiastic and dedicated acupuncture practitioners and teachers. A dozen of them took prominent roles in creating a second generation of acupuncture societies, each teacher following his special interest as this classical discipline was newly filtered through western perspectives. The society with which I was most allied, the French Medical Acupuncture Association, represented an ongoing juggle among the musculo-skeletal, energetic, and spiritualized purist interpretations of the available texts and techniques. Each approach was developed and promoted by a strong-willed and articulate teacher: Claude Roustan for musculoskeletal, Maurice Mussat for energetic, Jean-Marc Kespi for spiritualized purist.

The monthly meetings of this loose confederation of acupuncture societies took place in an overcrowded and smoke-filled auditorium at the Pasteur Institute. Several patients were presented in the morning, each one interviewed and examined by two or three leaders from different societies. The interstices between and after interviews—usually with the patients present—were filled with discussions comparing one approach with another. Afternoons turned into delightfully dramatic contests, where ego strength overrode rational debate, and none of the interviewing physicians was convinced to modify his approach. The finale always involved The Correct Analysis by Grand Master Nguyen Van Nghi. As I said, these were heady times, full of passion, hard work, scholarship, and extraordinary creativity.

Jean-Marc Kespi's approach to patient analysis and treatment, in public forums and private practice, consistently involved his search for the perfect single point or two to resolve the patient's health issues: physical, emotional, and spiritual. It is this very search that Kespi explores in *Acupuncture: From Symbol to Clinical Practice.* He does this by touring through important points along each channel, exposing his special understanding and appreciation for their qualities and capacities. Through brief case reports, he illustrates his relationship with the points, and the logic he uses to select just a point or two for each patient. The case reports give muscle and coherence to the theoretical skeleton of his approach. They reveal his observations and interpretations of his patients' problems, and his decisions about which factor or combination of factors define the core issue to be addressed. And then, which point, and why.

This is the work of a seasoned practitioner and teacher writing in his mature years, confident in his knowledge and the accuracy of his approach. The reflections on his cases sometimes read like a diary being generously opened for his students and their students, to share the intimate experiences of his extended family: his acupuncture points and his patients. He honors his fundamental principle throughout: to respond to the body's needs without preconception or anticipation, searching rationally and intuitively for the best points at the moment of each treatment session.

Acupuncture: From Symbol to Clinical Practice is not a book for beginners. Rather, it is a book for experienced practitioners who are still engaged in the quest for greater understanding and integration of the traditional tenets of acupuncture. It is unlikely that many readers will achieve the level of purity and confidence to select but one point in a treatment. Reading his synthesis of acupuncture theory, however, and studying the points and cases from his perspective, gives you a reference framework for reflecting on your own points and patients, building your own repertory, and expanding the thought processes and intuitive skills that you bring to your patients.

—JOSEPH M. HELMS, MD
President, Helms Medical Institute
Berkeley, California

PREFACE

Introduction

The Savage Mind (1963), by Claude Lévi-Strauss, maintains that the same logic underlies every thought, whether "primitive," dressed in magic and myth, or "civilized," based upon science and its technologies. This knowledge relies upon the work of ancient Chinese wise men despite the perception by some that their intelligence, vision, and logic are in some ways "simplistic." Simply because their vision and knowledge are different from ours does not make them any less valid.

Traditional Chinese medicine must be viewed with this in mind. This approach is illustrated by stories about Bian Que dating from the second century B.C.E. As of the second and third centuries C.E., works such as the *Inner Classic, Classic of Difficulties,* and *Discussion of Cold Damage* reveal a medical doctrine and cosmology that demonstrate that this medicine is not merely a collection of more or less magical recipes. The theories and concepts of this medicine have been further refined and developed over subsequent centuries, reflected in such important works from the Ming dynasty as the *Great Compendium of Acupuncture* and the *Comprehensive Outline of the Materia Medica.* Development continued unabated to the present, not only in East Asia, but all over the world.

Having completed my medical studies with great enthusiasm, my career began in 1962 as a general practitioner, the same year that I discovered acupuncture and began the study of Chinese medicine, a second type of medicine. At a time when acupuncture was often readily dismissed as archaic poetry, I had the privilege of studying Soulié de Morant's theories and of frequent interactions with Chamfrault, Nguyen Van Nghi, and Jean Choain. At any given moment they would punctuate their scholarly analysis of acupuncture texts with the same question, "Why?", intimating that there was something important to be understood there, a different view of life to be grasped, relentlessly urging towards a deeper understanding. I was immediately enthralled by this approach to medicine where you must observe, listen, palpate, and smell, while at the same time it permitted me to remain loyal to the clinical medicine that I had learned during my conventional training.

Gradually, I came more and more to appreciate the depth and validity of the Chinese tradition, which has not only considerably enriched my medical practice, but also altered my perspective on life, in particular recognizing the inter-connectedness among all living beings.

Purpose of This Work

This book has been written to transmit my understanding of acupuncture and Chinese conceptions of health and disease to English-speaking practitioners whose training is primarily based on textbooks derived from the conventional understanding of this material in modern-day China. My own perspective, based on the study of texts, learning from my above mentioned masters, and my training and experience is quite different. Consequently, this book will only treat concepts that lead either directly or indirectly to effective therapeutic applications, and will focus on those in which my own understanding differs from the conventional wisdom in modern China and acupuncture as practiced in the English-speaking world. I will specifically describe the manner that I use points in my everyday practice, through numerous case histories that illustrate their use and their efficacy.

My Path in Acupuncture

In December of 1962 I attended my first course of acupuncture, "Yin Yang," given by Jean-Claude Darras. From the beginning I found myself simultaneously both in another world and at home. This remains true today, except that regular immersion in the medicine, culture, and traditions of China has allowed me now to feel at home in both worlds. Not being born nor having grown up in China, I realized that I would never be a traditional Chinese doctor. On the other hand, being an outsider provided me with a different, but no less useful, perspective on traditional Chinese medicine and allows me to ask questions that only an outsider would ask.

In 1964, Chamfrault published the first translation of the *Inner Classic* in French, along with the groundbreaking *Traité of Médecine Chinoise*.[1] In these books he integrated acupuncture with the entire sphere of Chinese medicine, which includes manual therapy, herbal therapy and diet, relating all of them to cosmology.

In the early 1970s, Chamfrault introduced us to another major influence, Nguyen Van Nghi, who provided us with numerous French translations of other texts of Chinese medicine, usually with the help of Trung Yi Hoc. Van Nghi also helped us understand other tools for acupuncture practice, for example the study of the secondary channels. In this way he introduced supplementary rationality and logic to this medicine. Unfortunately, Chamfrault died around this time, but Van Nghi's writings expanded, enriched, and deepened our understanding of this medicine and its clinical practice. These two masters confirmed my belief that acupuncture is in and of itself an authentic and effective medicine.

As acupuncture achieved wider acceptance in France, a movement was launched which generated additional translations and more in-depth approaches to the medicine. The European School of Acupuncture (École Européenne d'Acupuncture) was founded in the late 70s by C. Larre, E. Rochat de la Vallée, and J. Schatz to encourage the translation and in-depth study of commentaries of medical and Daoist texts. Their analyses, and especially those of Père Larre, have always particularly inspired me. Chamfrault, Nguyen Van Nghi, and Larre were not only masters of sinology and acupuncture, but were also masters of life. All three helped me understand the depth and beauty of the traditional Chinese vision of life which is integral to the understanding of acupuncture.

In the 80s I was fortunate to study *taiji* with Gu Meicheng. This concrete experience of *taiji* allowed me to personnally get in touch with the reality of qi. It has also given me insight into the importance of the concept of "emptiness" in Chinese culture, as well as its place in the art of calligraphy and in the practice of acupuncture.

Influenced by their views, I have come to an understanding of Chinese medicine's vision about the structures and functions of the universe, and of all living beings, including humans. Chinese tradition asserts that there is a natural order of life, both celestial and terrestrial, and that all life—human, animal, plant, mineral, cosmic— is governed by the same laws, which are reflected in their structures as well as in their functions and relationships. This natural order is expressed in a symbolic language. Examples include heaven/humans/earth, water/fire, hard/soft, and the resonances of certain numbers.

As is often the case in the traditional sphere, symbols (象 *xiang*), myths and rites (禮 *li*) act as intermediaries between the symbolically "celestial" laws and their symbolically "terrestrial" manifestations. This has been true since the beginning of Chinese civilization, establishing, for example, relationships between the descriptions of earth and the human being as well as those between the functions of the human body and the government of the idealized Chinese empire. When we refer to this vision we are on a "celestial" level, not a "terrestrial," anatomical, or historical level. Thus it is unnecessary to describe terrestrial manifestations, such as the precise anatomy of the viscera; they express in symbolic language the celestial laws governing the function of the universe at all levels. These principles, establishing relationships between the macrocosm and the microcosm, between the human body and the idealized empire, have been held since the beginning of Chinese civilization.

These theories are discussed repeatedly in this book. For example, in the *Classic of Difficulties*, No. 42, it is said that the Small Intestine makes 16 turns to the left of the navel and the Large Intestine makes 16 turns to the right. The ancient Chinese acupuncturists knew their anatomy better than this; this is not a description of the physical anatomy but rather a symbolic language. Briefly, from a Daoist perspective on the body,[2] the Intestines are associated with "territory": the number four refers to boundaries. By using the number 16 (4 x 4) they tell us, as we will see later on, that the Intestines are the boundaries of all our territories, on physical, family, and professional levels. The *Classic of Difficulties*, Nos. 36 and 39, states that there is a pair of Kidneys, but fails to mention that there are two Lungs. Once again, this is a symbolic, not anatomical, description of the body: the number one symbolically refers to heaven, the number two to the earth. These symbols link the Kidneys to Earth with procreation (the meeting of male and female), and the Lung to Heaven, in connection with qi, which is the origin of all life.

Thus the practitioner must ask himself how to apply the various symbolic categories such as heaven/earth, water/fire, and heaven/human/earth to the human body. How does this help us to understand physiology and pathology? Also, since Chinese medicine presents an analogy between the empire and the human body, to which theoretical and practical understandings will this lead us? In fact, this book will establish that this symbolic vision has important clinical and therapeutic applications. The genius of Chinese medical tradition is that it demonstrates the continuity of this vision reaching from a symbol to a specific diagnostic and therapeutic action, to the inserting of a needle in a precise point of the body to relieve or heal, depending on the case.

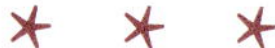

This medicine actually reflects a structure, a subtle architecture, where each component resonates with the primary and secondary channels and emerges to the level of the points. Thus, each is understood as the surface emergence of one or more functions and also as a means to act upon it; each point therefore responds to one or more of the functions described in the fundamental classics of acupuncture.

This vision is eminently practical as it affects at a very basic level how to use the points. For example, when studying any structure of the body, such as the Lung, I ask myself, which point controls its descent, its dissemination, its clarification, its relation to the autumn harvest? There are many similar questions that we must ask to reflect the clinical realities encountered on a daily basis. Which point records the events of adolescence, if that was a difficult period? Which points govern the diaphragm? Which point raises the qi of the Kidneys? Which points control the movement of the qi, yin, and yang to each part of the body? (These last have been named the barrier points.) This type of inquiry must continue at every step in the study of the physiology of Chinese medicine.

One interesting discovery during my own specific study of the points was the frequent ineffectiveness in my practice of formulas and treatments based on the five phases along with the main sets of points that are used within this framework. Thus, for over 35 years, I have researched and studied other points and their usages. As each living being is unique, our patients and their issues cannot be summarized in five categories and their relevant points. It is only by utilizing a variety of combinations of the hundreds of acupuncture points that we can treat each patient based on their individuality.

I continue to study the points in this context with the help of sinological colleagues such as Larre and Rochat de la Vallée; with the translations of Andres, Milsky, Guillaume Mach Chieu, Duron, and Laville-Mery; and with the help of the works of the Association Française d'Acupuncture and the dictionaries published by the Institut Ricci. An understanding of the names of these points, and their related signs and symptoms, can help us to appreciate more deeply their roles, and thereby use them more effectively in the treatment of patients. Through this study I have gradually come to understand that, in reality, there are no strictly local points.

In the same spirit, rather than treating the symptom, I find that acupuncture is most effective when it addresses the whole person. Consequently, it is often necessary to treat the disequilibrium found at the root level in order to make their clinical signs disappear. It is necessary to try to detect what the patient offers us, their somatic and psychological suffering, their traumas and difficulties, in order to get to their uniqueness and above all to understand what they need from us—whether or not they are able to express their needs consciously.

An investigation into all of their signs and symptoms, their history, their own attempts to understand what has created their suffering and causes it to continue, is necessary. In each case there are two or three troubled mechanisms that are at the root of all the symptoms and disorder, which should be able to explain their origin. This indicates a plan requiring few needles, to correct the original disturbances and disrupt the vicious circle that has arisen in response, which has prevented the person from healing by themselves. Fewer sessions are necessary, thereby reducing inappropriate harassment of the human body. The goal is simply to assist the body to recall the normal mode of functioning that it knew before, but has since forgotten.

The practitioner must work with the patient to trust in their own capacity to heal and to be restored, in both the somatic and psychological realms. This perspective enables the patient's own healing mechanisms, and does not attempt to substitute for them; we intervene only when the processes have passed beyond the limits of their own abilities to restore health. While this methodology contradicts the prevailing medical perspective in the West, it is in accordance with the spirit of Chinese medicine. The character 治 (zhi) means to rule or govern but also to treat or cure; it was used to describe how the legendary Yu the Great built the world as the Chinese knew it after the great flood. This means that each human being must develop him- or herself, and that all that we practitioners can do is to help the patient deal with their problems.

Let me give an example as an illustration. First, it is important to clarify one point. As often as possible, theoretical information is illustrated with case histories. I always choose exemplary cases. This approach runs the risk of making acupuncture seem miraculous and does not reflect the uncertainties and trial and error involved in clinical research, nor the need that often arises, in serious or chronic cases, for combining acupuncture with other therapies such as conventional allopathic medicine, homeopathy, osteopathy, or psychoanalysis. This is because the question that must be asked regarding each patient is: What are the best treatments available today, in view of our state of knowledge in various fields?

❖ Case History

A man came into my office with an acute debilitating pain that was centered in his left sacroiliac joint and radiated to the lateral side of the lower extremity. This problem had been labeled as sciatica. After my examination, I diagnosed the problem as being due to a blockage on the left, of the leg *jue yin* channel (Liver channel), and treated it by needling LR-11. The Liver corresponds to *jue yin,* wood, and the ethereal soul (魂 *hun*), which all speak to the continuity of circulation in much the same manner as the sap of the tree goes from its origin in the roots to the ends of the branches with flexibility and ease, and without interruption or discontinuity.

Furthermore the patient told me that he was born of an unknown father; he does not know his own son, his wife having left him when the baby was one year old. I tell myself that the attack on *jue yin* wood reflects a profound disruption at the level of the continuity of his genealogical lineage. This has weakened this channel and permitted a local blockage of LR-11. Based on this diagnosis I needle only one point, CV-18, the node of the *jue yin,* as this to me is particularly relevant for continuity in the transmission of ascending to descending. Forty-eight hours later the sacroiliac pain and radiating sciatica were gone.

Place of Acupuncture in Western Medical Practice

My views on the proper place of acupuncture derive from my own experiences as a physician. I believe that most of these comments are relevant to all practitioners of acupuncture.

AN OVERVIEW OF THE ESSENTIALS

The physician must determine, for each patient, which treatments will be the most effective, according to current knowledge. This might be conventional allopathic medicine, surgery, osteopathy, analytic psychotherapy or acupuncture, either alone or in combination with one of these other therapies.

The primary goal (and this is a return to the spirit of the "old-fashioned" clinical medicine that I learned in the 1950s) is to provide each patient with support but not to take over for them, to trust in their own capacities to return to somatic and psychic equilibrium, and to intervene more intensely only when their physical and/or mental resources have been exceeded.

The fundamental intent of acupuncture is to help the body remember how to function harmoniously, when, for a variety of reasons, it has lost this innate knowledge. Acupuncture is frequently indicated for both acute and chronic disease; it can also contribute to the treatment of critical illnesses, for example, by improving tolerance to chemotherapy or radiation therapy, etc. I must reiterate here that the aim of acupuncture is, to the greatest extent possible, to treat the patient as a whole, rather than just to treat a disease.

Contraindications

The primary contraindications for acupuncture are medical or surgical emergencies, since any loss of time can be fatal: consequently, it is crucial to know how to diagnose these conditions. Acupuncture is also contraindicated as the primary form of therapy for certain patients with serious or advanced physical or mental illnesses, if it interferes with other therapies. In such cases it is imperative to explain to the patient the place and limitations of our activities, for example, in the case of cancers or advanced infections, psychotic delirium or decompensation, and not allow them to believe that acupuncture is a panacea that can do everything. This does not mean it has no place in the treatment of such patients, because acupuncture can relieve a large number of symptoms, within limits. Anticoagulant treatments are not a contraindication because, since the acupuncture point is empty by definition, needling, if done accurately, should not encounter any vessels, nerves, tendons, etc.

Utility

How is a practitioner to decide whether acupuncture, alone or in combination, has a place in a given patient's treatment? First of all, acupuncture must be considered in relation to other possible therapies; to do this the practitioner must have a very broad grasp of what is available and a good grounding in conventional medical knowledge. Also, the better the practitioner understands acupuncture and the more experience they have, the better they will be able to utilize this form of therapy. Another important factor is the rational, as well as intuitive, understanding that we have of each patient; we all know that some patients are easier to understand than others, often depending on the quality of the relationship between practitioner and patient. Some examples follow.

No known diagnosis or effective treatment despite numerous investigations

Acupuncture is clearly indicated in such cases, often as the first line of treatment; it may even provide a diagnosis in "idiopathic" cases where Western medicine could not, thanks to its unique perspective.

Reversible organic lesions

Acupuncture can be used to help reduce or eliminate certain lesions such as fibromas, polyps, and cysts as an adjunct to any other appropriate overall treatment. The idea is to promote local circulation of qi in order to dissolve or reduce the mass in question. For example, I have had some good results with polyps in the nose or on the vocal cords.

❖ Case History

A woman, 46, had a leiomyoma that had been detected several years ago and that grew considerably after she learned that her husband had cancer of the left lung; it was the size of a grapefruit, which caused discomfort and urinary problems, so it needed to be surgically removed. This could only be done by laparotomy, and, because of its size, vaginal removal was impossible. GV-5, which releases and allows the qi to rise from the Kidneys and pelvis, considerably reduced the size of this leiomyoma, permitting a vaginal approach to treatment.

Note that while this may appear to be a local treatment, this point is concerned with fear and impotence through its connection with the Kidneys. Despite appearances and practices, there are no points with purely local effects, as all are rooted at a psycho-emotional level. Therefore, as we will see below, there are in reality no purely local treatments in acupuncture.

Irreversible organic lesions

Acupuncture can still often contribute to reducing pain or inflammation. In such cases the treatment is general, and specific to each patient: there is no all-purpose formula. Likewise, in certain serious psychiatric conditions such as schizophrenia, bipolar disorder, and obsessive-compulsive disorder, acupuncture can play an adjunctive role.

It may also serve as a means of diagnosis. If an organic lesion is associated with a symptom, it can be used to determine whether the lesion is responsible for the symptom.

❖ Case Histories

— For two months, a 32-year-old female presented with intense sciatica affecting the posterior aspect of the lower right limb. Due to an insufficient response to conservative allopathic treatment, and to the presence of a herniated intervertebral disk at L-5/S-1, surgery was presented as indicated. Given the association of this posterior (leg *tai yang*) pain with medial thigh pain, combined with numbness of the big toe on the right foot, sharp pain in right LR-11, the absence of neurological signs of compression of the root L5-S1, a moderate Lasègue sign and the small size of the disk problem on imaging studies, I decided to attempt acupuncture treatment. Needling of LR-11 and, in consideration of the combination of other *jue yin* Liver signs, BL-47, the gate of the ethereal soul, relieved the pain in three sessions following a 36-hour aggravation of the sciatica after the first treatment.

— A physician friend consulted for a sciatica of the same order combined with a severe herniated intervertebral disc. My treatment caused a distinct worsening of the condition for 48 hours with no ensuing improvement. There was no further question about which intervention was appropriate.

My experience has told me that, faced with any situation like this, I need to perform one or two acupuncture sessions in order to distinguish between a case of compression and inflammation from a different etiology. This diagnostic role of acupuncture is very important clinically.

Functional problems

In cases with no known organic, psychological, biochemical or other lesion, acupuncture is clearly indicated. The question is then: should it be used alone or in combination with other treatment? The age of the condition, the other related symptoms, the context, and the patient's overall life, etc., will help us decide. Logic is important in these circumstances. One should neither be too timid nor too aggressive.

Therapies should not be superimposed

This principle is extremely important. The patient should not be allowed to receive (except in emergencies) acupuncture and osteopathic treatments, homeopathic treatments (especially classical homeopathy) or massages in the same week. For example, a massage received shortly after an acupuncture treatment can markedly reduce its effectiveness by inadvertently working on certain points that are antagonistic to the ones used by the acupuncturist. Even when these treatments are complementary, it is important to allow acupuncture or osteopathy or other methods enough time to work and find their place. Furthermore, the elapsed time gives us a chance to get a better idea of what every therapy does: this is important in diagnosis and in the subsequent treatment. This time will also allow for a better interpretation of the classic interview question: "Has anything different or new occurred since the last session?"

The one important exception is acupuncturists working in a hospital unit. They need to participate in the unit's therapeutic and diagnostic activities as they should be able to contribute to the treatment of both acute and chronic syndromes by attenuating pain, and by stimulating the patients' natural capacities of defense and of somatic and psychological recovery. The acupuncturist may also help patients tolerate any required allopathic treatments. In preoperative situations, acupuncture can help reduce bleeding, improve healing and diminish subsequent pain. In the postoperative stage, it can alleviate a variety of discomforts, such as hiccups, pain, spasms, insomnia, etc. For a number of patients, the acupuncturist can also offer a Chinese medical diagnosis, which is particularly helpful for those cases where modern biomedicine has none, as we shall see in a number of case histories described in this book.

I would like to thank all the people who took the time to teach me, particularly A. Chamfrault, C. Larre, and Nguyen Van Nghi. I would also thank my friends in the French Association of Acupuncture from whose translations, lectures, and practices I have learned much. Their attitude, enthusiasm, and affection have continually inspired me. I would also thank Joe Helms, who has written the Foreword, and whom I hold in high esteem and affection. The work of the editors at Eastland Press helped me refine my message for an anglophone audience and is greatly appreciated.

CHAPTER ONE

INDISPENSABLE PRELIMINARIES

THESE ARE CONCEPTS WHICH, although further developed below, need to be stated at the beginning, as they underpin our approach to the subject.[1] There are two fundamental differences in the approaches of the West and China to understanding life and the universe that are necessary to understand in order for us to properly utilize Chinese medicine.

- There are two ways of looking at what makes light and matter. As the famous Nobel-winning French scientist Louis de Broglie described it in the 1920s, one is based on particles and the other on waves or vibrations. From this perspective we can see that modern biomedicine focuses more on the particle aspect of reality, while Chinese medicine emphasizes the vibrational aspect.

- As the sinologist François Jullien has noted, "classical Chinese has no verb 'to be.'"[2] Unlike the West, where the Judeo-Christian tradition has focused above all else on being and the relationship between the human and the divine, in China there was much less concern with the details of individualized being and much more on the relationships that make up the life of a being. The focus is on the relations of humans with the other beings around them, the cosmos, and the laws that govern these associations. A recently published book by Michel Bitbol, a researcher into the philosophy of science, posits that this approach is on the cutting edge of modern science. He writes, "Contemporary physics is less and less about things and more and more about relationships. ... How to understand relationships that pre-exist between objects or the properties that unite them?"[3]

Given this approach to Chinese medicine from a primarily symbolic perspective, when I refer to a traditional Chinese understanding of the body, I will generally choose translations that are as far as possible from precise anatomical terms.

Yin and Yang

> *"All the world knows beauty*
>
> *but if that becomes beautiful*
>
> *this become ugly.*
>
> *All the world knows good*
>
> *but if that becomes good*
>
> *this becomes bad."*

This is the warning in Chapter 2 of the *Daodejing*.[4] This principle of duality tells us that everything in the universe is *both* yin *and* yang, and not yin *or* yang. Each thing *and* its opposite (not *or* its opposite) inevitably coexist. It is Heraclitus' "To be *and* not to be", which is both the same *and* not the same, rather than Hamlet's "To be *or* not to be." Thus all of these pairs (beautiful and ugly, big and small, pure and impure, etc.) are in us to be explored, known and recognized both in ourselves and in others. From this we understand that it is necessary to simultaneously utilize both the yin and the yang of everything, including seeing the world as made up of both particles and vibrations and also utilizing both Western and Chinese approaches to medicine. Yin-yang is a principle of duality in its very definition as it involves duality and exchange, distinction and collaboration.

We can see this in the coexistence and the succession of inhalations and exhalations, day and night, contractions and expansions, movement and rest, heat and cold, inside and outside, masculine and feminine, fullness and emptiness, noise and silence, and so on. It reflects the inescapable duality of life. Whatever the function, structure, relationship or parameter considered, always and everywhere, two opposite and complementary aspects coexist. It inevitably gives two sides to the same reality, as the original concept of yin-yang related to two sides of the same hill.

Yin-yang is also a principle of alternation (inhaling and exhaling), of exchange (masculine and feminine), of transformation of the one into the other (day and night). It stresses the concerted action between these two elements: it is an exchange in which, in turn, one gives in to the other. As a principle of dialogue, union, marriage, it shows that the only purpose of distinction is to act in concert, unite and marry. Any opposition is necessarily relative and reversible; its goal is reunion. This is fundamental in our daily lives: it is permissible to separate only to reunite.

Yin-yang is a life lesson, a lesson of relativity, tolerance and prudence. It is a tool for learning about oneself and others. It induces the absence of judgment because we are all, without exception, built on the same contradictions. Life makes one aspect more visible at times while the less visible aspects are still present. We understand—and this is something that we take as fundamental in our everyday life—that the concept of yin-yang makes it impossible to truly judge the intrinsic value of a human being based on what one observes at any particular time, as we are made up of all the dualities inherent in life: the large and the small, the transient and the immutable, light and shade, the beautiful and the ugly, the pure and the impure ... which is everyone's lot, without exception, regardless of appearances. Especially because there is no hierarchy between yin and yang, since one is not superior or inferior to the other, their relationship is what matters.

Qi is the Difference in Chinese Medicine

Before discussing physiology and therapy any further, it is important to study the concept of qi. One of the merits of Chinese tradition is that it emphasizes and bases its theories on universal concepts like yin and yang, emptiness, etc., as well as defining an original reality known as qi. "All is qi." The word qi cannot be translated without betraying its basic essence. We will try here to examine what qi is from its various aspects.

Qi (氣) is the "vapor, air, breath, that which animates the human body, the most subtle of elements entering into the composition of all things, attitudes, anger, scents, or feelings."[5] Etymologically, qi consists of the "vapors that rise and form the layers of clouds above"; here, they are "rising from a hot, cooked grain."[6]

Qi, which animates and gives substance, is the mechanism by which a being emerges, takes form, and acquires a palpable, visible and perceptible appearance. Qi is linked to incarnation, to the process of taking form. Could it perhaps be in-*form*-ation? In any case, it is certainly trans-*form*-ation. When it examines living forms, Chinese medicine says that everything is qi, because it is with qi that a living being manifests, becomes perceptible: "The life of humans is the assembling of qi. When qi assembles there is life. When it disperses, there is death." (*Zhuangzi*, Chapter 22)

Qi is also the qi of the atmosphere, the air, odors, the breath of respiration that we inhale and exhale and that circulates, animates, constitutes and transforms life; that is, all that enables a visible, incarnate, and manifest being to continue to live. It is because this unique, original qi differentiates into the required infinite forms that it can manifest and maintain life, breath, blood and bodily fluids, yin and yang organs—in short, all of the structures and functions required for life.

Qi is important because everything that we have experienced since the time of conception, our pain, suffering, conflicts and joys, is written in our body, in different places for each one, depending on the type of aggression or emotion involved, the time it occurred and our hereditary weaknesses. Each of these effects, through excess or repetition, results in an obstruction of the circulation of qi and causes physical or emotional pain: this is the origin of disease.

Acupuncture addresses those locations of the body where the qi is blocked or obstructed and where its attendant suffering is located. After a successful acupuncture treatment that causes the qi to circulate more normally, the suffering is no longer attached to the area, and while the scars remain, they are far less painful. Moreover, when the suffering is released this way, and thereby detached from the body, it becomes more accessible to the psyche, possibly to psychotherapeutic processes.

Introduction to Symbolic Language

Chinese medicine, like any other traditional medicine, is based on a symbolic language. It is only through its study that we will grasp the original vision of man this tradition offers. Moreover, to go deeper in the understanding of Chinese medicine, including its clinical practice, it is necessary to delve deeper and deeper into the understanding of its symbolic foundations. In Chinese, the main word for a symbol is *xiang* (象), which means "symbol, to symbolize, image, looking like, to represent, appearance, elephant." The commentary adds: "It is the footprint of the elephant."[7] The elephant is no longer here; it is invisible. But its footprint tells us that he once existed and went this way. A very long time ago, before the sky or earth existed, there were only symbols *(xiang)* and no form *(xing 形)*.[8] The symbol, the archetype, the image is previous to the form, because *xiang*, the symbol, and *xing*, the form, are an indissoluble couple. Thus the symbols are the foundation of the life of the many, manifesting themselves under the forms.

Chinese medicine posits that there is an order to life, that some laws, some rules govern us. Symbols are intermediaries between these rules and laws and the infinite manifestations, forms, mechanisms and structures of life. Thus, the symbol, the mediation, links the visible and the invisible, the perceptible and the imperceptible: it links the mechanisms and the structures of the living to the archetypes and the laws that founded them.

On a symbolic level, Chinese medicine tells us that the human body is "the footprint of the archetypes." The clinical interest of symbolic language is both diagnostic and therapeutic, for it allows us to link mechanisms and structures that, *a priori*, have nothing to do with one another. Here is a clinical example of how these concepts can be utilized.

❖ Case History

A tall, slender, elegant 40-year-old woman who, at times, suffered from diarrhea with an intense burning intestinal and urinary pain came to my practice. She also had a very intense heat sensation in the gums, the tongue, the palate, and the feet. The symptoms were therefore located in the lower part of the face, the abdomen and the legs. The only common medical references were the three earth areas, located at the lower part of the head and trunk, and of the lower limbs. The attacks of diarrhea, recurring twice a month, had started at puberty;

at that time, she could not but face the reality of her own body and femininity. "What are your roots?" I asked. "I do not have any. I have no flat. I live in a hotel. I am a foreigner; I have no country of my own. I'm only passing through. There is no place where I feel at home," she explained. Without a body, without a home, without roots, I can understand the suffering of the earth areas. ST-27, in the lower abdomen, each side of CV-5, which is a foundation landmark, reduced the intensity of the attacks and their frequency.

CHAPTER TWO

INTRODUCTIONS

Introduction to the Channels of Acupuncture

There are three ways of studying these, which we will describe below.

■ Channels (*jing* 經) and Vessels (*mai* 脈)

Jing is translated as a "road from north to south, channel, acupuncture channel, constant rule, warp (as opposed to woof), or canonical books."[1] All of these things—the rule, law, warp, and canonical books—transmit fundamental truths, the immutable laws. To understand what *jing* means in the Chinese tradition, one should read Robinet's book *Méditation taoïste,* because what she writes about *jing* (books) can be applied to *jing* (channels), as it is the same character. "*Jing* reveals the laws of the world, *jing* is the path, the way; it guides, shows, reveals. … *Jing* are the foundations of the world; originally, they coexisted with the original Breath and were produced at the same time as the original Beginning; … they are manifestations of the *dao*: it is thanks to the *dao* that *jing* were brought into life, and it is thanks to *jing* that the *dao* was revealed."[2] This passage stresses how archaic, how cosmic the *jing* are. But they need to be embodied, and this is what the *mai* do.

Mai are their medium. They embody them and give them colors. *Mai* means "seam, vein, mountain range, genealogical lineage, vessels, veins of a leaf, pulse; it is a powerful vital force (it moves mountains), which has a direction, which is oriented (seam, vein, mountain range, genealogical lineage)."[3] The *mai* are connected to the Heart: "The Heart rules the *mai;* the *mai* are the abode of the spirit" (*Divine Pivot,* Chapter 8). *Mai* are the medium of *jing,* they give colors to each being, according to their essential nature, and according to *xing* (形), their specificity of form.

■ Warp (*jing* 經) and Woof (*luo* 絡)

The channels can also be seen as the warp and woof of a weaving loom. The warp is made up of the *jing,* which transmit laws, essential rules, fundamental information, for we have seen that Chinese medicine takes for granted that there is such a thing as a natural order in life with laws ruling us all. The symbols are intermediaries between these laws and the infinite manifestations, forms, mechanisms and structures of life. Trinh Xuan Thuan speaks of "the incredibly precise regulation of the physical constants of the universe, which allows massive stars to be born and heavy elements necessary to life and consciousness to be produced."[4] The woof is the shuttle that goes through the warp and corresponds to the connecting vessels (*luo*); they rule all the relationships of a being from the inside to the outside, at each and every moment. This is an important feature because, from a Chinese perspective, human beings rely above all on relationships.

The channels and vessels consist of three groups:

- The six main channels and their subdivisions
- The eight extraordinary vessels
- The sixteen connecting vessels

The connecting vessels are not considered channels (*jing*) because they are the fabric of the cloth, which is linked to the shuttle that weaves around the direct chains that are the channels.

■ Vibrations and Resonances

All of the information, structures and functions that make up life reverberate in the channels, which I see as having a vibratory nature. As noted above, there are two ways of looking at life, one vibratory and the other particulate, just like the natures of light and matter. It seems to me that Chinese medicine has a vibratory perspective whereas Western medicine and sciences have an approach that emphasizes particles. Therefore, all the activities of the body and the psyche impact the channel system so that it can receive information and in turn coordinate and regulate.

Introduction to the Points of Acupuncture

The most commonly used word in Chinese for an acupuncture point is *xue* (穴), which originally referred to a cavern or a dwelling dug in the earth.[5] In a mountain, a cavern is the empty space where exterior winds and underground air streams gather, where the qi of heaven and the qi of the earth join and transform themselves. It is most probable that the specific anatomic structures of an acupuncture point can never be revealed, for they embody emptiness; the fullness of the point is pathological and linked to the obstruction of qi.

Symbolically enough, there are approximately 365 acupuncture points, as many as the days in a year, even if their number changes as time passes. In fact, most books describe 361 points: 218 on the six main yang channels, 91 on the six main yin channels, and 52 on the Governing and Conception vessels. All the principal points are located on the 12 main channels and the two median vessels.

We do not yet know the mechanism of action of acupuncture. It seems very likely that it must work through the neuroendocrine systems, but we cannot explain the diversity of the effects of millions of different possible combinations. We must look to the Chinese tradition and return to the concept of qi. Qi linked to form, in the event of a form, in the appearance of a form, is for me in-*form*-ation. A point is the emergence on the exterior of one or more sets of information and these reflect the functions of the organism as understood by Chinese medicine. From the perspective of Chinese medicine, all the information that ensures the functioning of our lives emerges at the acupuncture points. Thus each one is a focal point of information of various types and thereby has a specific set of functions.

For example, ST-25, lateral to the navel, is at the same time a reunion in the body of heaven (corresponding to above the navel) and earth (below the navel); home to both the ethereal and corporeal souls; the alarm point of the Large Intestine; and, according to the *Classic of Difficulties,* No. 31, the alarm point of the middle burner. The problem is to know how to choose among these four actions. In the same vein, HM-6 is both the connecting point of the hand *jue yin* channel and the opening point of the Yin Linking vessel. CV-5 (*shi men* or "stone gate") is the alarm point of the Triple Burner and also a point that relates to the gestational envelopes, both of which are associated with the maintenance of our lives and our lineage. Furthermore, by its location it mediates between the primal qi (*yuan qi*) of the Kidneys that emerges at CV-4 and the qi that the body produces that is related to CV-6, the "sea of qi" (*qi hai*).

Both CV-5 and GV-5 are mediators and are always in dialogue. As the channel point following GV-4 (*ming men* or "the gate of the mandate of our life"), GV-5 makes the qi of the Kidneys ascend toward the other yin organs, starting with the Spleen. The Kidneys are the roots of the five yin organs and are tied to the prenatal *(xian tian,* literally "former heaven") and the Spleen is connected with the postnatal *(hou tian,* literally "later heaven") at GV-6. The point below GV-4, GV-3, is linked to the Large Intestine, the Kidneys and the gestational envelopes, and grasps the qi that is propelled downward by the Lung via CV-20. What wonderful interlocking architecture!

Moreover, we have seen that for Chinese medicine all kinds of pathologies are the result of an obstruction of the circulation of qi. For me this means an obstruction in the circulation of information that has been forgotten or blocked somewhere in the body, due to somatic or psychoemotional traumas.

Needling an acupuncture point is a way to help the organism recall this forgotten or blocked information. This is why we should not needle numerous points in one session, as the organism can only hear and understand what we want to tell it if a limited and consistent set of information is provided. It cannot do so if it is drowned in a flood of information given by many needles. It is also crucial that all the information supplied, on a local, regional, and systemic level, is matched and in a coherent stream.

Moreover, considering that an acupuncture point is the emergence of several different pieces of information, one piece of information will be favored according to which other points are associated to the chosen one at a given time in a patient. For example, if you puncture HM-6 by itself, you will mostly be engaging its function as a connecting point. If you puncture it in association with KI-9, which serves to unobstruct the Yin Linking vessel, then it will function in relation to the extraordinary vessel. Trust the body to switch the point's function to whatever is appropriate.

The problem is to understand, for each patient, which type of qi—that is, which functions or pieces of information—has been forgotten or obstructed; which vicious cycles are making the illness chronic and preventing healing; and which points will have to be stimulated, updated, or activated to improve circulation again to break these vicious cycles. To determine this, one must know the location of each point, its symptoms, functions, and indications, which mechanisms it embodies, and the needling method required to reset it.

In addition there are times when a patient unknowingly, and, provided his relationship with the practitioner allows it, asks through his symptoms, his speech or his dreams that a specific point be treated. It is our task to recognize this particular point, to recognize what knowing it implies. It is important at this stage not to anticipate but to humbly follow the requests of the body.

CHAPTER THREE

PATHOPHYSIOLOGY AND THERAPY

Now we will revisit some of the fundamental concepts of Chinese medicine that will help us to further utilize clinically the concepts noted above.

Placement of Structures and Functions in the Human Body

Chinese medicine, with its special and symbolic viewpoint, describes the mechanisms of life in human beings. I will describe these first as a whole.

- To begin with, our body is perceived as being administered by a government consisting of ten organs. At the center, the Heart presides; it is surrounded by the other organs, which are its ministers: Lung, Liver, Kidneys, and Spleen. Under the command of the Spleen, the yang organs (Gallbladder, Stomach, Intestines and Bladder) manage all of our personal territories (physical, familial, social, etc.), beginning with the body. We will return to this concept.

- Next, our life is maintained: to this end it is nourished, in every way, and perpetuated. The Triple Burner is in charge of our nutrition. Its three upper, middle and lower burners, which are subdivisions of the Triple Burner, produce the qi, blood and fluids, an emblematic ternary system encompassing all that nourishes us.

   The six extraordinary organs (奇恒之腑 *qi heng zhi fu)* ensure our durability and perpetuation. Their three pairs (brain and marrow, bones and vessels and Gallbladder and gestational envelopes) perpetuate our existence. Among the six extraordinary organs are the vessels, which conduct qi, blood and fluids. The first of these, the qi vessels, are the acupuncture channels that contribute to our durability.

- Moreover, we communicate with all that surrounds us through the orifices: the eyes, ears, nose, mouth, anus and urethra which, in turn, organize our being.
- Situated in the cosmos, we are also paced by various influences including the alternation of day and night, the four seasons, the phases of the moon, etc.

Yin and Yang Organs

The organs such as the Heart, Lung, Kidneys, and Gallbladder do not encompass the same concepts in Chinese medicine as in modern biomedicine. These two viewpoints are like yin and yang in that they both differ from each other and yet complement one another. From a purely functional viewpoint, in Chinese medicine there are yin organs (*zang*) and yang organs (*fu*). The yin organs—Heart, Lung, Liver, Spleen and Kidneys—store up the qi and essence of the corresponding organs. The yang organs—Gallbladder, Stomach, Large and Small Intestines and Bladder—are places of transit and transformation; they receive, transform and cause to bear fruit. Some of their descriptions in the classics appear to be anatomical but in fact are symbolic. For example, Chinese physicians knew perfectly well that, anatomically, the large intestine and the small intestine do not "wind sixteen times to the right and left of the navel", as stated in the *Classic of Difficulties*, No. 42.

In this spirit, all living structures reflect various forms of the same fundamental architecture, the same principles and laws: the archetypal structure of microcosms corresponds to that of the macrocosm. The construction and functioning of the idealized empire are also superimposed on that of the human body. To illustrate, we will use the example of this image of the administration, according to the same model, of the idealized empire and of the human body. To avoid weighing down this work, I will not review the paths of the channels here nor the locations of the points, which the reader will find in basic texts.

EMPIRE AND BODY

The government of the idealized empire, like that of the human body, should aim ideally to bring the empire and the body into conformity with the cosmic and natural order of life. The emperor, at the center, administers the empire. His ministers act under his authority. The human body is governed according to the same schema.

- The Heart at the center, plays the role of emperor. The other organs are the ministers. This is a schematic description of the roles attributed to each one in Chapter 8 of *Basic Questions*.
- The Lung is the prime minister. Located with the Heart/emperor in the thorax, it is the master of qi that breathes, circulates, incarnates, takes form and is transformed with each breath, as we are recreated with every respiration. It is the prime minister because it is closest to the emperor.

- The Liver is the general that is the issuer of strategies and planning. A good general wins a war without going to battle. He sees and anticipates, far in advance. It is through the Liver that the qi, blood and fluids circulate without obstacle or hindrance, flexibly and easily, like the sap in a tree that flows freely from its origins in the roots to the tips of the branches. In the same spirit, the Liver builds up stores in anticipation of the future and provides defenses. Since it is in charge of anticipating what might come, it evens out and regulates the qi, blood, foods, emotions and feelings.

- The Kidneys are the seat, the foundation where all of man's creations originate. Emergence of the visible in the invisible, procreation, spiritual, psychological, artistic and literary creation are all rooted in the Kidneys. Moreover, the Kidneys are said to be the only double organ; this "double" here is functional, in that creation required both a masculine and a feminine, both a paternal and a maternal aspect. A passage in Chapter 8 of the *Divine Pivot* states: "Therefore the arrival of life is called essence and the interaction of two essences is called spirit." The Kidneys are connected with the origin of life. They store up the essence of the qi for the organs. As Nguyen Van Nghi noted, they are the root of production of the five organs. They are therefore affected in all chronic or serious illness, regardless of its location.

- The Spleen is the minister of the granaries in charge of nutrition, transformation and transportation, in close cooperation with the Stomach. It is in charge of the yang organs that manage our regions or territories,[1] that is, the Gallbladder, Stomach, Intestines and Bladder.

These organs are controlled by general points, which treat their qi or essence deficiencies, which purify them, respond to their seasonal aspects, govern the ascending or descending movements of their qi, and by other points that provide special functions for each of the five organs.

The following clinical case will help the reader perceive this view of the organs, in this case, of the Liver.

❖ Case History

A 35-year-old female civil servant, slim, active, who spoke quickly as if she were afraid of taking up too much space or time, had, since the age of fifteen, endured a case of generalized eczema, which was very itchy at night. Three years of psychoanalysis, which was incidentally very beneficial to her, did not help with this condition. She also complained of heartburn, nausea, intolerance of dietary fats and of headaches related to digestion. A sleepwalker as a child, and subject to night terrors, she experienced difficulty falling asleep and awoke frequently at night. She was highly animated and did everything quickly, out of fear she would not manage; she had always felt forced or restrained in her studies and her choice of profession (she wanted to be a midwife). It is apparent that the Liver is involved, with its power over the comings and goings of spirit and the free, unobstructed circulation of qi, which should flow flexibly and with ease, and which suffers when they are blocked. One of the points of the Liver, BL-47, which manages these comings and goings, brought about a cure in three sessions.

POINTS FOR DEFICIENCIES OF QI AND ESSENCE

Qi is the circulating breath of an organ and is immediately available to it. The essence of the qi of this organ constitutes a sort of reserve. For various reasons, such as physical or psychological trauma, disease, or overwork, the qi of an organ may become deficient. If this effect is brief, superficial and recent, as in the case of an acute, benign illness, only the immediately available qi will be deficient. This will usually result in signs of cold. We restore it by the corresponding associated points on the back, located on the inside branch of the leg *tai yang* Bladder channel. If the impairment is chronic, profound or severe, the reserve qi will be affected: this is the essence of the organ qi. This impairment usually manifests with signs of heat. We treat these *essence* deficiencies by the points located on the outer branch of the same *tai yang* Bladder channel at the same level as the associated points of the corresponding organs. These are the deficiencies that we encounter most frequently in the West.

The diagnosis of organ impairment is made from the association of visceral, somatic and psychological signs that may affect the corresponding organs (e.g., muscles and Liver) or problems along the lines of the corresponding channel. Furthermore, it is not always easy to tell whether the origin is in the organ or the channel. The choice can often be guided by small pathognomonic signs. I will mention the most typical organ symptoms (they are not exclusive and not always present). We should always take into account their respective positions on the radial pulse as well as the examination of the tongue.

- Heart: functional cardiac signs, precordial pains, emotional lability, melancholy, depression, insomnia, memory impairment, heat and pain in the palms. We will have to choose according to the signs of the associated channels between the Heart—arm *shao yin*—and Heart Master (Pericardium)—arm *jue yin* (BL-15 and BL-44 or BL-14 and BL-43).

- Lung: respiratory signs, sorrow, melancholy, insomnia, heat in the palms.

- Spleen: anorexia, indigestion, diarrhea, flatulence, intolerance of raw ("cold") foods, fats and alcohol, intense physical fatigue with sensation of heaviness, edema, pain at the root of the tongue.

- Liver: dyspepsia, nausea, vomiting, intestinal and urinary disturbances, testicular pains, feeling of oppression, insomnia, cramps or muscle spasms, visual disturbances, anger, anxiety, or fear.

- Kidneys: physical or mental fatigue, general decrease in libido, urinary disturbances, frequent sexual dysfunction, low back pain, pharyngitis, heat in the soles of feet, difficulty in concentration, insomnia.

- Stomach: gastric signs, drooling, precordial pains and palpitations, runny nose.

- Gallbladder: digestive disturbances, bitter taste in mouth, frequent sighing, headaches, vertigo, visual disturbances.

- Small Intestine: diarrhea, intolerance of raw ("cold") foods, periumbilical pains sometimes extending to the lumbar region or testicles, urinary disturbances, swelling of the jaws or submaxillary region.

- Large Intestine: thirst, runny nose, epistaxis, pharyngitis, painful intestinal disturbances that may extend to the lower back, milk intolerance.

- Bladder: urinary disturbances (incontinence or retention), runny nose.

Qi problems

The related points on the medial branch of the Bladder channel are BL-13 for the Lung, BL-15 for the Heart, BL-18 for the Liver, BL-20 for the Spleen, and BL-23 for the Kidney.

❖ Case History

A young woman, age 28, with a severe neurological disease that was momentarily stabilized, arrived in tears and highly agitated, saying, "I am terribly worried; my psychotherapy this week has brought back the fears of death that plagued me throughout my childhood and that I had managed to hide." In the face of this emergency, with the recent resurgence of symptoms, BL-15 seemed to be indicated, in order to restore the Heart qi. Half an hour later, she was relaxed and peaceful.

Essence deficiencies

The related points are level with the associated points corresponding to each organ, on the outer line of leg *tai yang* Bladder channel: BL-42 for Lung, BL-44 for the Heart, BL-47 for the Liver, BL-49 for the Spleen and BL-52 for the Kidneys.

❖ Case History

A 51-year-old woman consulted me for repeated pneumothorax over the last three years. Surgery was planned. She had no pulmonary history, but had previously undergone an operation for sciatica caused by a herniated disc. She was now complaining of slight low back pain and constipation. She had not experienced any grief or major emotional blows: she was not sad. Her pneumothorax occurred after a case of bronchitis that lasted two months, during a period of extreme overwork. The pulse, empty in the right distal position, confirmed my supposition of an essence deficiency in the Lung. I decided to puncture BL-42, hoping there would not be an immediate recurrence, so there would be time to restore her essence that had been depleted by intense overwork. The first two sessions were followed by forty-eight hours of thoracic pain, although without relapse, which was a good sign. After the third treatment, the pneumothorax healed spontaneously in one week. A slight relapse, the last one, healed in two days after the sixth session. After the eighth treatment, there were a few persistent costal pains but these gradually faded.

Note the potential for acupuncture intervention in organic diseases: it can reinforce the defenses and the body's capacities for restoration.

❖ Case History

A 58-year-old man, measuring 170cm (a little under 5'7"), with a sturdy, squat build, and a serious, quiet demeanor, was a financial officer in a large company. He consulted me for uncharacteristic anxiety, which had been troubling him for a few months. His sleep was relatively good. He admitted to a decrease in drive and endurance, with moments of fatigue around 3 p.m. He had considerable professional worries (his business was about to be taken over) and his wife had just undergone surgery for a craniopharyngioma.

Physically, there was not much to report: low back pain, particularly in the morning. Prior history included a herniated intervertebral disk that caused sciatica on the right, healed by osteopathy. There was also intellectual and sexual fatigue. His tongue appeared normal. The pulse indicated essence impairment in the Heart and Kidneys.

It should be noted that there was a deficiency in both the Kidneys and the Heart, so this was not a case of dissociation between the Kidneys and Heart in which there is a deficiency in the Kidneys and excess in the Heart. With this simultaneous deficiency, what could it be? Exhaustion of the essence of the Kidneys and Heart is associated with worry and stress and the wear and tear they can bring. Wear is an important term; it is often the cause behind essence deficiencies. The physical, psychological, intellectual and sexual nature of the exhaustion corresponds to impairment of the Heart and Kidneys.

When I asked him, "Have you recently experienced a situation that wears you out?" he answered, "Yes; two kinds." First, there was a professional "war of nerves" because he had to present the company balance sheet to each potential buyer, knowing that he would be losing his job; moreover, the atmosphere at the company was very tense. And also the "sword of Damocles" hanging over his wife's head increased his anxiety.

Which points should be punctured? BL-44 and BL-52. These points restored the essence of these two organs. The results were very good after three sessions. The patient was to return whenever he felt the need, depending on the circumstances, usually about every eight weeks.

❖ Case History

Mr. D., 46-years-old, consulted me for sensations of epigastric blockage, accompanied by intense fatigue and occurring after meals or at 11 a.m. and 5 p.m. These sensations produced a great deal of anguish. They began nine months earlier and had not been alleviated by any treatment. This man, who had not presented any other symptoms before, was physically exhausted by an overload of work. Psychologically, he still had plenty of drive and will to work, but he no longer had the physical strength. Intellectually, he had difficulty concentrating. His fatigue had little influence on his sexuality. He did not describe any other symptoms. His pulses were weak. An examination of his tongue confirmed the deficiency of Spleen essence, as it was pale with clear indentations from the teeth. We should note that essence deficiency in the Kidneys leads to mental and sexual impairment, which was not the case here, and does not produce hypoglycemia. We punctured BL-49. There was a distinct improvement from the very first treatment. After the third session, this patient was essentially cured.

POINTS FOR DRAINING ORGANS

In order to function well, the qi, blood and fluids of the organs need to be drained and purged properly. Otherwise, toxins accumulate, resulting in symptoms of damp-heat that are variable depending on the organ concerned.[2] These mechanisms are involved in a number of immune, allergic, and autoimmune disorders, but also in all toxic overload syndromes.

The draining points are KI-26 for the Lung, KI-23 for the Heart, KI-18 for the Spleen, KI-20 for the Liver, and KI-15 for the Kidneys. Because these points drain toxins, they are also known as points of purification.

❖ Case History

Mr. N., 40-years-old, consulted me for respiratory allergies (nasal, pharyngeal and bronchial), foul-smelling diarrhea, burning during urination and tinea of the groin and feet. The foul-smelling stools and tinea immediately brought to mind a toxic overload of damp-heat. He experienced anxiety, sleep disturbances, heat sensations and excessive perspiration. He was overly sensitive and took everything to heart. He mentioned respiratory problems in his childhood. His right distal pulse was rapid and deep; his tongue was red, with a yellow coating, which confirmed the presence of excessive dampness and heat. We immediately discussed the need for draining mechanisms and I chose to work on the Lung, because of the childhood vulnerability, the respiratory allergies, and the cutaneous signs, and on the Kidneys, because of the combination of symptoms of diarrhea and the burning sensation during urination. Needling KI-15 and KI-26 had a good effect.

❖ Case History

Ms. C., age 15, was brought in by her mother for skin problems that had been progressing since the age of four, with recurrences approximately every two months. The eczematous lesions, mostly dry, although occasionally seeping, were always located on the extremities or the face. They began on the left thumb and had reached the feet, the right orbital region, and the chin. On the limbs, the lesions were selectively located on the dorsal (yang) sides. The previous summer there had been an uncustomary outbreak of vesicular lesions on the left (yang) half of the body. This coincided with the mother's hospitalization for a nervous breakdown; and the outbreaks were associated with visits by the grandmother, with whom she had conflicting relations. There were no climatic or seasonal influences. Ms. C. also complained of insomnia with difficulty falling asleep, beginning one year before, along with a sensation of excessive heat over the entire body. She was visibly emotional, anxious and given to nervous attacks. I noted oppression and tachycardia. Her menstrual periods started six months earlier, were relatively profuse, and would last for six days. Our discussion did not uncover any other organ signs. The anxiety, intense emotions, tachycardia, oppression, and profuse menstruation enabled me to locate the initial anomaly in the Heart, master of the blood.

I punctured KI-23, which was, incidentally, painful to the touch. To stimulate the skin's externalization functions, I selected SI-7, the connecting point that governs the skin, located on the channel (arm *tai yang*) paired with that of the Heart (arm *shao yin*).[3] Note the consistency in the choice of the second point. A session of twenty minutes per week for two weeks followed by two sessions at thirty-day intervals were sufficient. Preventive treatment was recommended, with sessions scheduled every six months.

The following case history illustrates a method that consists of translating our perceptions of the patient or his own sensations into acupuncture points: I see a lot of potential in this approach because it helps us get outside the box of limited, stereotyped syndromes.

❖ Case History

Mr. G., age 61, came to see me about periods of fatigue, feeling drained, with considerable qi fluctuations. His sleep was normal. These periods were accompanied by pain in the limbs, muscular trembling, and a feeling of heaviness. Physical labor tended to bring improvement. In addition, he reported some constipation, burning during urination, and vulnerability of the ears, nose and throat, with recurring nasopharyngitis. His pulses were tense. His tongue had a white coating. He could not determine when these problems had begun, and they were a part of a general physical and psychological malaise that had led him to begin psychotherapy three years earlier.

As we continued our conversation, the patient told me that he "was not eliminating toxins," which seemed plausible to me, since a toxic buildup can produce the muscle trembling, nasopharyngitis and low qi levels of which he complained; note that when they were eliminated by physical effort there was an improvement. So I decided to treat the alarm point of the lower burner, CV-7, which governs elimination, and to add KI-20, which has the functions of draining and decongesting the Liver. The muscular implications of the signs and the tense pulses led me to choose this organ. There was a distinct improvement following the first session. By the third session, the improvement lasted a month, and then two months after the fourth session. This trend of increasingly marked and lasting improvement continued.

OTHER HEART POINTS

Here I will consider CV-14, CV-15 and CV-16, which are all connected with the 'Heart fire', the central fire comparable to the sun, source of life (moreover, the Sovereign Heart[4] is said to be the 'sun of man'); and two spirit points, BL-44 and GV-24. The fire is Heart qi (just as wind is that of the Liver) and the Heart is the home of the spirit (神 *shen*). This should convey the importance of these two elements in the physiology and pathology of this organ.

Pathologically, a patient can be in a state of deficiency (addressed by CV-14), which corresponds to an eclipse of the sun, causing symptoms of deficiency and cold, or in a state of excess, either because it cannot externalize (CV-15 is used, which rules the expressions of the Heart), or because it cannot return to its home, the Heart, remaining blocked outside (addressed by CV-16).

❖ Case History

Mr. J., age 65, sought help for depression, anxiety and insomnia. Two of his sons had died, fifteen years and one year before, in a car crash and a boating accident, respectively. His symptoms had worsened only recently, after he had finished staging an exhibition of his younger son's paintings; "something has come to an end here," he said.

He felt dispirited, had no drive, and lacked his usual energy. The anxiety attacks, close to panic attacks, included a sensation of oppression in the chest with palpitations, and of knots in the chest; he then became prostrate and unable to move. He often woke up during the night and could not go back to sleep; he did not have nightmares but frequently dreamed that he was asking for help. On several occasions, he said that he could not settle down, that he was "no longer connected with his deep self" and that he "could no longer reach his innermost self." "There is a voice in me wanting to speak," he added, understanding this as a need to express his own creativity now that his son's has been made public.

The Heart pulse was weak and deep. The proximal pulses were normal.

Having needled CV-19 and GV-24, I decided to needle CV-14. The difference was obvious: "Perhaps I can make out a light," he said after this point has been needled. He noted that it allowed him to perceive the "uncertain light of the free and open air" (he was referring to Henry Bauchau's marvelous book *Oedipus on the Road*); CV-14 perhaps brought him to perceive his own deep self, to settle in it and maybe then "someone hidden in himself will be able to speak." The results were excellent.

❖ Case History

An austere, reserved, bright-eyed man complained of severe insomnia; he had difficulty falling asleep and was frequently awakened by nightmares. Furthermore, he mentioned attacks of tachycardia, extreme anxiety attacks in which he could not sit still, and intense internal nervousness: he felt "like a pressure cooker with no outlet for the steam." The Heart pulse, deep and tense, confirmed the symptoms and the impairment of this organ with the compression of its fire qi inside. The reason was that he felt helpless because he could not understand his wife's decision to divorce him. He could not bear to leave his two children, ages six and eight, but also could not think of separating them from their mother. Needling CV-15 helped him provide an outlet or expression for the Heart fire that was blocked inside, providing noticeable symptomatic relief so that he could gain some perspective on his situation, take charge of it, and make plans for undergoing psychotherapy to understand his part in this painful failure.

❖ Case History

A 38-year-old nurse described herself as being off-centered, scattered, unable to concentrate, flitting from one task to another, insomniac, anxious, and agitated, all of which began with surgery and chemotherapy for cancer in her right breast. Prior to that, she had suffered from occasional sore throats and rare cases of painful diarrhea connected with stress. She observed that recently her face became quickly congested in case of heat, emotion or after consuming alcohol. The Heart pulses were weak. We therefore needed to return the fire, which was in excess on the exterior, to its home in the Heart; in other words, to internalize it. Puncturing CV-16 considerably reduced her symptoms. She said that it was "as if she had been re-rooted in her heart."

BL-44, named *shen tang* or "hall of the spirit," is a connection with the Heart spirit, and can contribute to the treatment of major mental disorders such as manic depression. It is difficult to provide examples because, in such cases, it is only a modest but useful adjunct. We saw above how it was used in a case of worn-out Heart essence. These points on the lateral branch of the Bladder channel actually store the essence and spirit of their corresponding organs.

Another important spirit point for certain types of depression is GV-24. Cranial, in the midline, between two other spirit points to the right and left—GB-13—which bring to mind the right and left brain, GV-24 seems to unify and pacify the person, while stimulating their mental qi.

❖ Case History

A man, age 57, who was 190cm tall (almost 6'3"), slightly stooped, and a merchant by profession, came to me in 1991 for a long-term case of depression, including some severe episodes where he lost interest in everything. He was constantly apathetic. He could not pinpoint the origin; he was already that way as an adolescent. He would become "worried over nothing," but did not present with major pharyngeal, thoracic or solar plexus anxiety attacks. He slept poorly, awoke around three or four in the morning and took a long time to fall back asleep. He reported a few attacks of tachycardia and emotional outbursts (he was highly emotional and sensitive), although without cause. There was a slight case of psoriasis on the elbows and head. That was all, in terms of physical symptoms.

Psychologically, he described himself as being "poorly armed"; he felt constantly insecure; he did not know his father (who died before his was born) or his grandfather; nobody had ever protected him.

His tongue appeared normal and the Heart pulse was weak (and deep in the left distal position). The diagnosis: a deficiency of Heart spirit: depression, anxiety, insomnia, tachycardia, intense emotions, and typical pulse. The psoriasis could be connected to this impairment. How to treat this syndrome? It seemed clear to me that I should work on the Governing vessel, because of the stooped posture and especially because of the lack of a father and grandfather: *tai yang* and the Governing vessel relate to the father. GV-24 is clearly indicated as the spirit point that corresponds to the Heart. The results were excellent: by the fifth session he declared himself healed. Considering the length of time he had been suffering, the causes and the absence of any analytic work, I advised him to schedule additional sessions every quarter for a year, and then every six months thereafter. He is still following this treatment.

On each side of CV-19 is KI-25, the name of which is *shen cang* 神藏, "storehouse of the spirit." The word *cang* (storehouse) defines both what occurs during winter and the functions of the organs. Its symptoms show that there is counterflow of both the Lung and Stomach qi. Soulié de Morant adds two important signs: "lingers on the unpleasant side, does not like life."

❖ Case History

Mr. D., age 73, once came to my practice. He was a small, stocky, retired policeman, both a father (one son) and a grandfather (one grandson); he was withdrawn and taciturn. His wife told me of his depression, his lack of drive, of desire and enthusiasm. His anxiety, mainly felt in the throat, made him unable to move, paralyzed him so that he was unable to leave his bed. It did not help that he also was having problems sleeping.

He had always been an emotional and pessimistic person, brooding endlessly, and had difficulties coping with his emotions. His condition was further aggravated by the onset of Parkinson's disease; he had no tremor but a significant rigidity which made his staring look even more obvious. He was taking the antidepressant escitalopram (Lexapro) as well as levodopa (Madopar) for the Parkinson's. This man of strong moral principles had been extremely shocked when, four months earlier, he had been told that his grandson had stolen a record in a large music shop.

On a physical level, he had suffered from asthma during his teens and had a painful sensation of tension in the neck related to his anxiety. His tongue was normal, if a little stiff. The pulses were wiry, but the Heart pulse could not be felt. The involvement of the Heart was obvious. During the first four sessions, I needled CV-14 and GV-24. At the fifth session his wife stressed his basic pessimism, in that he had always thought the worst would happen. "Does he stick to the unpleasant side of things?" "Exactly. He's always done this." KI-25 needled once a month was quickly efficacious, albeit followed by a nauseous reaction in the throat (from counterflow). This man was then livelier and less anxious. After four treatments using this point, his walk had improved and was less shuffling and stiff. The Parkinson's disease symptoms were largely improved, which showed that they had been greatly amplified by his depression. With one treatment every three months, he gradually improved without any change to his drug regimen.

OTHER LUNG POINTS

I will discuss four points here: LU-2, KI-22, CV-20, BL-42.

LU-2, under the clavicle, is called the "cloud door" (*yun men*). This governs expression, the outward escape of qi, which we also refer to as externalization, from the chest and Lung. It often carries latent, repressed anger.

❖ Case History

An elegant woman, age 51, an artist and painter, complained of burning eyes. Her eyes were red and watered copiously: "They are incontinent," she said. "My lachrymal glands are exasperated. My eyes are going to pop out of their sockets." She reported that, for two years, there had been neither improvement nor aggravation. Nor had she noticed any triggering factors. The only other symptom she reported was fatigue, especially psychological fatigue. She lacked drive and enthusiasm, saying that she had "no future." Furthermore, she said that, emotionally, she could not take any more ("it's overflowing") nor express herself, not even the latent anger that she acknowledged was present. She was married and a happy wife and the mother of two children, with no major worries. But there was one event which had seriously disturbed her: her mother had married the father of her husband. Her tongue was normal and her pulse was deep: the qi was blocked inside.

I thought of using *tai yin* channels but there were neither respiratory nor digestive signs, nor any pains on the corresponding channels. I was puzzled, and decided to puncture two local points: M-HN-7 (*yu yao*) and GB-14. After two sessions, seeing little effect, I replaced the M-HN-7 (*yu yao*) treatment with BL-1. On her next visit, she reported a small improvement, the death of the father-in-law, and the reappearance of pain in her thumbs and big toes on the *tai yin* channels, which she had forgotten about.

In the absence of other *tai yin* symptoms and because of the unexpressed anger, I decided to puncture LU-2. The improvement in the ocular signs and in the thumb and toe pain was quite significant for a period of three weeks. Since I could not tell how much of this was due to the death of the father-in-law and how much to the needling of LU-2, I punctured this point again. Once again, the improvement was even more remarkable. She asked me to explain it. I mentioned *tai yin*, which both receives and opens to the outside, and LU-2, which expresses emotions, often in the range of rage or anger. "What is it called?" she asked me. "Cloud Door," I answered. "I will be back in half an hour," she said. When she returned, she explained: "You know that I am a painter. It so happens that, six months before the onset of the symptoms, as a way of presenting myself, I decided to print some post cards with a reproduction of a painting that I did entitled *"Terre"* (Earth); it represents a "door in the clouds"! I painted it in late 1999 or early 2000. The crying started during 2000!"

KI-22, in the fifth intercostal space, governs the dispersion function of the Lung; it is linked to fairness and judgment or justice[5] and therefore, pathologically, to injustice.

❖ Case History

A man, 51, had been suffering from bronchitis for four months. He had not improved despite all of the usual treatments nor had other tests revealed a different diagnosis. I immediately asked him the classic acupuncture question for such cases: "During the three months that preceded the onset of this bronchitis, did you feel that you were subjected to a serious injustice?" He was surprised, and replied, "Yes indeed, I was running a prosperous agency, and a con artist cheated me out of a lot of money, so the director fired me, without taking any account of my past performance." I later learned that he had invested a lot in this older man, since his father had died when he was only three. I explained the origin of the bronchitis to him and punctured KI-22, which cleared up the ailment within 48 hours. This is a classic case in acupuncture and a good illustration of what Chinese medicine can contribute in diagnostic as well as therapeutic terms.

CV-20 governs the heavenly function of the Lung, which is the "canopy of the organs." The name of this point—*hua gai*—means the canopy that covers the emperor's chariot. This point has a very profound descending function and complements the physiologic actions of KI-27, which directs the Lung qi and the fluids that converge there downwards.

This case history illustrates the fact that any persistent pain should incite us to search for the overall underlying and sustaining cause. Often, as in this case, a treatment that focuses on the general condition is sufficient.

❖ Case History

Mr. G., age 36, came to me in October 1991 for acute lower back pain that occurred after a fall from a height of two meters during a climbing expedition, in which he twisted his back. The pain began at the level of the lumbosacral ligaments and radiated in an intense and diffuse manner through the lower left limb at unpredictable and variable movements. It was neither improved nor worsened by cold, heat, coughing, or habitual movements (flexing, extending). He often experienced stiffness in the morning and felt better when standing. No trigger point could be found on examination. Among the antecedents was a deep, acute pain in the sacrum in April 1991, which disappeared after one session with GV-1, and sacroiliac pain on the left side that appeared in August 1991 and disappeared with needling LR-11. The pulses were normal. The Heart pulse was deeper than that of the Lung. He said he felt well otherwise, without any complaints, except that he was "not connected to his body and feelings."

After three unsuccessful sessions using regional points, I started questioning the patient again. The gentleman said he had always had difficulty breathing; his stomach always felt tight and full so he could not breathe deeply. Since the pulse in the proximal position was tense, I decided to release the pelvis by needling GV-5, which caused qi to rise from the Kidneys. I completed the treatment with CV-20, which brought the qi down from the Lung. I did not puncture any local points. From that moment on, the improvement was spectacular and lasting. After the third session, there was still some lumbar weakness. The entire problem cleared up after two more treatments at one-month intervals. I recommended that he follow up with a session every three months if there were no symptoms. One year later, all was well.

BL-42 (*po hu*), the door of the corporeal soul, apart from controlling the Lung essence, is connected with this organ's spirit, that is, the corporeal soul (*po*), which, as described in Chapter 8 of the *Divine Pivot*, "matches the essence as it goes in and comes out", beginning with what is referred to in Chapter 50 of the *Laozi* as the "coming out into life and entry into death."

❖ Case History

A woman, age 51, petite and slim, reserved but energetic—even aggressive—came to see me for asthma and rheumatism in her hands. The asthma was already present in her childhood but had worsened over the last three years. Up until then, it had been relatively well managed by means of allopathic and homeopathic treatments. The attacks, occurring either at night or triggered by effort, caused impeded inhalation and exhalation, wheezing, along with phlegm and a sensation of tightness in the thorax. In addition, every year she had two or three cases of infectious bronchitis from which she had a hard time recovering. The rheumatism in her hands was painful, although not too deforming. In my experience, this type of joint problem is often seen as related to trouble with the Lung or Heart. In this case, the Lung appeared to be responsible. On examination, the pulse for this organ was deficient. The woman confided in me about an exceptionally difficult period in her life that brought to mind problems with the corporeal soul:[6] following childbirth she had experienced murderous impulses towards her daughter for several weeks. She was terrified, feeling unsure that she could control them; this lasted for a month and then disappeared.

As I listened to her, I noticed how mismatched her clothing was, as if she had simply dressed by chance. Because we had a good relationship, I was able to bring this to her attention after the fifth session. She replied that she never bought anything for herself; that she had no such desire, so when she needed a jacket or skirt, she would choose something as quickly as possible, which explained the mismatched results. The problems connected with the Lung seemed evident, with the concurrence of asthma, pain in the hands, the episode of murderous impulses and the lack of interest in her personal appearance. I punctured BL-42 monthly, as points that are this important should not be punctured too often. After the third session, there was some improvement in the respiratory issues. This was confirmed in subsequent sessions, which became bimonthly. After the tenth session (approximately a year and a half after the beginning of treatment), her asthma attacks were less frequent, her hands less painful, and I noticed a change in her manner of dressing, with some attention to harmony. Noticing that I was looking at her, she smiled and shyly said, "For the first time in my life, I had the urge to buy myself something just for the pleasure of it, so I did." The name of BL-42 is the "door of the corporeal soul" and, as noted above, this aspect of the psyche relates to "coming out into life," and its use had something to do with this change.

OTHER KIDNEY POINTS

I consider KI-11 through KI-14 and then BL-52 in the aspect of the resolve, the essence of the Kidneys.

Points KI-11 to KI-14 define various Kidney functions, with KI-15 in charge of draining.

KI-11, at the upper edge of the pubis, governs the Kidneys in their role as the root of production of the five organs. This manifests with the signs of a deficiency in the Kidneys: a lack of sperm (the essence of the Kidneys) or amenorrhea, along with symptoms of exhaustion of the four other yin organs, that is, the Heart, Lung, Spleen and Liver. This is an indicator of the intensity of the fatigue.

KI-12 acts on the genitals and on sexuality. Therefore: lack of virility, impotence, and genital diseases in both men and women.

KI-13, the meeting point of the Conception and Penetrating vessels, protects and favors pregnancy and controls the ebb and flow of the Kidney qi.

KI-14 regulates the pathways of water[7] while controlling the storage function of the Kidneys and bone marrow.

BL-52 also stores up the Kidney essence and spirit, that is, the resolve (志 *zhi*, sometimes translated as will or ambition) connected with the survival instinct. It is the quality of our resolve that enables us to survive in physically or psychologically difficult conditions. Without it, we are physically, intellectually, and sexually fatigued and, above all, lacking in drive and will to live. The following example concerns a deficiency of the essence of the Kidneys caused by wear and tear.

❖ Case History

A 57-year-old married woman, with two children, and clearly overweight, consulted me for depression, anxiety, and insomnia. She had been taking the antidepressant escitalopram (Lexapro) for a year with little result. She lacked drive and had no desires. Her anxiety was not somatized in any specific location, but it paralyzed her. Her insomnia presented with difficulty both falling asleep and staying asleep, and was being treated with the hypnotic zolpidem (Ambien). These symptoms had been present for a long time and were aggravated by the illness and death of her mother three years before, followed by a serious problem with her only brother.

In addition, she complained of crippling joint pains in both knees. Indeed, she had carried a lot of weight in her life, including her husband, children, and mother. This suggested BL-11, the meeting point of the bones, for knee pain in those who carry too much, either physically or psychologically.

Her tongue appeared normal. The distal pulse on the left and the proximal pulse on the right, corresponding to the Heart and Kidneys, were deficient. This implied a deficiency in these two organs, either simultaneous or one being caused by the other.

In addition to BL-11, I started by treating the Heart, using GV-24, a frontal spirit point, particularly effective in cases of depression arising from the Heart. This improved the knees but not the other signs. So I considered the possibility of an essence deficiency in the Heart, caused by wear, and replaced GV-24 with BL-44, but this did not work much better. Thus I told myself that the cause was in the Kidneys, particularly in the resolve, considering the long duration of the problems. I punctured BL-52. After three sessions, the improvement was impressive. We continued this treatment with quarterly sessions.

The next case history also deals with the resolve of the Kidneys.

❖ Case History

A 55-year-old man, austere-looking and slightly overweight, sought help for a depression which had started one year before, two years after having been treated by radiation therapy for prostate cancer. He lacked liveliness, had a diminished libido and suffered from panic attacks with sensations localized in the solar plexus. Very soon after undergoing a therapy that consisted of using sleeping pills to keep depressed people asleep for a prolonged period of time (many days), he was prescribed Zoloft (two 50mg tablets per day), which made it impossible to really know what his sleep was like. He was becoming increasingly tired and tended to be more easily fatigued. Moreover, he complained of tendonitis mainly in the shoulders, elbows and adductor muscles. Following the radiation therapy he also started suffering from difficult urination.

The tendonitis started when he was 40. In fact, at this age, he began to feel less lively and to have a phobia about being constrained or enclosed; he also had severe panic attacks before leaving home or when on a plane. He had no clue why these symptoms appeared and never considered undergoing psychotherapy.

He was a solitary person, the fourth of five children. He suffered a lot from the aggressive behavior of his eldest brother, who had epileptic seizures and died at the age of 18. His wife, undemonstrative, had gained a lot of weight in the last 14 years. He had two children. His proximal pulses were weak. His tongue was normal.

Because of the prostate cancer and the urinary symptoms, I first needled CV-3. Two sessions did not make any difference. I therefore diagnosed a disorder of the resolve, which corresponds to the creative will, the desire to live, the life instinct, and I needled BL-52.

The improvement was then noticeable. The man has been cutting down the Zoloft and planned to stop it completely after six acupuncture treatments. He has continued to do well and now comes for treatment every six months.

OTHER LIVER POINTS

I will discuss LR-10, KI-21 and BL-47.

❖ Case History

Mrs. R. was 84 years old. She was a fine-looking lady, full of energy but not to the point of being eccentric, cultured, elegant and somewhat flirtatious, self-assertive but tolerant. Her husband had been diagnosed with Alzheimer's disease a few months before. They had been very close to each other (she was 13 and he was 16 when they had first met) until the husband's first symptoms appeared. The situation demanded that she both accept that her husband was ill and that she needed help, which required that she master her fits of anger and to "no longer feel she wanted to be rebellious." She wanted me to help with her constipation, work on controlling her temper, and also enable her to take better care of herself.

She had been suffering from constipation for years and said it was "difficult for her to eliminate." She sometimes suffered from insomnia. Her nose was either stuffed up or constantly running. She mentioned that she had recently lost her voice temporarily, which was followed by an attack of bronchitis with a high fever (40°C). Ever since, she had been complaining of feeling weak, especially after 6:30 or 7:00 p.m., she was coughing a lot, and she had the impression that her eardrums were swollen. She felt as if there were no longer "any muscles between her knees and her hips." Her pulses were short and wiry.

All this pointed to an attempt by the body to get rid of its toxins. To facilitate this evacuation, I needled LR-10 to help with this function. On the following day she was unable to work in her garden because of severe lower back pain; she could not even pick up things from the ground. Her ankles were also painful. The next day she developed an itchy rash on both sides of her legs, and two days later, she woke up with torticollis. Again this was a reactive elimination, which, this time, had blocked the psoas muscles. LR-10 is a major point for detoxification, especially in the springtime. The psoas muscles are the wastebaskets of the body, as somatic, chemical, and psychological toxins have a tendency to accumulate there, and are also related to LR-10.

After a while all of these clinical symptoms had disappeared and when I saw this lady for a third treatment in June, she told me she "had regained her energy." She was in much better spirits and was more understanding and patient with her husband. Her sleep was also better. The cough had receded but she still had a hoarse voice. She no longer had pains but experienced a discomfort in both shoulders (she confessed to having been gardening the day before). Clinical examination showed a deep Heart pulse and a normal posterior tibialis (KI-3) pulse. The tip of the tongue was slightly red. I concluded that Heart fire could not descend. Mrs. R. asked me to "help her to learn how to live and get older with wisdom." I then needled CV-16, as it allows centering and anchoring on the Heart. It proved efficient for this lady who had to accept that she no longer was the child "spoiled" by life and by her husband, as she had been previously.

LR-10 and CV-16 are both related to the center; they correspond to a letting-go attitude that requires discarding and dismissing previous values.

KI-21 releases Liver qi and loosens contractions. It treats qi constraint affecting this organ. It controls the hepatic function of evening out and regulating the qi of the body, and the functions of the yang organs (it is an important point for vomiting and motion sickness), emotional lability (particularly bad moods, aggravated by anger), and poor memory.

❖ Case History

Mrs. N., age 64, a legal advisor, came to see me in September 1987 for two types of symptoms that she had experienced "for so long that she could not remember when they started." First of all, she complained of muscle pains with contractions, spasms and pulling, located in her back (between the shoulder blades), in the neck, in the superior muscles of the orbit, occasionally extending to the upper eyelids and eyebrows. These pains were alleviated by heat and aggravated by any nervous tension. No other factors had any effect. She also reported nocturnal cramps in her feet. There were several possible causes: *shao yang*, constraint of Liver qi, or *yang ming*.

She also complained of digestive difficulties, stomach cramps or heartburn or both, which would wake her at half an hour after midnight or at 5 a.m., regard-less of what she ate. Her digestion was often slow; she reported soft or liquid stools accompanied by epigastric pains and frequent flare-ups of hemorrhoids. The laboratory tests were all negative. A fiberoptic endoscopy revealed a large quantity of stagnant fluids. Her history did not reveal anything else about this recently menopausal woman, who had three children, and there was nothing of significance in her medical history, apart from an appendectomy. Her menstrual periods had been normal.

Psychologically, she was preoccupied with doing right and described herself primarily as tied up in knots, tight and anxious. Her only stress was work-related, and due to the very nature of her profession. Her sleep was normal when not wakened by stomach trouble. She was not tired and felt good on waking. She often expressed anger about the tension she experienced. Her pulses were tense and her tongue presented tremors (a sign of wind release).

Was there a disturbance in the *shao yang* axis? An examination did not reveal any signs pointing towards *shao yang*, such as vertigo, signs of dampness, aggravation of pain with rotation, impact on the Gallbladder or morning difficulties.

Could this be explained by a constraint of qi in the Gallbladder? No, because in this case, the tension, anger and feelings were expressed, unlike cases of constraint related to GB-23 or GB-24.

Could it be clumping of the Liver qi from tension and constraint? This seems probable, judging by the pulse, the behavior and the muscular and digestive implications: the sign of dwelling on one's worries (part of the symptomatology of BL-18) can be a part of this clumping in the Liver qi.

How should we treat this Liver qi clumping tension, with its impact on the stomach or *yang ming*? LR-6, an unblocking point, and KI-21 are the most appropriate and will be most effective: we alternated treatment using just one each time. The treatment cleared up this dual symptomatology.

BL-47 controls the Liver's relationship with its spirit, the ethereal soul that ensures all of the "comings and goings," day and night, muscular and energetic, etc., like tree sap that flows readily and freely, with ease, from the furthest ends of the roots to the tips of the branches.

❖ Case History

A young woman, age 34, could not manage to overcome her alcoholism. After six years of psychoanalysis, she was "just a hair away from quitting." While I was taking her history, she revealed the right point to puncture with her own words: "Alcohol lets me come and go freely, in every way—it is something I cannot do without." She finally stopped drinking for good after the second time I punctured BL-47, the gate of the ethereal soul. She now felt a sense of freedom and ease without alcohol that she had never known before.

OTHER SPLEEN POINTS

Here we will consider KI-17 and BL-49.

KI-17 handles the transport functions of the Spleen. When this is deficient, there is an accumulation of Stomach qi in the abdomen with hernia from excess, hiccups, stomachache, abdominal accumulation and uterine congestion.

BL-49 controls the Spleen's relationship with its spirit, the intention *(yi)*. According to the sinologists at the Institut Ricci, this aspect of a person "takes action in every moment, in everyday life, with adaptation to the changes required."

❖ Case History

A 35-year-old man consulted me for a case of physical, sexual and intellectual asthenia, accompanied by hair loss. This constant weakness reached a peak one or two hours after the noon meal. It was aggravated by any prolonged physical or intellectual effort. It had begun seven years earlier, after an unwanted change in his job assignment. It could not be explained by his lifestyle. He worked ten hours a day and his profession as an engineer did not require physical effort. He led a regular life. Other symptoms that appeared at the same time were loss of memory, difficulties with concentration (signs of a cerebral essence deficiency) without any changes in behavior, character or thinking. He did not suffer from anxiety, depression, irritability or anger and he slept well. He did not shiver, tolerated cold and heat well and his fatigue was not influenced by the climate. He did not sweat, particularly not in his feet and hands.

The history was unremarkable. To my repeated question, "What is your weak point?" he answered, "Difficulty with change: examples include going through adolescence, marriage, the work life."

The history-taking also revealed a fronto-occipital headache that had appeared along with the fatigue, which was dull and deep, without any special characteristics (probably due to the cerebral essence deficiency) and also a history for many years of postnasal drip.

The origin of this trouble with the Spleen, which was responsible for the general and cerebral essence deficiency, and the phlegm, was most likely related to the difficulty with change and in particular with "digesting" his last job transfer. We tonified the intention *(yi)* and reinforced the essence in the Kidneys (because the Spleen essence is derived from that of the Kidneys, and because of the hair loss and the decrease in his libido) with BL-49 and BL-52. This man was fully cured in three sessions.

Qi Movements in the Organs

It is relatively common to see that organ pathology is linked not to problems with its qi or essence, disturbances in one of its functions or draining, or disturbances of its alarm point, but rather to a defect in the ascending or descending movements of its qi.

The qi of the Lung and Heart descends, like that of the yang organs, while that of the Spleen and Kidneys ascends. The Liver qi, which regulates and evens things out, flows in all directions, like the wind with which it resonates. A disturbance in one of these movements can generate symptoms and is corrected by special points: BL-16 for the Heart, KI-27 for the Lung, SP-17 for the Spleen and GV-5 for the Kidneys. The treatment is to bring together the two "window-of-heaven" points (discussed later) that bring down qi from the Lung (LU-3 for nasal allergies) or blood from the Heart (HM-1 for head congestion).

Indications for BL-16 (which has the alternate name of "high canopy" 高盖 *gao gai)* and KI-27 (which is located on either side of CV-20 and which also has the word "canopy" *[gai]* in its name), are evidenced on the one hand by signs of excess above in the organ in question (hysterics, dizziness, precordial pain and hair loss for BL-16 to address the Heart; and sneezing, dyspnea, agitation, cough, and thoracic pain for KI-27 to address the Lung); and deficiency further down (stomach trouble, abdominal pain for BL-16; or difficulty eating, vomiting and bloating for KI-27).

❖ Case History

Mrs. C., age 34, a choreographer, came to see me in November 1993 for attacks of lightheadedness accompanied by rapid breathing, tachycardia, hot and sweaty hands and excessive heat all over her body. She was unable to explain the cause; it did not seem to be related to her menstrual periods, nor to her emotions or eating habits. The occurrences were random. In addition, there were benign cysts in both breasts and she suffered from premenstrual syndrome. The patient had a four-year-old son. She often dreamed that she was flying (a sign that some qi is not descending, regardless of its origin or characteristics: Lung, Heart, or one of the three yang). She was emotional and sensitive and prone to nervous attacks. When I examined her, I observed scoliosis that was not painful at present, a slight redness on the tip of her tongue, and a deep Heart pulse.

The lightheadedness can be seen to correspond to inversion or *jue* (厥) as described in *Basic Questions* Chapter 45, often due to a counterflow (逆 *ni*) of qi that is ascending rather than descending, for example. These attacks seemed to originate with the Heart. This diagnosis was supported by the tongue, the pulse, the tachycardia with hot and sweaty hands, and the overall heat. Considering the heat in the hands and the rapid breathing, one could diagnose a Lung problem, but there were no other corroborating signs (cough, corresponding pulse, etc.).

I opted for the diagnosis of Heart qi ascending instead of descending. I hesitated between HM-1 and BL-16. After two sessions using HM-1, the patient had a new attack of lightheadedness; she felt "irritated, sleepless and off-center." It should be noted that she had just lost a close friend. I decided then to puncture GV-1 (considering the scoliosis), connected to somatic and nervous strength, and BL-16. Forty-eight hours after the first treatment, she was feeling better: she felt "centered" again. After three monthly sessions, she reported no attacks, not even the early signs of attacks. We then reduced the treatments to once every three months. Since then, she describes herself as cured, even though the cysts in her breasts have remained unchanged. The other symptoms, including emotional lability, nervousness and PMS have substantially decreased.

KI-27 is an important point for perennial allergic rhinitis, asthma, and dyspnea with sensations of high, short, superficial breathing, etc.

❖ Case History

Mrs. B., age 36, president of a company and mother of two, came to see me for an allergy that was distinctly worse in May, June and July, with red, watery eyes, sneezing with a serous nasal discharge, itchy throat, and coughing. She presented with intermittent eczema that had recurred for years on her fingers and eyebrows. In addition, she reported a tendency to retain water, with edema of the hands, feet and face. She was slightly constipated, with normal urination. Her pulse was deep in the proximal position and normal at KI-3: there was qi, probably of the Lung, that was either failing to descend or was not being properly received. I had to choose between the arm *tai yin* window-of-heaven point, LU-3, and KI-27. I began by needling LU-3, even though this allergy occurred outside of the usual hay fever season. The symptoms remained unchanged. So I then punctured KI-27. The results were spectacular, with a 90 percent improvement. This failure of the Lung qi to descend should be taken into consideration for cases of edema, which should be treated with KI-27 along with other relevant points.

SP-17 brings up the pure Spleen qi.

❖ Case History

A 39-year-old man, a high-ranking official, had already consulted me for depression, insomnia and anxiety that had been treated by allopathic methods. "I haven't had any drive or enthusiasm for years, I do not want anything, and I have trouble falling asleep, wake up often, and feel anxious, especially at dusk. I am always insecure and am afraid of everything. I guess my background explains it all; I have been HIV-positive for 14 years; both my father and grandfather committed suicide. As a homosexual, living in a difficult relationship, I regret not having any children. Death is always at hand; I have trouble dealing with everyday life."

I interpreted the symptoms as expressing constraint in the thorax and Heart, linked to the disturbances in the family tree (grandfather, father, children), which I treated effectively with CV-18. This point is considered to link to the *jue yin* as a kind of node (based on Chapter 5 of the *Divine Pivot*) and permits flexible, easy flow in all areas and all planes, including from our ancestors to our descendants and along the various axes of the body.

Several months later, when he was doing well, he suddenly asked for an emergency appointment. For 18 days he had been very tired, with little physical endurance. He had episodes of dizziness accompanied by feelings of malaise and instability, such that he felt he was about to lose consciousness. He also had muscle pains and prickly sensations in the extremities; he became quickly out-of-breath, suffered bloating with an overwhelming desire to unbuckle his belt, flatulence, and nausea. Otherwise, he was well, slept well, and had little anxiety, even at dusk. His pulses were weakest at the middle and proximal positions.

I interpreted these signs as an indication of a counterflow. The flatulence was a sign of excess due its aggravation by pressure.[8] Also, the pulses seemed to indicate qi accumulating under the diaphragm, unable to rise. The culprit might be a blockage of the diaphragm, a failure of qi to rise from either the Kidneys or the Spleen (qi from the Lung, Heart and yang organs was descending; that of the Liver was rising too fast and strong, a pathological excess). Since there were no hiccups or belching to give relief and no sense of constriction around the lower thorax, I surmised that the pure Spleen qi was failing to rise and treated it with SP-17. The symptoms disappeared after two sessions.

What is the connection between these two scenarios? I perceived that they were both evidence of the same type of difficulty with turning towards life and turning away from the death of the father and grandfather. Of course, to be HIV-positive is to feel a constant threat.

GV-5 brings up the Kidney qi.

❖ Case History

Mrs. R., age 46, consulted me for uterine bleeding that had persisted continuously since the removal of her IUD 18 months previously.[9] Up to that time, her menstrual cycles had been perfectly normal. She had given birth to five children; the third child had died 14 years before, at the age of three months, a case of sudden infant death syndrome (SIDS). She still cried when talking about it, although she believed she had finished her grieving. Suddenly, she realized: "In fact, I gave birth every four years; the bleeding began four years after the birth of the last baby! But I did not want more children; neither did my husband." I told her about the body's memory. "Do you believe that my body periodically remembers that little girl who died so suddenly?"

Furthermore, the history revealed feelings of oppression, palpitations, feelings of constriction around the lower thorax, intense physical and mental fatigue attributed to anemia, insomnia with difficulty falling asleep, and nasopharyngitis that had persisted for five months with runny nose, pain in the right side of the forehead and pharyngeal discomfort. This tall, slender woman with long fingers was simultaneously energetic and reserved; at times, her face lighted up with a smile. Her tongue appeared normal. There were no symptoms of deficiency or blood stasis. The pulses, mostly full, were much deeper in the distal positions. It was clear that this was a general problem rather than a local or regional one.

Based on the pulses and thoracic symptoms, I first thought there might be a deficiency in the upper burner that would explain the fatigue, insomnia and flow of uterine blood. I punctured CV-17, the alarm point of the upper burner. Despite a worsening on the fifth day (which is late for a reaction to a session), none of the symptoms had changed by her second visit two weeks later. No older signs had reappeared. However, this young woman shyly spoke up: "You told me that I should pay attention to any wild dreams. Well, I had one: there were two wooden snakes fighting a duel." This made me think of a point that includes a reference to "snake dreams" and I told myself that I must have misinterpreted the pulses; instead of the upper pulse being deficient, it was the lower one that was excessive. In fact, the qi was blocked in the bottom of the pelvis and unable to rise to the thorax. The point to puncture was GV-5 which, when blocked, can result in an obstruction of Kidney qi in the pelvis,[10] preventing it from rising to the other organs, the Heart in particular. So I punctured this point: the bleeding stopped for good after 12 hours.

Yang Organ Points

A common way of presenting the five phases is with the Spleen at the center and the other four phases at the four cardinal directions. It "receives the seed and gives the harvests" (*Basic Questions,* Chapter 9). It is in charge of the yang organs, which have the function of managing our emotional, social, professional, family and other territories, beginning with the body. The yang organs define, irrigate, seed, nourish, bring to fruition, drain and coordinate.

There are two sets of yang organs. The first central set includes the Stomach and the Gallbladder. The second set includes the ground, corresponding to the Lung, Heart and Kidneys—the Large and Small Intestines and the Bladder.

IN THE CENTER

The Stomach/Gallbladder pair is governed by CV-11. Note that these are the only two yang organs that have points on the outer branch of the Bladder channel, BL-48 and BL-50.

❖ Case History

Mrs. C. came to see me with symptoms that, on the one hand, pointed to the Gallbladder (nausea, bitter taste in the mouth, dizziness, pain in the area of the gallbladder) and, on the other hand, to the Intestines (intestinal spasms with malodorous gas, pain in the right hand and shoulder along the Large Intestine channel). Which of these two is the cause? "Spiritually, I am moving forward, I am constantly seeking my true self. But I do not get any recognition from my husband and my son. I am afraid of being left out. This is a problem in my everyday existence." I asked, "An existential problem involving ones territory?" "Exactly," she replied. I successfully punctured a point that governs the middle regions of the Gallbladder, Stomach and Spleen, CV-11.

The Stomach receives, cooks and digests foods. It is central, the "sea of water and grains", and "provides in all seasons", that is, to the entire body: this makes it the "root of all the organs and yang organs"[11] and the "sea of qi and blood." It is the source of qi for the Kidneys. It governs the ability to fill up, for getting nourishment for oneself, for being empty, for fasting and for depriving oneself.

Apart from the associated and alarm points, the Stomach is governed by BL-50 and by ST-20 and ST-21.

❖ Case History

A 56-year-old woman had been suffering for more than 30 years from intense migraines on the left side that pulled her eye down into the socket. They did not respond to any therapy. She also complained of light sleep that was rarely restful and, unless she restricted herself to small meals, of a stomach that would not empty. She knew the reason for this. "Until I left home at the age of 25, family meals took place in a climate of hatred." From an acupuncture perspective, these three symptoms were connected: they originated in the Stomach, which was confirmed by an excess of tension in the Stomach position of the pulse. I punctured ST-20, the name of which means "receiving fullness" (承滿 *cheng man*), which is indicated when the Stomach cannot be full. For the migraines, I also added a Stomach channel point (leg *yang ming*) located on the head, ST-8 on the left. The improvement in the three symptoms, which began to appear after the third session, was distinct after the fifth session, including a problem with hay fever that she had neglected to mention and that, of course, also responded to puncturing the same channel.

The Gallbladder, in the middle region, is dedicated to initiative, to launching transformations (digestive and otherwise). Chapter 9 of *Basic Questions* states that "All of the organs take their orders from here." Many take its description in Chapter 8 of *Basic Questions,* as the 中 正 *zhong zheng* organ, to mean that it is "just and moderate." Larre in his commentary notes that it is the "judge that decides and condemns" and that it governs all beginnings. It ensures that these occur in the right time and place, like the emperor who initiates the beginning of the year in the east, in the spring, bringing together the corresponding time and space. The Gallbladder is associated with courage and aggression, which are necessary for good beginnings and decisions. Gallbladder dysfunction causes dreams of battles. In Chinese, someone who takes risks and is very bold is referred to as having a "big Gallbladder" (*da dan*).

❖ Case History

A sculptor, 48, suffered from headaches that recurred two or three times a week, for the previous two years, on the left side, extending laterally from the outer canthus along the pathway of the Gallbladder channel. There was no clear cause identified in the environment or food. Digestive disturbances appeared at the same time, with nausea, post-prandial indigestion, bitter taste in the mouth, and intolerance to coffee and chocolate, all of which indicated a Gallbladder problem. He had never been sick and could not stand to have any sickness among those surrounding him. This had all begun, inexplicably, a few months after he moved to Switzerland. I gave him some texts to read about the Chinese view of the Gallbladder. At the next visit, he explained, "I always wanted to be a sculptor. In order to earn my living, I was an international financier from the time I was 25 until I was 45. Since I was successful, I was able to retire and pursue my true vocation. As a financier, I was able to give ample expression to my aggressive nature, my decision-making powers, the ability to choose and to take initiative. But before I can begin to do this with sculpture, I have to go through a long phase of learning the technique. This repression of my assertiveness and aggression is blocking my Gallbladder." Meanwhile, puncturing GB-23, the alarm point that releases this constrained qi, gave symptomatic relief.

As the only "pure" yang organ that does not come into contact with foods, the Gallbladder is also a part of the extraordinary yang organs, which are in charge of perpetuating existence: thus it responds to BL-48 on the external branch of the Bladder channel; we will return to this.

THREE "GROUNDS"

The second group of yang organs encompasses three "grounds": the Small Intestine ("ground of the Heart"), the Large Intestine ("ground of the Lung") and the Bladder ("ground of the Kidneys").

These three grounds are in charge of the transformations necessary for the life of our territories, those of the food bowl as well as everything that nourishes us in every way. The grounding functions of these areas are to receive, realize and act upon the information and orders coming from the three corresponding yin organs. Considering relationships such as these between the yin and yang organs, it is understandable that Chinese medicine pairs them and their channels in an exterior-interior relationship.

The Small Intestine has the functions of harvesting, fulfillment and prosperity.

"Matter emerges from it transformed." It receives that which comes from the Stomach, transforms it and causes it to bear fruit under the influence of the Heart fire that it receives: it is that organ's "ground." It also receives the Heart spirit; if it cannot do this, this unanchored spirit becomes volatile and detached, leading to anxiety, insomnia, difficulty with centering and concentration, emotional lability and, naturally, intestinal complaints. There are two points that respond to these earth functions, ST-23 and ST-24. The first of these is only connected with stress and anxiety. The second is also connected to problems with certain foods, especially cold foods and raw vegetables. ST-23 fixes or treats Heart spirit, and ST-24 fixes Heart fire.

❖ Case History

A little girl, age 7, was brought to me by her mother, who thought she was fidgety, temperamental, irritable and impatient. The girl was thin and restless, and complained of three warts on her feet and hands, pains in her right wrist resulting from a traumatic fracture, sensitive to humidity, and possibly to barometric pressures, and she suffered from painful abdominal spasms without diarrhea but always connected with fear. She was highly emotional. Her agitation masked her anxiety and nervousness, which were evident at school. She did not stutter, which eliminated choosing GV-15. Her tongue appeared normal. Her deep Heart pulse may have been explained by the medical examination itself, as she was afraid of doctors.

Her behavior suggested an excess of yang that was not linked or fixed to the corresponding yin. The cause appeared to be in the Heart, more because of the emotional lability, anxiety and nervousness than because of the pulses, which seemed relatively insignificant in this context. Possible causes of volatility in the Heart yang may be a dissociation between the coupled channels in the interior/exterior relationship, the Heart and the Small Intestine, which is best treated by puncturing the connecting and source points because the qi is not flowing from the connecting point on the yang channel to the source point on the yin. Alternatively, it may be a failure of the Heart spirit to be rooted in the Small Intestine. A dissociation between the connecting and source points by necessity concerns the exterior-interior paired channels which respond to the Heart, the arm *tai yang* Small Intestine and the arm *shao yin* Heart channels; and the arm *shao yang* Triple Burner and arm *jue yin* Heart Master (Pericardium) channels. The warts and intestinal pains suggested SI-7 and therefore a dissociation between arm *tai yang* and arm *shao yin* (HT-7). This suggested TB-5, and therefore a dissociation between arm *shao yang* and arm reversing *yin* (*shou jue yin* HM-7), and the barometric cause of the wrist pains eventually became clear. The agitation was more of an indication of TB-5, the emotional lability and nervousness of SI-7. The behavioral signs of these two connecting points are insanity, apprehension, nervousness, overexcited speech for SI-7, and excitation and tremors for TB-5. I first punctured SI-7.

One month later, nothing had changed. In children, responses are quick. I then thought of the second mechanism, the volatility of the Heart spirit when it is not anchored to the Small Intestine. The abdominal pains under stress favored this hypothesis. I chose ST-23. (I would have chosen ST-24 had the intestines been more sensitive to raw vegetables and cold foods, and if the Heart fire had been involved.) There was an immediate, substantial improvement in the abdominal and joint pain, as well as in the anxiety and agitation. This result was confirmed in a second session, three months later. The warts had not changed after these three sessions. I did not see the child again for eight months, but her mother told me that she is well.

The Large Intestine, the "ground" of the Lung, receives all the qi, fluids and information sent down by this organ, which is like a canopy over the organs. It transmits, conveys and coordinates. The role of transmission and coordination brings it to bear on the functioning of the nervous system and, according to the literature, in some types of paralysis. GV-3 controls the Large Intestine in its role as the "ground" of the Lung.

❖ Case History

Mr. D., age 36, a physiotherapist, was stocky, energetic, enthusiastic, easily in-fluenced and sometimes aggressive. He came to see me to "correct his general condition and treat an isolated transient problem." In terms of general condition, he had suffered from respiratory weakness with bronchitis between the ages of 12 to 19, frequent nasopharyngitis from November to February, hay fever in May and June, intestinal problems with alternating diarrhea and constipation and severe low back pain when standing. These symptoms suggested Lung qi that was not descending and was not properly received below by the Large Intestine. When I saw him he was feeling disoriented, scattered and destabilized after a series of relationship and professional trials. I punctured one of the points that brings qi down from the Lung, CV-20, and the Large Intestine point that receives it below, GV-3. This treatment, first monthly and then bimonthly, brought improvement on all fronts.

One reading of the relevant passage in Chapter 8 of *Basic Questions* has the Bladder in charge of "organizing territories and cities." It marks them (in the way that a cat will urinate at the borders of its domain), lays out channels through it and drains these. In order to do so, it receives the organic fluids that come from the Small Intestine and the Kidneys, then sorts and circulates them: it is the "ground" of the Kidneys. For me, ST-28 (*shui dao* "water pathways") regulates this territorial function of the Bladder.

❖ Case History

A female patient, age 41, who was highly energetic and easily outraged, had always lived alone. Two years before she had become romantically involved. Six months later she was living with her friend in an efficiency apartment of 41 sq.m. (about 441 sq.ft.), where she quickly started to feel cramped. From that time on, the cystitis that she had occasionally experienced became more frequent and intense, with urgency, a deep burning sensation, a feeling of heaviness in the pelvis and occasional incontinence. The relationship between this worsening of her condition and the territorial problems was evident. ST-28 was very helpful in this case.

GOVERNING VESSEL ORGAN POINTS

We have previously considered GV-3, which treats the Large Intestine as the "ground" of the Lung, as well as GV-5, which causes qi to rise from the Kidneys. The other corresponding points are GV-4 for the Kidneys, GV-6 for the Spleen, GV-7 for the Gallbladder, GV-8 for the Liver, GV-11 for the Heart, and GV-12 for the Lung. Each point simultaneously controls and governs the related organ and expresses its internal qi, such as wind in the case of the Liver. At the posterior midline, each point is located at the level of the associated point on the back of the corresponding organs.

Let us illustrate these concepts with a case history involving GV-8, which shows how a Governing vessel point can express a qi anomaly in an organ, such as wind in the Liver.

❖ Case History

A man, age 30, was brought to the office in 1986 for hysterical attacks. During these attacks, he exhibited violent behavior, going so far as to destroy all the objects and furniture in a room. The attacks occurred as he was emerging from a depressive syndrome, with dejection and insomnia, due to relationship and emotional problems. He had shaking hands, red eyes, a trembling tongue and tense pulses, denoting a constraint of Liver qi with a disruption of wind, which culminated in the hysterical episodes. The origin in the Liver was probably due to a family weakness, with a history of an episode of icteric hepatitis around the age of 19, as well as the Liver's participation in emotional control.

I began by stimulating LR-6, an unblocking point that is particularly indicated in cases of acute psychological blockages, without results. I next turned to GV-8. There was an immediate, spectacular effect on the hysterical attacks.

The central functions of the Gallbladder, as described in Chapter 8 of *Basic Questions*, is as the 中正 *zhong zheng* organ. There is some controversy about the meaning of this term. It probably refers to the official charged with ranking and classifying men in their jurisdiction for higher office. Another interpretation is that it means to "correct the middle territory", and above we have noted that Larre thought that it meant "just and moderate." To me, the Gallbladder refers to the "inner teacher" in everyone, who always knows what is right, as this interpretation is congruent with all of these interpretations. The one point that corresponds to these functions is GV-7 (中樞 *zhong shu*), the "central pivot," the only point related to the leg lesser yang Gallbladder that has the word 'center' or 'middle' (*zhong*) in its name. The word *shu* means pivot and refers to what is cardinal, essential. The point has an alternate name, "central pillar" (*zhong zhu*), which I believe refers to a column, pillar, or support, that which shores up. It is along the midline, under the spinous process of the 10th thoracic vertebra, at the same level as two Bladder points that relate to the Gallbladder, BL-19 and BL-48. It improves visual acuity and appetite for life, treats gastric problems, hepatitis and cholecystitis (all of which are related to the Gallbladder), pains connecting the chest and back (attributed to its relationship with the Heart), low back pain and spinal stiffness.

According to Chamfrault, this is the starting point of the Governing vessel qi, in dialogue with CV-20, the point relating to the Lung, which is said to be the starting point of Conception vessel qi. This brings us back to the Gallbladder-Lung relationship that concerns the management of all beginnings.

❖ Case History

A notary clerk, age 27, tall, thin and slightly stooped, complained of digestive problems: pains of the right hypochondrium, heartburn, slow digestion, fatigue and post-prandial somnolence, alternating hard and soft stools, intolerance of fats, coffee and chocolate. The origin is either in the Liver or in the Gallbladder; the latter seemed more likely, which was borne out by the rest of the examination. In addition, he reported repeated episodes of bronchitis (slight fever with productive cough), frequent obstruction of the nose and ears, although it was not clear whether this respiratory vulnerability was due to weakened defenses, discharge of toxins that had not been eliminated, or a disturbance between the Lung and Gallbladder in connection with trouble getting started with things. The second hypothesis turned out to be the most likely. There was also some low back pain on the right. He did not report feeling tired despite irregular sleep. His tongue had a yellow coating. The pulses were tense. Introspective, emotional, anxious, indecisive, he reported frequent sighing and a sense of rage that was explained by his life: an absent father, an overbearing mother, a spouse who had taken the mother's place, and a professional status that did not reflect his capacities. I had needled various points of the Gallbladder with good symptomatic results, but without a significant change in the underlying situation. During one of his visits he began by saying, "I do not have many symptoms now," then suddenly, almost taking himself by surprise, he added, "I cannot stand this mediocrity any more, my indecision. My relationship needs to change, for her and for me. I need to find a job that measures up to my abilities. I need a little help." GV-7 was now the obvious point to puncture. A month later, he was standing straighter: "I felt as if my head came out of the water; I now have confidence and determination." Two more punctures of this point at three-month intervals helped him change the direction of his life.

The following case history, involving GV-11, illustrates a Governing vessel point in its role of governing the corresponding organ, in this case the Heart.

❖ Case History

A 35-year-old woman with scoliosis who had a 5-year-old boy spoke to me of her depression and functional cardiac disturbances, with tachycardia and precordial pains. She had lost her drive and her joy in life. She was constantly bogged down in a conflict with her mother, which had led her to return to psychotherapy a year earlier. She now felt incapable of "running her own life." The pulses confirmed a Heart deficiency. Puncturing GV-11, selected on the Governing vessel because of the scoliosis, helped bring about a considerable improvement in her depression.

CHAPTER FOUR

MAINTENANCE OF LIFE: NUTRITION AND TRANSMISSION

THERE ARE TWO MAIN functions that maintain life: nutrition and transmission. I nourish myself and recreate myself with each breath, and I transmit, in one way or another, the life that has been given to me. Both of these evoke the interaction of clouds and rain: vapor rises from the earth to the sky to form clouds, which condense, forming rain that falls on the earth and renders it fertile.

Nutrition depends on the Triple Burner, the perpetuation of the "six extraordinary organs."

The Triple Burner is the channel that supports all nutrition, respiration, food as well as emotional, intellectual, artistic, spiritual and any other type of nurturing. It is simultaneously cosmic, human and even cellular, as there is a Triple Burner in each being, universe or cell. The *Classic of Difficulties,* No. 25, states that the Triple Burner is the minister and emissary of the gate of vitality, and No. 38 states that it is the source of primal qi.[1] This means that it brings the Kidneys' potential into action, brings the invisible into the visible, something which is at work throughout all creation. It is controlled by two points: CV-5 and BL-22. CV-5, along the midline, which we have already seen,[2] is below the navel. BL-22, on the back, is at the level of GV-5, between the first and second lumbar vertebrae.

THREE BURNERS

The Triple Burner (TB) is made up of three burners: upper, middle and lower. Their "anatomical" distinctions and locations are, as always, symbolic.

The upper burner receives the food that is ingested and the air that is inhaled.[3] In return, it receives the transformed products, encompassed by the designations of qi, blood and fluids, distributing and circulating them to warm and nourish the body. Linked to the ancestral qi (*zong qi*), it expresses both the unique, singular being that we are, and the culmination of a line of ancestors (*zong*), which we also are. CV-17, on the midline and in the center of the chest at the level of the fourth intercostal space, controls this upper burner.

The symptomatology of the upper burner is, in case of excess: a feeling of fullness in the thorax, oppression, dyspnea that improves with effort, anxiety, and full, strong pulses in both distal positions; and, in case of deficiency: intense physical and psychological fatigue, depression, insomnia, dyspnea during effort, weak voice, palpitations, anorexia, and small, thin pulses in both distal positions.

❖ Case History

A physician, age 51, was suffering from intense physical and psychological fatigue: he had no drive, no desire or appetite for food or for life in general. He slept poorly, unable to fall asleep or awaking after only three or four hours of sleep. Anxiety, centered in the solar plexus, exhausted him. This had begun in adolescence, with peaks that could last for weeks. Anxiolytics and antidepressants had little effect. He refused any psychotherapy. This doctor, a social and professional success, said he was dominated by the memory of his father, a "tremendous man" and great attorney who he could not see as being "like everyone else," with strengths and weaknesses. The pulses confirmed a deficiency in the upper burner. The treatment—CV-17 supplemented by HT-7, HM-7 and LU-9—brought notable improvement.

The lower burner separates the pure from the impure in our nutrition and determines what to keep and what to eliminate,[4] and above all puts everything in its place (the pure above and inside, the impure below and outside). The pathology does not lie in the existence of the impure, which, based on the principles of yin and yang, must coexist with the pure; it is the impure not being in its proper place that is the problem. CV-7, along the midline at one inch below the navel, controls it.

Its symptomatology includes intestinal, urinary and lumbar signs: bloating under the umbilicus, a pelvic region that is failing to breathe, a white or yellow coating on the root of the tongue, an ample, tense pulse in the proximal position (if there is an excess) or fine and empty (if there is a deficiency). The patient has difficulty sorting things out and putting things in their place in every sense.

❖ Case History

A young (age 38) attorney suffered from constipation and had urgent urination with occasional incontinence; her periods were far apart and scanty. She described her life as disconnected: without a commitment, she had difficulty sorting things out or harmonizing or prioritizing her instincts and feelings. The weaker pulse in both proximal positions revealed a deficiency in the lower burner and explained her problem with sorting, situating and connecting. Needling CV-7 brought about "a sensation of heat in the middle of the spine," and after the fourth session, there was noticeable improvement in her symptoms.

BL-39, which "releases the heat of the lower burner," is useful in certain cases of cystitis or diarrhea with burning during urination and/or in the intestines, if the pulses in both proximal positions are deficient. It may be indicated in a case of insufficient draining of the blood in the lower burner resulting in either skin diseases (eczema) or gynecological problems featuring particularly malodorous menstrual blood (painful periods, sterility, gynecological infections, etc.).

The middle burner ensures the "cooking and digestion" of foods, the extraction of essence of all our nourishment and the distillation of organic fluids. It has the role of accomplishment and completion, including of the person. Indeed, between heaven above (upper burner) and earth below (lower burner) is the realm of man, whose function is to symbolically reunite heaven and earth.

The symptomatology of the middle burner suggests gastrointestinal problems, epigastric pain, digestion that is too slow or too fast, a coated tongue, a middle pulse that is ample and strong in cases of excess and fine in case of deficiency.

CV-12, at the midline, the epigastric area, halfway between the sternum and the navel, controls this accomplishment function of the middle burner. It is also indicated in essence deficiencies in the middle burner caused by overwork or exhaustion (in this case, the signs include intense fatigue, digestive problems, especially epigastric problems, and a brief, hard-to-locate pulse in both the proximal and distal positions).

❖ Case History

A man, age 57, who worked as a car mechanic, was dressed in very elegant clothing when he came to see me for pains and digestive problems. The pains were electric, unbearable, starting at the base of the skull, at the occiput at GV-15, and descending along the spinal column to the middle of the back. At the same time, he could not digest anything. The slightest indulgence led to indigestion, nausea, heartburn, regurgitation and insomnia. This made it impossible for him to see friends or have a social life. And that was all he had left! "My relationships have been a disaster; I am not married and have no children. I am only a garage mechanic even though I went to college. My life is a failure. Anyway, it already started out all wrong, since I have had no father or mother since I was five." The pulse confirmed a diagnosis of a middle burner issue: without a father (heaven) or mother (earth), this person had a profound sense of having accomplished nothing. He rejected psychotherapy, believing that it "would not do any good, considering the context." To me, his lack of accomplishment indicated a middle burner deficiency and, secondarily, led to an imbalance between the two midline anterior and posterior vessels, the Conception and Governing vessels. I punctured CV-12 and GV-15. The pains cleared up very quickly. His digestion improved markedly, for one to three weeks, which gave him a chance to resume his social life. For unknown reasons he did not return after the fifth session.

QI, BLOOD AND FLUIDS: PRODUCTS OF THE TRIPLE BURNER

The qi that is allotted to us at birth, responsible for the apparent, visible manifestation of our shape, further differentiates into an infinite variety of forms of qi that concern all the structures and functions required for life. These forms include ancestral qi (*zong qi*), original qi (*yuan qi*) and essential qi (*jing qi*), nurturing qi (*ying qi*) and protective qi (*wei qi*), as well as the qi of the organs, extraordinary organs, primary and secondary channels, and so on.

The fluids (*jin ye*) are in charge of fertilizing all areas of the body and participate in managing all of our territories.

The blood (*xue*) is connected to the specific characteristics and nature of each individual. In connection with the Heart, it is the medium of our individuality and individuation.

The pathologies of the qi, blood and fluids are due to insufficiency, stagnation or to abnormal circulation outside of their regular pathways. Let's look at an example of headaches to differentiate the way they manifest.

- Qi headaches are of a wrenching, burning type.

❖ Case History

A young woman, age 32, had been suffering for years from intense splitting headaches at the top of her head. They were often triggered by stress or emotion, but had no connection with her periods (blood). Note that pain associated with blood is usually influenced by the menses, alcohol and heat. Tests did not reveal any organic causes. She felt torn between the Eastern Orthodox faith inherited from her parents and the Jewish faith of her husband: this contradiction had a connection with her headaches, as if there could not be a harmonious communication between the two hemispheres of her brain. GV-20, at the top of the skull, called the "Hundred Meetings," reduced the headaches considerably.

- Blood-type headaches are pulsatile or vise-like, aggravated by menses or by alcohol.

❖ Case History

An employee in a law firm, age 53, with a congested face, presented with pulsatile headaches that made it impossible for him to drink any alcohol. He said that he had failed, professionally and especially personally; he felt as if he had been "passed by." GV-22 produced an 80 percent improvement in the headaches.

- Ophthalmic migraines with characteristic visual disturbances, sometimes accompanied by difficulty in speaking and numbness of the tongue or of an upper limb, are frequently due to phlegm related to stagnant fluids. These are often connected to digestive problems; they may be due to an excess of blood in the head, but in that case the context is different, as we have just seen. GV-18 has an excellent immediate curative and preventive effect.

QI PATHOLOGIES

Overall Disturbances of Qi

All overall qi disturbance implies to me the involvement of the Kidneys, the "roots of production of all organs," which, after a certain period of development, are always concerned. We will put aside those major deficiencies due to malnourishment and serious or terminal illness and limit our discussion to cases seen in everyday outpatient care.

Overall Deficiencies of Yin or Yang

In both cases, there is intense fatigue accompanied by nighttime sweating, feelings of heat and insomnia (for yin deficiencies), and daytime sweating, cold and hypersomnia (in deficiencies of yang). As always, the most important priority is to find and treat the etiology.

Overall Stagnation of Yin or Yang

CV-4 sets the body's yin in motion and GB-25 does the same for the yang. These are two alarm points (募 *mu*). CV-4 corresponds to the summer, to setting yin in motion, and to the Small Intestine. GB-25 is connected to the winter, to setting yang in motion, and to the Kidneys. Further on, in the chapter on alarm points, I recount a case history involving this point. Stagnation, either general or local, is improved with heat, movement and massage. Like a global deficiency, a global stagnation of qi relates to the Kidneys; it is treated by GB-25, the alarm point of the Kidneys, along with CV-4, which counts "gate of vitality" (*ming men*) as one of its secondary names.

❖ Case History

A woman, age 41, consulted me for headaches and excessive sweating. She could not pinpoint when the headaches had begun. With no apparent cause, they occurred in attacks that lasted for four days. The weather, menstrual periods, digestion and emotions did not have any connection to them. The pains were deep, endocranial, severe and vise-like. Local application of cold provided momentary relief. Pressure on the eyes did not affect them, and they were accompanied by a marked sensation of fullness in the head.

The yang type signs—alleviated by local cold, accompanied by a feeling of fullness—correspond to an excess of endocranial yang. The first point to consider is BL-8, which releases this. In this case, it brought rapid relief. BL-7 would be the next point to puncture if BL-8 had failed to produce results. It is difficult to make a clinical distinction between the two.

The perspiration, which had begun four years before, was mainly at night. It also occurred during naps. In the daytime, it was localized in the axilla. The patient could not say whether it was hot or cold. It was abundant at night and had increased during the past year. Normally, night sweats suggest a yin deficiency. The etiology can be determined by examining the overall condition of the patient.

A young woman, she said that she was always tired. She was rarely cheerful or energetic, and reported that this "horrible" fatigue was worse in the mornings and had increased over the years. She did not suffer from sudden exhaustion during the daytime. The main causes of morning fatigue are stagnation of the Gallbladder qi, general stagnation of yin (CV-4) or of yang (GB-25), or an insufficiency of the "morning audience" of the Lung (LU-1). This last Item refers to a disruption in the Lung's beginning of the diurnal circulation of qi each morning between 3 and 5 a.m., as noted in *Basic Questions*, Chapter 21. In this case, yin stagnation seems likely. She felt chilled to the bone and reported sometimes experiencing heat in her head. Her sleep had been poor for a long time; she had difficulty falling asleep, but did not have nightmares. Sensitivity to cold contributed to the stagnation. Any generalized yin stagnation is accompanied by a leakage of yang; this explains the feelings of heat, headaches and insomnia. As the leakage of yang increases, it reveals the blockage of cephalic yang at BL-8.

This patient was an accountant, an orderly person, who smoked 60 cigarettes a day and paid little attention to her diet: she did not like meat or fruits. She did not report any cardiac or pulmonary symptoms, coughing, spitting or shortness of breath despite her tobacco addiction. She digested all foods well. She often had gas and had been constipated for a long time. Her urination was normal. Her periods occurred every 28 days. She constantly had a white vaginal discharge. She had a son who was 18 years old and, just eight months before her visit, she had given birth to a second child, after spending three years trying to conceive. She had been bedridden for the last six months of the pregnancy. Three-and-a-half years previously she had miscarried. Her sexual relations were satisfactory. Apart from an appendectomy and breast enhancement surgery, she did not report any significant surgical history.

As a child, she had been sent to boarding school; she stayed until the age of ten, when her father died. She tried to escape the material and emotional difficulties of her childhood by marrying at the age of 17. She quickly became pregnant and then found herself alone with her son; she stayed alone for ten years. For the last several years, everything had been going better.

CV-4 was the right point to treat. It proved highly beneficial.

Regional or Local Circulatory Problems

These are acupuncture treatment notions that have been particularly developed or emphasized in the West. Here, I will address windows of heaven, breakdowns and the diaphragm. The barrier points are discussed in the section on qi after the acupuncture points.

"WINDOWS OF HEAVEN"

These points govern certain relationships between the head, the "heaven" of the body, and the thorax below. Mainly located on the front and back of the neck, they were categorized by Chamfrault under the name of "windows of heaven," also the name of one of the points, TB-16. They are described in Chapters 2 and 21 of the *Divine Pivot*. There are ten of them, and apart from GV-16, their names all include the word *tian* 天, which means heaven or firmament.

- On the neck, from front to back, ST-9, LI-17, SI-17 and SI-16, TB-16, and BL-10.

We do not consider, as do Duron and his colleagues,[5] LI-18 to really be a window-of-heaven point. While it does act in the role of emitting the protective qi out of the trunk,[6] this does not make it a window of heaven. That is the role of LI-17, the name of which also contains the character 天 (*tian*, heaven), and with which the symptomatology of "sudden muteness" is more connected with that of the other nine.

- At the base of the skull, GV-16, and at the exit of the trunk, CV-22.

GV-16, under the occipital protuberance, where the qi of the Governing vessel enters the brain, is a wind point that mobilizes all of the brain qi. Its indications include, among others, certain types of headaches, vertigo, convulsions and insanity, torticollis, and stiffness of the neck with pain radiating from this point to the two shoulders. CV-22, in the hollow of the throat, governs the relationship between the thorax and heaven. It is effective in aphonia, in certain cases of dyspnea or spasms of the diaphragm; the patient's face is often ruddy and very hot.

- In relationship to the qi and blood are LU-3 and HM-1 (*Divine Pivot*, Chapter 21). HM-1 comes up from the middle burner and governs qi and blood. Arm *tai yin*, related to the Lung, corresponds to qi while arm *jue yin*, linked with the Heart Master (Pericardium), corresponds to the blood. So LU-3 of the arm *tai yin* serves to facilitate qi exchanges with the head. HM-1 serves the same role with the blood. "The Liver and Lung contend with one another," wrote Nguyen Van Nghi regarding arm *tai yin*.[7] This means that *jue yin* and *tai yin* contend with each other, and therefore that the qi and blood are fighting each other. Signs of bleeding from above and below will occur, as noted in Chapter 21 of the *Divine Pivot*.

- BL-10 on the leg *tai yang* favors the descent of yang from the cranium downwards. If this window does not function properly, it results in a cranial excess of yang with a deficiency below; some examples from Van Nghi are "vertigo with weakness in the legs, extreme pain at the top of the skull, weak legs that cannot support the body." By contrast, ST-9 facilitates the ascent of yang from the body to the head. A dysfunction of this point therefore leads to an excess of yang in the thorax and a deficiency above: "excess in the chest, dyspnea"; the reference to the "vocal cords" evokes the throat exit of yang from the trunk, like "problems with the tongue and throat, goiter, platysma muscles."

- SI-17 governs the ascent of yin from the body to the head, which explains the symptomatology of cephalic yin deficiency with an excess below: "excess in the chest, dyspnea, chest pains, nausea and vomiting, inability to speak, (yin exit), scrophula" … "ringing in the ears, deafness [due to a yin deficiency]."

- SI-16 on the arm *tai yang* suggests affliction "of the face and head by cold and wind," and an impact on eye and ear function.

- LI-17 on the arm *yang ming* includes "sudden muteness, loss of voice."

- TB-16 on the arm *shao yang* implies "deaf, poor vision, swollen face, strange dreams, stiff neck, internal congestion headaches"; and "dreams of standing on head."

Frequently, SI-16, TB-16 and LI-17 are effective for acute torticollis and cervicobrachial neuralgia radiating along the *tai yang* (for SI-16), *shao yang* (for TB-16), and both the anterior and posterior aspects of the shoulder (for LI-17).

Here we will provide a few typical examples of how these points are best utilized.

External origin

❖ Case History

Mrs. H., age 56, consulted me in 1988 for a syndrome that had appeared in 1975. The circumstances were astonishing: she had been talking on the telephone during a storm at her country home and was suddenly struck by lightning in the right ear! This produced the following syndrome, which had persisted up to the present: hemicrania continua headache on the right along the *shao yang* channel, always accompanied by ipsilateral facial pain, both aggravated by wind; and visual disturbances with blurred vision and photosensitivity. The symptoms were improved by sweating. The incident resulted in permanent amenorrhea. In addition, there were seemingly spontaneous attacks that featured bradycardia, a sensation of tightness in the heart, lightheadedness, coldness in the extremities and weakness in the legs. Since that time, this woman had suffered from anxiety and insomnia, with difficulty falling asleep and a tendency to awaken easily. She did not have nightmares or recurring dreams. Moreover, the history taking revealed some Yang Linking vessel type pains in response to changes in barometric pressure, rare emotionally-triggered diarrhea and pelvic phlebitis following the birth of her second child. Her tongue was normal and pulses were deep and tight.

In acupuncture terms, what was the impact of this lightning strike? I immediately thought of using a window-of-heaven point, but which one? It was likely to be located on the *shao yang,* both because of the pathway of the hemicranias and the effect of wind. The TB-16 point is strongly suggested, especially because the arm lesser yang divergent channel starts at GV-20, goes to TB-16 and then down into the thorax. TB-16 also happens to bear the name of "Heavenly Window" (*tian you*). So I decided to puncture it, and, given the circumstances, I also punctured TB-5, a connecting point that deals with relations with the outside world, on the right side. I also considered HT-1, which treats yin stagnation in the chest, for the thoracic attacks and tightness in the Heart. It is connected to the Heart, which in this case received a physical and psychological shock. In the end I decided to use this point at a subsequent visit. So I began by stimulating TB-5 and TB-16 on the right. An upsetting aggravation of symptoms followed (the patient had been forewarned of this possibility) for 36 hours, then a slight improvement. At the second session a week later, there was a lesser reaction followed by a more distinct improvement. By the third session, the symptoms began to disappear quickly. After the fifth session, the hemicrania, facial pains and visual disturbances had disappeared; they only reappeared marginally in situations with a high level of tension or during storms.

The thoracic attacks were less frequent and less intense but did not disappear. I added HT-1 on the right and reduced the treatments to once a month. By the eighth session, the patient was cured. I recommended semiannual maintenance sessions around the spring and fall equinoxes.

Internal causes

❖ Case History

A 49-year-old woman presented with migraines that had occurred since adolescence, of various types (wrenching, burning pain, in different parts of the skull) but always highly debilitating. They were always preceded by a loss of voice (which suggests using one of the window-of-heaven points on the neck), and they improved during her two pregnancies. In addition, I noted some digestive problems related to the Gallbladder, and extreme fatigue partly due to depression and partly to overwork. Puncturing SI-17, a window-of-heaven point on the neck that is also connected to the Gallbladder, and BL-48, the Gallbladder point connected with the father (both because it is on the *tai yang* channel, which relates to the father, and because the Gallbladder itself is associated with fire), brought a considerable improvement after six sessions.

BREAKDOWNS OF QI AND OF THE PERSON

I have repeatedly mentioned those times when a person's entire life seems to crumble for emotional, professional or other reasons. This breakdown leaves psychological and somatic traces, especially in the pelvic area (it is the floor that caves in), and shows up in the pulses as a weakness in both proximal positions. I refer the reader to the two case histories related above, in which I punctured CV-5. Here I relate a third case.

❖ Case History

Mr. P. consulted me for pain caused by a trauma to the right knee, sustained in a motorcycle accident. His knee was hot and swollen. The pain was located at the inner side of the joint; it extended to the groin. It was intense and debilitating, aggravated by both fatigue and rest, and improved by pressure and heat. It was accompanied by a sensation of a "loose rubber band" with a loss of strength in the knee.

The pain was of the yang type (heat). It was not stagnation (aggravated by rest) or excess (aggravated by fatigue): GB-31, a wind point, which has a good effect on stagnation in the knee, was not indicated. When the pain Is located on the inside of the knee, it is often advisable to puncture LR-7, the "knee barrier" (*xi guan*).

Following an accident in 1997, Mr. P. had also complained of a left cervical pain that limited rotation and radiated along the *shao yang* to the shoulder. A window-of-heaven point located on the *shao yang* channel, namely TB-16, seemed to be strongly indicated. Moreover, it was very tender.

This hyperactive man slept no more than six hours a night, described feelings of instability, extensive muscular fatigue, prior episodes of somnambulism and healthy digestion, provided that he avoided fats. He was always highly stressed, even for no valid reason, and his muscles were extremely tense: "My muscles are as knotted as wood." Of medium, stocky build, he did everything quickly but precisely and meticulously. He appeared to correspond to BL-47, the point whose name means the gate of the ethereal soul, that is, a constraint of qi that cannot "come and go" easily, freely, flexibly. We know the relationship between ethereal soul, sleep (somnambulism), the muscles, the Liver, and the Gallbladder. This constraint may be a primary or a secondary reaction. BL-47 notably improved the terrain and the symptoms. Mr. P. did not present signs of dysfunctions affecting the Yang Linking vessel (pains due to barometric pressure) or Yin Linking vessel (dissipation, low back pain). Treating the terrain with BL-47, there is no need to add symptomatic points such as LR-7 or TB-16. The progress made justified this choice.

In the patient's history I noted an operation for a urethral stricture at the age of 8, and intestinal fragility since childhood, with attacks of painful diarrhea that were rarely caused by food and more often due to emotions. The man, who divided his time between Greece and Paris, was very reserved about his difficult childhood.

His tongue appeared normal; his muscles were very contracted; the proximal pulses were tense and broken down. The tense pulses corresponded to an ethereal soul type of qi constraint. Yet the deep pulses in the proximal positions indicated that there has been a breakdown at some point: he answered that there had been a very painful breakup of a relationship six years before. Considering the history of painful diarrhea, I wondered whether this breakup had not caused an earlier childhood breakdown to resurface.

So, in addition to BL-47, I punctured CV-5 to treat the breakdown, which may lead to or contribute to knee pain or foot pain, since the feet and knees are also the "footing" and foundations of a person. The knee pain disappeared two hours after the first treatment and then returned even stronger 18 hours later, this time located on the inside and outside of the knee, on *shao yang* and *jue yin* (corresponding to ethereal soul). He experienced diarrhea without pain for the first three days. The neck pain disappeared. He felt much more relaxed.

I punctured the same points during his second visit, which was only four days later because he was leaving for Greece. After the second session, the knee pain disappeared for six weeks. His stools were still soft but there was no more intestinal pain. He was not nearly as stressed and felt more at ease; he even indulged in reading for three hours over the weekend. He experienced a marked reduction in cramps in the morning.

I repeated the same treatment twice every half year, during his visits to Paris, which alleviated all the symptoms for a few months. In this case, once again, it was important to ignore the symptom.

BLOOD PATHOLOGIES

In general, blood disorders can be classified as related to deficiency, excess, stagnation or an issue with the elimination of toxins.

- Most major deficiencies (e.g., anemia) or excesses (e.g., erythremia) are not readily treatable by acupuncture. However, herbal medicine and diet can be an effective complement to allopathic treatment. By contrast, acupuncture has a place in the treatment of moderate chronic anemia, where it can stop repeated bleeding or improve the absorption of iron or vitamin B-12, etc. The treatment in such cases is a purely etiological approach.

- It has an important effect on stagnation. This is due to cold or to deficiency of qi. The tongue is purple; the patient feels cold and tired and presents atrophic and circulatory disorders in the extremities, the integuments and the two membranes, which will be discussed shortly. The treatment should, in general, be aimed at the etiology, but one of the remarkable points in this case is BL-17.

- What we refer to as "impurities" are related to an accumulation of toxins, for which we need to define the cause. The symptomatology is of the heat or fire type. Heat manifests in the form of eczema, pruritus, urticaria, herpes, or even local bleeding (the heat pushes the blood out of its normal circulatory passages). Fire often manifests on the skin (furuncles, acne, purulent wounds), with foul-smelling sweat or menses. As always in Chinese medicine, the correct approach is to treat the cause. KI-23 is often useful in purifying the Heart blood, and SP-10 is another important point.

❖ Case History

A man, age 42, was suffering from a long-term case of eczema on the face and hands. His face showed congestion, which was aggravated by heat, emotion or alcohol consumption (typical of KI-23). He was highly emotional and sensitive, although he tried to hide it. He grew tired quickly and lacked vitality. The pulses were generally deep and that of the Heart was deficient. I chose KI-23, a point on the *shao yin* channel, because of the fatigue and lack of vitality, in connection with the Heart because of the pulse and the emotionality, which would also purify the blood. This choice produced a remarkable result.

Local

The most likely places for blood disorders to manifest are the Heart envelope[8] (which contains the coronary circulation) and gestational envelopes, or sacs, of the pelvis (胞 *bao,* which encompass the uterine and prostate circulation), the brain (*nao* 腦), and the blood vessels (血脈 *xue mai*), which include the arteries, veins and capillaries. Note that I am using such words as "contain, include, encompass" on purpose, as these terms are not strictly limited to the structures mentioned, but go beyond the coronary, uterine, or prostate structures to include related circulatory and lymphatic structures.

This is often a case of local blood stasis, which manifests with fixed stabbing or sharp pains that are aggravated by cold. Problems due to deficiency become worse after menstrual periods or alcohol consumption. The tongue is dark red to purple. The pulse is fine and rough in general or in particular positions.

Blood circulation in the Heart envelope is governed by BL-43; that of the pelvic envelope by BL-53; and GV-22 controls the circulation of blood in the head.

Huang points

The word 肓 *huang* refers to a kind of nutrition that is linked to activity (alimentary, intellectual, spiritual), which we call nutritive heat. There are four points that have this character in their names—BL-43, BL-51, BL-53, and KI-16—and two Conception vessel points that are connected with it—CV-6 and CV-16. Here we will briefly discuss this concept of nutritive heat and how these points reflect it.

BL-43, named *gao huang shu* (膏肓俞), supplies the Heart with both its noble fats (*gao*) as well as nutritive heat (*huang*). It is indicated in cases of exhaustion with an internal sensation of cold due to chronic illness, in neurasthenia with memory loss, in malnutrition and in broken relationships, and, like the previously mentioned KI-23, it is highly useful for certain types of coronary insufficiency.

❖ Case History

A 49-year-old man had undergone an angioplasty in 1996. Unfortunately, a stenosis had recurred, necessitating a bypass. Despite this surgery and medication, he continued to experience chest pains when cold. Single, lonely, in a difficult profession, tense, anxious, irritable, and in need of a vacation, he decided to turn to acupuncture. BL-43, a point which is known for nourishing the affective aspects, punctured every three weeks, was one of the points that best reduced his pain.

Point BL-53 is named *bao huang* 胞肓 (*bao* means envelope, an organ surrounded by a membrane, a bladder or a vesicle). It is located on the outer branch of the *tai yang* channel at the level of the second sacral foramen. The symptomatology of BL-53 is mainly pelvic, with significant genital implications. This point is related to the pelvic envelope, the balance between qi and blood in the pelvis, and, as a result, the uterus. Its pathology is connected to a blockage of qi and blood in the pelvis, and this blockage is closely linked to the genitals, the prostate, menstruation, and pregnancy.

❖ Case History

Mrs. D., age 46, presented with classic attacks of spontaneous muscle contractions, known as spasmophilia, ever since an abortion performed when she was 27. She reported that the abortion had gone well, physically and psychologically. The attacks were more frequent and intense around her menstrual periods. In addition, she reported difficulties with concentration and memory, substantial hair loss, which could be a deficiency of blood in the upper body, and insomnia, both of difficulty in falling asleep and waking up early. Her periods occurred every 23 days. They started slowly, lasted a long time and caused a marked sensation of heaviness in her lower limbs. Ever since puberty, the patient had cystalgia with clear urine. Her tongue was purple. The proximal pulses were deep. This young woman had been faced with relationship and affective problems throughout her life; this probably explains the blood nature of her disorder. I diagnosed a blockage in the blood in her pelvis and lower limbs and tonified BL-53 and SP-6. After four bimonthly sessions the improvement was considerable in every respect. Because this patient moved with her husband to the United States, I was unable to complete the treatment and do not know of the ensuing outcome.

Below are two additional cases concerning other points with *huang* in their names. These are KI-16, *huang shu* ("Nutritive Heat Transport"), located on either side of the navel, and CV-6, *qi hai* ("Sea of Qi"), which has the alternate name of *xia huang* ("Lower Nutritive Heat") and is the sea of the membranes.

❖ Case History

Ms. I., age 22, was a lively, slender, intelligent and generous lady; she was unmarried and had no children. She consulted for severe fatigue caused by hypochromic anemia. In fact, she always went to sleep very late, talked loudly in her sleep and woke up tired. She sometimes fainted. She had been a sleepwalker when she was a child. She suffered from constipation and could not stand eating fats, which made her nauseous. She frequently had cystitis and vaginal mycosis with pruritic vaginal discharge. Her periods were irregular, very often late and prolonged. She had intense headaches, although not very frequently. She was irritable and quick-tempered. She often had night terrors. Her proximal pulses were wiry and deep. Her tongue was normal.

It was obvious from the sleep problems, the abdominal disorders, and her behavior, which betrayed a compressed and at times explosive energy, that the ethereal soul was disturbed. Biological tests confirmed that there was a slowing down of the liver's stocking of ferritin.

Four monthly sessions using BL-48 greatly improved her condition. A fifth session, three months later, reinforced this result.

The patient returned seven years later, having become pregnant a month earlier via an embryo transplant. She complained of drowsiness (which was normal), of very sensitive areolas, and of irritability and anxiety (justifiably enough). I needled KI-9, which is known to be useful at the beginning of a pregnancy. She came again a month later. Her obstetrician had diagnosed a placental abruption detected by ultrasonography, the clinical symptoms of which were brown spotting and a sensation of heaviness in the lower abdomen along with contractions. Moreover, she had experienced diarrhea with abdominal pain for the previous seven days.

She was thirsty. Her sleep was light. Her pulse was rapid and slippery on the right distal position, confirming her pregnant status. I needled KI-16, a *huang* point near the navel, bilaterally, as it is related to pregnancy. After the first session the spotting stopped, the contractions and the pelvic heaviness diminished, and the bowels were normal; she experienced reactive yang sciatica on the right side 48 hours later. From that time, I gave her three weekly treatments using these same points. After the third session, the clinical signs receded and the ultrasonography examination showed the placental abruption had disappeared. She had a normal pregnancy thereafter.

❖ Case History

Mrs. C., age 41, consulted for constant allergies dating six years. Her allergies affected the nose (sneezing, serous rhinorrhea) and the skin of the forehead, upper lids, and upper limbs, with pruritus aggravated by heat (e.g., while in bed). The antihistamine Zyrtec controlled these symptoms rather well. These allergies were of a heat type and were located in the upper part of the body.

The history also revealed that she had diarrhea secondary to anxiety with a sensation of cold in the abdomen, as well as cold feet that contrasted with her hot hands. This energetic lady was passionate, impatient, irritable and quick-tempered; her emotional nature no doubt pertained to fire. There was an imbalance between the upper and the lower parts of the body, between the heat in the upper part and the cold abdomen and feet. Her behavior, weak proximal pulses and symptoms suggested that the fire, constrained in the upper part, was unable to descend. CV-6, which makes fire descend into water, seemed the best choice. After the second session, the improvement was perceptible. The symptoms had markedly decreased. Within a fortnight, she was only taking a half tablet of Zyrtec. As far as the heat signs were concerned, "fire was going down." She was calmer and more balanced. However, the pulses were not yet completely back to normal. I therefore added CV-16 because this point governs the return of fire to the Heart. The symptoms totally disappeared after the second needling of CV-16. The sessions then became less frequent as the improvement progressed (once every six, then eight, then 12 weeks).

❖ Case History

A 50-year-old man with a stocky build came to see me for a stuffy nose that had lasted for some six years. The condition had developed gradually and then worsened. He did not report any significant events occurring at the time other than some professional and marital difficulties. At present, the obstruction was permanent, although there was a slight improvement in the winter. It was accompanied by a strange impression that the nose was swollen, "like a sponge," and alcohol ingestion brought relief. These last two signs suggested blood stasis in the head. Treating GV-22, which governs the blood in the head, with moxa (because the heat promotes circulation) healed this patient.

FLUID PATHOLOGIES

A deficiency of fluids produces dryness or, when more advanced, dehydration, stagnation, phlegm caused by congealing;[9] and an accumulation, such as edema, either local or regional.

Deficiencies of organic fluids, that is, dehydration, are not primarily within the province of acupuncture, even though CV-9 and KI-7 can be useful for edema. Herbal medicine and diet are important here, as in systemic edema of a cardiac or renal etiology. Local edema is a good indication for acupuncture, as internal or external dampness is often the cause. In any case, the principle is to promote local circulation of qi in order to dissolve the accumulation. Points like CV-9 and KI-7 have a valuable diuretic effect.

Likewise, phlegm *(tan yin)*, derived from the condensation or desiccation by heat of stagnating fluids, is treatable by acupuncture alone or in combination with herbal medicines. It may be of the cold type (white and easily expelled, with a white coating on the tongue) or heat type (yellowish and difficult to expel, with a yellowish tongue coating). In both cases, the pulses are slippery. They always result in an obstruction in the flow of qi and/or blood in some part of the body. They can be a cause for certain digestive or respiratory disorders (which is close to the understanding of Western biomedical pathology), but also sometimes for cardiac disorders (some coronary diseases), psychological disorders (mental illness, confused or distraught states) and neurological disorders (some cerebral vascular accidents, loss of consciousness, epilepsy or ophthalmic migraines).

- ST-40 is the point that dissolves phlegm regardless of where it manifests: it may be punctured or, preferably, tonified with moxa.
- LU-7 has a pulmonary effect. GV-18 has a cerebral impact which makes it very useful in the treatment of ophthalmic migraines, as a cure during an attack, or as a preventive measure.

In all cases, the right approach is to find and treat the general mechanism responsible for the formation of phlegm.

❖ Case History

Mr. H., age 48, a construction foreman, complained of constant discomfort in the hollow of the throat, without hoarseness or coughing. He felt the urge to clear his throat and spit, but could not expel anything except during physical effort, such as riding a bicycle. Even then, the spitting did not give lasting relief from this sensation. It had appeared gradually about two years before. Cold or damp weather did not alter this symptomatology, nor did the seasons, or cold or warm air. Only nervous tension seemed to aggravate it. Athletic activities provided momentary relief, by enabling him to expectorate. The discomfort was permanent, although it varied in intensity. It was not accompanied by gagging.

Mr. H. was a small, solid man with a rigid, square appearance who held his chin tucked into his chest. His complexion was congested and his ears were red. He was a straightforward, direct man who only believed in what he could see, did not want anyone to touch his possessions and did not like to give.

The symptomatology did not fit into any of the eight parameters and was not external in origin. It was located at CV-22, at the exit of the trunk. The only factors that influenced this symptomatology were nervous tension and activity. I could not find any mechanical causes (dental, vertebral, or scars). All of this suggested that there was a problem with the circulation of phlegm in the throat, which is a transition zone.

The patient had undergone surgery 20 years before on his ankle for a fracture following a motorcycle accident, and had never had any major illness. He had lost his mother to asthma over 30 years before and his father had died of a heart attack at the age of 74.

Mr. H.'s digestion was slow and he suffered from flatulence. He was irritable and felt nervous and tense. At work he had good relations with other people; he knew his business well. He described himself as demanding, severe and sometimes harsh at work; he was a real stickler for principles. He said he would like to go out more, but he was obliged to visit his mother-in-law every weekend, and this annoyed him a bit.

He was married and had a 15-year-old daughter. He had good relationships with his wife and daughter and said that he had a normal sex life. He worked very hard. He had grown up in the countryside, during the war. His tongue had no coating, and looked slightly pale and thick. The yang pulses were slightly weaker than the yin pulses, which were tense.

So far, I had little to go by, other than the slow digestion and flatulence. I therefore used a two-pronged treatment. Physical exercises to open up the trunk seemed to be indicated, considering his appearance: small, solid, rigid, stocky, with his chin tucked into his chest. This physical therapy would treat the local factor, which was the poor circulation in the neck and throat, which explained why the illness had manifested in this part of the body.

This case history is a good example of a patient who does not show many symptoms. In such cases, it is important to carefully examine the patient's physical constitution and morphology for the clues they can provide, at least about the location of the disease, if not the actual cause. The acupuncture treatment aimed, first, to treat the phlegm with CV-13, a digestion point that governs phlegm, and ST-40, a connecting point that is said to be one of the major phlegm points, especially since it is also said to govern the throat; and second, to treat the throat and the exit of the trunk with CV-22, a window-of-heaven point that favors the exit of yin and yang from the chest towards the neck and the head.

This produced excellent results. There was already a marked improvement immediately after the first session, and after the third treatment, Mr. H. was cured.

DIAPHRAGM

PHYSIOLOGY

The diaphragmatic dome that stretches between the thorax and the abdomen, the principal breath muscle, the diaphragm:

- separates and joins the thorax and abdomen. It is analogous to the base of the cranium which separates and joins the face (with its orifices) and the neck with the cranium. The latter, which contains the brain, enclosed in a case of bone, is comparable to the thorax, which is contained by the rib cage and contains the Lung and Heart. A disturbance in one of these can cause a disturbance in the other.

- as a filter, it allows the clear qi to rise to the thorax and head while preventing the turbid qi from rising, keeping it in the abdomen instead; it keeps each type of qi in its place. Pathology does not reside in the existence of the turbid qi, but only when it (or the clear qi) is not in its proper place. That which is clear should be above, irrigating the Lung, Heart and brain, which I consider noble in part because they are protected by the thorax and cranium, and going inward. The turbid qi should be below and going outward, where it is handled in other ways, including by evacuation.

Symptoms and Pathology

My clinical experience has shown that this structure is often involved in pathology that produces a wide variety of symptoms. This is especially true because, as noted above, each of the several diaphragms influences all of the others. (*See* Table 1.)

ETIOLOGY

In my experience, the etiology of diaphragmatic problems is usually psychological. This includes:

- a sensation of being "cut in half," torn between two irreconcilable forces (so the person cannot, symbolically, connect their thorax and abdomen);

Table 1: Diaphragms and their Symptoms	
LOCATION	SYMPTOMS
Diaphragm	• A sensation of a tight band at the level of the xiphoid process and/or at T-7 • Hiccups, belching, discharging yawns, burning spasms or epigastric pain • Frequently accompanied by a feeling of oppression or short, superficial breathing
Thorax	• Palpitations, tachycardia, precordial heaviness, sudden surges of high blood pressure • Dry cough, deep intrathoracic pains, apparently pulmonary or pleural • Back pain (centered at T-7) that may extend to the neck or lumbar areas, painful shoulder (particularly subdeltoid bursitis) • Pains are often unilateral
Head & neck	• A feeling of congestion in the head, with headaches, dizziness, stuffy nose, hot flashes, etc. • Lightheadedness or vasovagal episodes • A sense of blockage and tension in the muscles of the cervicothoracic junction
Abdomen	• Tension and knots in the solar plexus • Nausea, indigestion, flatulence, belching and aerophagia; if there is a preexisting hiatal hernia, the spasmodic state of the diaphragm often leads to the appearance of the relevant symptoms
General signs	• Difficulty in getting to sleep and/or early awakening • Physical or mental fatigue

• both a need to cry and an inability to do so, incapacity for expressing a powerful emotion located in the chest (such as terror, sorrow), resulting in a respiratory blockage.

It may be post-traumatic. But the emotional factor is preponderant in these cases.

POINTS RELATED TO THE DIAPHRAGM

The following points are the most often used. In each case, we have to choose one or two according to the symptomatology and typology of the patient. I classify them:

According to the Centers

- Stomach and Spleen, middle burner: CV-11 (Stomach and Gallbladder in the middle region controlled by the Spleen), CV-12 (alarm point of the Stomach and the middle burner), LR-13 (alarm point of the Spleen), BL-20 and BL-21 (associated points of the Stomach and Spleen), SP-17 (brings up pure qi from the Spleen), KI-17 (transport function of the Spleen), ST-36 (sea of the Stomach), SP-3 (stream point of the Spleen)
- Heart: CV-14 (alarm), CV-17 (Heart and alarm point of the upper burner), points on the arm *shao yin* channel (particularly HT-5)

Diaphragm Points

- The *huang* point BL-43, a point that nourishes the Heart
- Points with the word "diaphragm" (膈 *ge*) in their names: BL-17 (*ge shu*) and BL-46 (*ge guan*)
- Another point that is effective in my experience, although I know of no reference for it, is GV-9, at the same level.

In Relation to Qi Phases

- Spring: GB-24 and LR-14, alarm points of the Gall Bladder and Liver that encompasses a movement from the abdomen towards the thorax (*see* section on the alarm points)
- Clavicular: ST-11, ST-13, CV-22, which, in this area, governs movement in and out of the thorax

The channels and points that are most often concerned:

- arm *jue yin:* HM-6, HM-7, HM-8
- arm *yang ming:* LI-5, LI-6, LI-9
- leg *shao yin* (less frequently): KI-3 and KI-5

There are also two connecting points that cover the diaphragm in their symptomatology, as described in Chapter 10 of the *Divine Pivot*, which are highly effective: HT-5 and LI-6.

The three case histories that follow illustrate three different and typical causes of blockage in the diaphragm.

❖ Case History

Mr. B., age 39, consulted me in January 2000 for a painful sensation of tension under the navel that extended to the perineum and had occurred spontaneously, over five years before, with no apparent cause. Neither a pelvic support device, local applications of cold or heat, nor urinating or defecating brought any relief. No intestinal or urinary disorder could be detected. He also reported periodic sensitivity in the lower back. I otherwise noticed that he had shallow and high breathing, which I attributed to a constraint in the diaphragm, evidenced by hiccups, attacks of aerophagia relieved by belching and the sensation of having a tight band around the base of the thorax at the level of CV-16. Mr. B. reported an intermittent epicondylitis in his left elbow and forearm, along the arm *yang ming*, a few episodes of tracheal cough, but nothing more. How are these symptoms tied together? The tension under the navel is related to the failure of respiratory qi to descend to the pelvis, which could be the cause of the blockage in the diaphragm.

The tongue appeared normal; the radial pulses were weak in both proximal positions but the pulse was strong at the KI-3 points. This confirms that some type of qi was not descending, in this case from the Lung. Why? If the proximal pulses and the KI-3 pulses were both weak, it would imply a weakness in the lower half of the body (e.g., of the CV-5 or Yin Heel type) or a general deficiency of yin and yang in the Kidneys. The normal pulses at KI-3 ruled out this diagnosis. So it had to be a failure of qi to descend to the pelvis. This illustrates the importance of comparing the radial and peripheral pulses. What might cause this non-descent? A blockage in the upper part of one of the three yang channels: *tai yang*, *shao yang*, or *yang ming*. Otherwise, the origin might be thoracic, with a failure of the Lung and/or Heart qi to descend; or pelvic, with these types of qi not being received below; or along the midline, with an epigastric or diaphragmatic blockage. In this case, the origin seems to be in the diaphragm, due to the hiccups, aerophagia, and tight sensation around the base of the thorax, as noted above.

In Chinese medicine, the potential causes of a diaphragmatic blockage are numerous. Often, the arm *yang ming* and *jue yin* channels are involved. Because of the absence of symptoms suggesting the other etiologies, and the occurrence of episodes of left-side epicondylitis and of coughing, arm *yang ming* seemed the most likely channel. Incidentally, it should be noted that sometimes only a minor sign or symptom points to the answer. The points most often involved along arm *yang ming* are LI-5, LI-6 (the connecting point), and LI-9. Mr. B was very glib and described himself as impatient and short-tempered. "If someone comes looking for trouble, I will give it to them."

To the question, "Have you had a lot of cavities or gingivitis?" he answered, "I am constantly getting treated for cavities." It so happens that the symptomatology of LI-6 includes, in a person who reacts quickly and easily:

• painful gums, cavities and toothaches, cold sensations in the teeth and gums
• grinding of teeth
• sudden deafness
• impairment of the diaphragm

• mental disturbances, and excessive talking

From the first session, bilateral puncturing of this point resulted in improvement after a 48-hour reaction that included epistaxis on the left, anal itching and low back pain. Since these symptoms appeared on the left side, from then on I started needling the LI-6 point on the left. The second session, ten days later, reinforced the improvement after a reaction that consisted of a tracheal cough and thoracic pain on the left with blockage of the ipsilateral shoulder. It should be noted that a number of cases of shoulder pain originate in the diaphragm. The third puncture six weeks later confirmed this overall improvement. Occasional anal itching persisted. I saw the patient again ten weeks later, after he had been in a car accident. The shock of the trauma and of the seatbelt had led to a blockage on the left side of the diaphragm, with shortness of breath, which he immediately diagnosed by himself based on his earlier sessions with me. Puncturing LI-6 on the left was effective within 36 hours. Six months later, he was doing well and, after a final treatment, I agreed that he would return only when needed.

❖ Case History

A woman, age 60, tall, slender and reserved, consulted me for a case of asthma that had appeared nine years prior following an assault as well as the death of her mother. She suffered from nocturnal inspiratory asthma. Her respiration was blocked at the clavicles although she did not feel any weight or any tightness around the thorax. The attacks ended with the difficult expectoration of white sputum. Moreover, she noted that her breathing had always been shallow, and did not usually descend into the epigastric or pelvic areas. Other symptoms appearing at the same time were sensations of blockage in the diaphragm, independent of the asthma attacks, with a tight band at the base of the thorax, a sense of oppression, and aerophagia. She rarely had hiccups. In fact, this blockage preceded the asthma. She pointed out, in connection with this, that she had been born feet-first, with the umbilical cord wrapped around her.

In addition, she reported alternating constipation and diarrhea, without pain or flatulence, although she could not connect it with any specific foods. She had never had spontaneous menstruation, but had only experienceed periods in response to hormonal treatments. She had never been pregnant, and said that she was not troubled by a lack of children. She was neither tired nor sensitive to cold, and slept well. Her pulses were full. Her tongue appeared normal.

I planned to start by puncturing BL-17, which both treats the diaphragm and governs the blood: it is the "meeting point of blood." She was well for two days, then the asthma and diaphragm problems returned. But she observed other symptoms during these two days: she awoke at four in the morning, experiencing tachycardia and cardiac auricular pain on the right side, radiating along the arm *shao yang*. On examination, I found point BL-43 to be very painful on the right side: this point, often involved in cases of emotional shock and separations, corresponds to the diaphragm and the blood. I decided that I needed to also look for a point on arm *jue yin,* which has an exterior-interior pairing with arm *shao yang*. Which was the right point to choose on this channel that treats the diaphragm—since this was characteristic of most points on arm *jue yin*, in particular HM-1, HM-5, HM-6, HM-7, and HM-8—as well as the menstrual problems? Only HM-5 meets these criteria. Moreover, its symptoms include sorrow and fear, which corresponds well to the death of her mother and the attack experience. So I punctured BL-43 and HM-5 on the right. This session was followed by a marked improvement in the asthma and of the spasms in the diaphragm, as well as a pain in the right middle finger, which corresponds to the Heart Master (Pericardium) channel.

At the next visit, she said that she was much better. She craved sugar in the evenings and noticed the day after the treatment that she had pain in the left big toe on the leg *jue yin* channel, which I attributed to the session. I saw her seven months later for back pain at the level of the diaphragm, allergic rhinitis and insomnia at four in the morning. She said that she felt stressed and held back by her husband, who was uncommunicative. I treated her again with HM-5. Eighteen months later, she was still doing well.

❖ Case History

A young Chinese man, age 24, a computer specialist, came to me in December 1998 for an acute blockage of the diaphragm, which manifested as deep thoracic pain on the right side, radiating toward the nape of the neck, to the lumbar area and the upper right limb, and accompanied by a strong feeling of oppression. A few attacks of the hiccups at the beginning signaled this impairment of the diaphragm. All of the laboratory tests were normal.

This blockage occurred following the breakup of a relationship that caused profound sorrow; this had been a very important relationship to him and he had been completely surprised by its end. Otherwise, he was in very good health. He exhibited a tendency to easily become anxious, as well as a lot of nervousness. His tongue was normal. The Heart pulse was so deep as to be imperceptible.

Impairment of the Heart was evident in this case. As there were no Lung symptoms and the Lung pulse was normal, we could eliminate the Lung, which is often affected in irreversible separations. The indicated point seemed to be HT-5, the only arm *shao yin* point that acts on the diaphragm, confirmed by the high degree of nervousness. This produced rapid results on the diaphragmatic symptoms. The second and last session confirmed this result and, according to the patient, enabled him to gain some detachment from his breakup.

Human Transmission and Perpetuation: The Extraordinary Organs

DEFINITION

In Chinese, the extraordinary organs is written 奇恆之腑 *qi heng zhi fu*. The word *qi* here means extraordinary, surprising and wonderful. It refers to the emergence of a life, the conception of a being, the differentiation of a being from the undifferentiated, a creation. *Heng* means durable, permanent, constant, perennial, and to make something last. *Fu* refers to the yang organs.

The six extraordinary organs, which govern the perpetuation of the being, consist of three pairs.

- brain and marrow

- bones and vessels

- Gallbladder and gestational envelopes

These three pairs correspond to the symbolic nature of heaven, man, and earth. Chapter 10 of *Divine Pivot* offers us the key to comprehension by noting that brain and marrow are of the order of heaven, while bones and vessels are of the earth.[10] The purpose of the brain and marrow[11] is, in order to perpetuate life, to reflect the natural order of life, the secret vein of all that exists within our bodies (like a vein of jade), in which they trace out the design for opening the way for qi, blood, nerve impulses and so forth.

Bones and vessels carry, support, transport and actualize that which is reflected by the brain and marrow. Bones, which are solid, contain marrow and are linked to the ancestral tablets and thereby to our personal lineage. The vessels, which are flexible, transport qi, blood and fluids. They specify and color the essences, according to our individual nature, rooting us into a cosmic lineage.

The Gallbladder and the gestational envelopes are of man, between heaven and earth, and are that which accomplishes this perpetuation. These two yang organs ensure the transmission of life, within our lineage and ourselves. They are the locus of therapeutic applications, in cases such as functional infertility in men or women, the impact of sexual assaults, certain gynecological problems and so forth, with such points as BL-48 (on the outer line of the Bladder channel, level with the associated point of the Gallbladder) and CV-5 (alarm point of the Triple Burner).

THE THREE PAIRS

As stated above, the three pairs are brain and marrow, bones and vessels, Gallbladder and gestational envelopes. The gestational envelopes include but are not limited to the uterus; they govern all types of gestation, from the most material to the most subtle, from the fetus to the spiritual embryo. Examined in greater detail:

- The brain, "home of the *yuan shen*" (original spirit), is linked to the Heart, which Chapter 8 of the *Divine Pivot* states "contains the spirit." But while the Heart spirit, characterized by inspired or spontaneous knowledge, tends toward unity (one is referred to Heart intelligence or coherence), the spirit of the brain tends toward duality, with reflection (thought and mirror), and the right and left brain hemispheres which have been well studied by Western medicine. The brain is the "sea of marrow" and it is the Kidneys that "produce the marrow." Marrow forms and nourishes the brain. In Chinese the same word, *sui* (髓), is used to refer to both the marrow of the bones and the spinal cord, as both play a very valuable part in the perpetuation of life and are within the bones and spine. At the same time, the marrow conveys messages traveling in both directions. The brain and marrow are celestial and convey the cosmic laws and rules of life; in this way, they contribute to its perpetuation.

- The bones, governed by the Kidneys, constitute a rigid structure that contains the brain and marrow (skull), Lung and Heart (thorax), and protect the internal genital organs (pelvis). In Chinese medicine, the bones, which endure after death, are linked to the ancestors' tablets and therefore to our genealogical lineage and perpetuation.

- The vessels (脈 *mai),* governed by the Heart, convey the qi, blood and fluids throughout the body. They disappear after death. We will come back to these later. Bones and vessels are of the earth and are the medium for ancestral and personal laws and rules.

- The Gallbladder, as an extraordinary organ, is in my opinion the beginning of all creation through its relationship with fire. Since our creation is recurrent (in Chinese medicine, we are recreated with each breath), it participates in conception and in each breath.

- The gestational envelopes are the place of the origin of life. Along with the Gallbladder, they ensure the perpetuation of each being and of the species, by taking part in the various types of gestation and in the transmission of life.

I only have clinical experience with BL-48, CV-5, and BL-11 (the meeting point of the bones).

BL-48 governs the Gallbladder as an extraordinary organ, that is, as a participant in the perpetuation of our lineage.

❖ Case History

Mrs. V. came to see me for a problem with functional infertility. Everything was normal: her periods, ovulation, compatibility with her husband's sperm, as well as other diagnostic tests. She reported other symptoms that drew my attention to the Gallbladder: nausea, indigestion, intolerance of coffee, chocolate and eggs, headaches along the trajectory of the leg *shao yang,* and difficulties with starting things and making decisions. Confronted with this combination of infertility and problems related to the Gallbladder, I thought of a possible dysfunction of that extraordinary organ, particularly since I sensed in this woman, a practicing Christian, a feeling of controlled aggression of which she did not seem fully aware. I punctured BL-48. Twenty days later, she was pregnant.

CV-5 governs the gestational envelopes. These are involved in cases of infertility and in certain sexual dysfunctions, including the after effects of assaults. As we have already seen, this is also the alarm point of the Triple Burner and therefore corresponds to all that maintains life, nutrition and perpetuation.

❖ Case History

Mrs. H., age 41, an executive assistant with a stocky build and a pale complexion, had been suffering for four years in her shoulders and hips, especially on the external side of these joints. The pains were not joint pains. They were not influenced by weather, movement, rest, cold or heat. They were constant, although they sometimes became worse for no apparent reason. She did not have pains in the back of the neck, the trapezius muscles or in the elbows.

The fact that she did not have pains in the back of the neck or in the lumbar region eliminated any mechanical, static or energetic cause of vertebral origin and any disturbance in the flow of yang energies into the trunk. An obstruction in the return of yin energies would manifest at the inside facets of the shoulders and thighs. So it had to be a poor exit of qi from the trunk to the root of the upper and lower limbs.

What mechanisms and points may be implicated? It could be a lack of distribution of the middle qi via CV-12 or LR-13, but in that case there would be symptoms affecting the middle part of the body, such as the solar plexus and epigastrium. Or it could be a failure of qi to exit the trunk along *tai yang* or *tai yin* with the symptoms that correspond to these main channels. A lack of distribution of qi from the chest via LU-2, which would cause pains in the proximal aspects of the four limbs, is another possibility but in that case there would be signs of excess in the chest.

The patient said that she often sighed and felt oppressed. There were no tachycardia or palpitations, no epigastric symptoms, no digestive or urinary problems, nor any other pains, in particular along *tai yang* or *tai yin*. The only other complaint that she had was insomnia, with awakening at around 3 a.m. She had difficulty falling back asleep, but did not have nightmares.

Everything pointed towards an excess in the chest, with a sense of oppression in the chest caused by non-distribution of the qi through the "cloud door," LU-2, which includes the symptomatology of awakening at 3 a.m.

Her tongue was normal, with tense distal pulses and deep proximal ones. The pains had begun at the time of a highly conflicted love affair; she was very torn between an intense sexuality and a poor affective and intellectual relationship, which led her to have an abortion, in violation of her moral principles.

The proximal pulses were deep, showing the energetic imprint of the abortion. CV-5 was the point indicated: it would alleviate the pain associated with this physical memory. After the first treatment, she had a strong reaction for 48 hours, with increased pains and complete insomnia. The symptoms began to diminish slightly on the third day. The second treatment brought a spectacular result: a week later, the pains, pulses and insomnia showed a marked improvement. After a third treatment, one month later, everything had returned to normal. Four months later when she came for a fall check-up, the symptoms had not returned.

BL-11 is the meeting point for the bones, an extraordinary organ.

❖ Case History

Mrs. X., age 65, came to see me for rheumatoid arthritis, from which she had been suffering for fifteen years. The pains appeared shortly after her daughter experienced a bout of depression. They fluctuated along with the condition of her daughter. In fact, the mother said that she only lived for her daughter. The pains began in the right ankle and shifted, over three years, to the left, then to the left wrist and shoulder, cervical area, and finally to the left knee.

The pain was chronic, piercing and dull at once: it was of the yin type and accompanied by swelling of the joint. However, it should be noted that at the beginning of an attack, the superficial pain was an acute burning sensation; then it became yin. It was aggravated by pressure and by cold, improved by heat, movement and massage. She felt better in the evenings.

Based on these findings, I concluded that this pain was either due to stagnation or an excess of yin, as movement improves stagnation by promoting circulation and alleviates excess by expending qi.

In addition, she reported:

• a sensation of swelling in the throat, with difficulty swallowing, mostly at night and in the mornings
• hemithoracic pain with a sensation of thoracic oppression; it was better when she unhooked her bra, and she said she thought this was linked to the shoulder pain.

She also reported some dizziness.

The clinical examination revealed some swelling in the anterior aspects of the painful joints.

Her tongue and her pulses were more or less normal.

This was a case of deep pathology with a long history. In such cases, it is necessary to seek another factor in addition to the local yin excess or stagnation. One cannot implicate a water movement, a water phase, a problem with body movements, a *shao yang*, Yang Linking or Girdle vessel problem in the absence of corresponding signs.

This woman lived only for her daughter, her descendant. She was suffering from an impairment in her own perpetuation. In acupuncture, what are the mechanisms behind perpetuation? These are the extraordinary organs, namely the gestational envelopes, Gallbladder, brain, marrow, bones, and alarm points. In this case, there was an impairment of the bones, not in their structural role but as an extraordinary organ, although both functions are interlinked. Moreover, they are controlled by the same point, BL-11, which I tonified.

I circulated the yin with GB-41, a key point of the Girdle vessel, and associated point of *shao yang*, the yang that causes the yin to circulate; and with KI-1, an essence point that sets yin in motion, the action of the *shao yin*. Furthermore, *shao yin* is also connected with the bones.

Mrs. X's condition improved after five weekly sessions; we then switched to monthly sessions. She is now under regular treatment. There has been no recurrence of pain. She described her condition as satisfactory. This case history is interesting because it illustrates an aspect of pathology of the extraordinary organs.

CHAPTER FIVE

CHANNELS

WE HAVE SEEN THAT the vessels (脈 *mai)*, regardless of their type, must be included and understood within the context of the extraordinary organs. Considering their importance in Chinese medicine, I will elaborate on the vessels of qi *(qi mai)*, known in the West as channels or meridians. While we have introduced the fundamental concepts of the channels above, I want to emphasize these crucial concepts here to make it clear that the channels should not be conceived of as qi tubes or pipes. They play a vital, even cosmic role.

The word 經 *jing* can be translated in many ways, including main road from north to south, channels, constant rule, immutable law, warp (as opposed to weft), and canonical books. The rule, the law, the warp, the canonical books all have in common the fact that they transmit fundamental truths, archetypes or immutable laws. That is the fundamental role of the channels in acupuncture. But they need to be incarnated, within our bodies: that is the role of the vessels.

The *mai* serve as their medium. *Mai* means a seam, vein, mountain chain, a genealogical lineage, vessels, the veins of a leaf, or a pulse. As a powerful vital force (it moves mountains), *mai* is directed and oriented (e.g., seam, vein, veins of a leaf, genealogical lineage). The *mai* are connected with the Heart and therefore to our specialness, our uniqueness. Chapter 8 of the *Divine Pivot* states that the Heart governs the vessels and that the vessels are where the spirit resides. They are the supporting medium of the channels; for each individual, they color it in a special way, according to their essential and specific nature. So it is even clearer now that they contribute to our perpetuation.

These vessels comprise three groups: six main channels (*jing mai*) with their subdivisions, the eight extraordinary vessels *(qi jing ba mai)* and the sixteen connecting vessels *(luo mai)*, which are not called *jing* because, to use a weaving metaphor, they are the shuttle that weaves the weft and runs on the warp of *jing.*

Six Main Channels

The main channels *(jing mai)* described in Chapter 6 of *Basic Questions* number three yin and three yang. The founding elements, to me they engender all the energetic structures and functions of a being. To begin with, they are the origin of the five phases and therefore of the yin and yang organs, at the center of the four directions. Next, by dividing in two, they engender the twelve primary channels, the twelve channel divergences, and the twelve channel sinews as well as the eight extraordinary channels. They can be considered the original channels.

THREE YIN

The three yin are called *tai yin, shao yin,* and *jue yin.* Related to the interior, they are connected with the five yin organs. Their diagnosis depends on the presence of symptoms that correspond to one of the six main channels, located simultaneously on that of the hand *(shou)* and of the foot *(zu),*[1] and on the disturbance of one of their functions. This is why it is important to know them. Once one has identified which main channel is disturbed, the next step is to choose the indicated point or points along its path.

Tai yin pertains to the surface, in connection with yang. *Tai yin* is "mother," welcoming and receptive, as stated in Chapter 79 of the *Divine Pivot*. It is related to the Lung and Spleen, and schematically to respiration and nourishment.

❖ Case History

A patient who was in psychoanalysis told me that she "needed to be freed of the qi of her old-fashioned, possessive mother."[2] The combination of digestive and respiratory problems that she showed—slow digestion with intolerance of sugar, fats and alcohol, diarrhea with soft stools, occasional asthma attacks influenced by humidity, periodic shortness of breath during effort, and negative diagnostic tests—made me think of *tai yin*. SP-15 of the leg *tai yin*, located at the level of the navel, helped clear up her symptoms. Note the combination of digestive and respiratory symptoms as well as the relationship with the mother.

Shao yin is deep vitality; we know that it corresponds to the Kidneys and the Heart. The mandate of life (命 *ming*) is linked to the Kidneys. One's proper nature (性 *xing*) is linked to the Heart *shao yin,* which relates to an inner actualization. An earlier case history illustrates this.

Jue yin is an "ending," a "servant" *(Basic Questions,* Chapters 7 and 79), precisely, the servant of the Heart, along with the Minister of the Heart, which according to Larre is "that by which the Heart commands";[3] and the Liver, the "general of the armies," who seconds and protects the Heart. The two require the free, flexible and easy circulation of qi, blood and fluids all the way to the extremities, just as the sap of the tree in spring-time runs from the tips of the roots to the ends of the branches without obstruction.

❖ Case History

A 32-year-old woman was suffering from endometriosis with gynecological pains in the left iliac fossa radiating to the thigh along the *jue yin* channel; these occurred at the end of her periods, but also at unpredictable moments throughout her menstrual cycle. She was knotted, tight, and tense, and prone to anxiety. She said that nothing was easy for her. LR-9 relieved these pains.

Note the pain along the trajectory of the channel and the knotted, tight, tense feelings that indicate difficult circulation of the qi within.

In addition to their relationship with the five yin organs, the fundamental laws established and governed by the three yin include receptivity, the mother, deep vitality, servants of the Heart, and internal free circulation.

THREE YANG

The three yang are called *tai yang, shao yang*, and *yang ming*.

Tai yang is described in *Basic Questions* as being the ruler (Chapter 49) and the father (Chapter 79). It is the outermost on the arms, the topmost on the head, and the furthest back on the neck, the trunk and the lower limbs. To me, it marks the north of the body (traditionally in China the emperor always sat facing south); the aspect related to the laws of earlier heaven (the prenatal state); and the mark of the unseen made visible on the body.

❖ Case History

A young man, age 22, consulted me for generalized eczema, and intense headaches along the lines of *tai yang*, starting at the nape of the neck at point BL-10. While he had rejected the rules of his father and of all social and religious orders, he had not yet achieved his own set of rules. Puncturing BL-10 and BL-40 relieved these symptoms and the comments about *tai yang* enlightened him about their causes.

Shao yang is described in *Basic Questions* as relating to regulation (Chapter 79), the hinge (Chapter 6) and to wandering (Chapter 79), or the free circulation of the yang to the exterior—the surface of the body and of the outside world. So its course, which is on the lateral aspect of the limbs, head and trunk, makes incursions both onto the surface (*tai yang*) and into the depths (*yang ming*). It means 'wandering' in a positive sense of psychological and physical freedom; it corresponds to the skin, muscles, and vessels. It is often involved in people who feel knotted, tight, and tense. *Shao yang* plays the role of mediator in the yang and in the body as a whole in relation to what is external, our self, as well as with heaven and the archetypes that are the foundation of our existence.

❖ Case History

A 37-year-old woman came to see me in 1999 for headaches that had started after a phase of considerable nervous tension in the summer of 1984. The pain started in the eyes, radiated to the temples, to the top of the head, the nape of the neck and, in rare cases, to the ears, with a superficial trajectory along the *shao yang* channel. These dull headaches were neither improved nor aggravated by pressure on the eyeballs. However, they were accompanied by a distinct feeling of fullness in the head.

Local application of heat gave some relief, which suggests stagnation and confirms *shao yang* involvement. So I looked for the general mechanism, in relation to *shao yang*, that maintained this local disturbance.

During my interview of the patient I learned that she had been married for ten years and had an eight-year-old child. She had never had any surgery; she reported some digestive problems and nasopharyngitis triggered by dampness and cold. She had trouble falling asleep and complained of muscle pain, especially in the morning, after meals, and in damp weather. She was impulsive, irritable, knotted and tense, particularly when she was stressed.

In this case, the *shao yang* axis was implicated. What had happened in the summer of 1984? It was something important of which she could not speak. I punctured the root of *shao yang*, GB-44, and combined this with GB-15 on the skull, which helped her significantly.

Yang ming is described as protective in *Basic Questions* (Chapter 79) and focuses on nutrition, in the sense of internalization of nutrients. It is also, in the interior of the person, connection (Chapter 79) and closing inwards (Chapter 6). It closes toward the yin, toward *tai yin*. In this way, it contributes to wholeness. It circulates on the front of the face, the trunk, and the lower limbs, and on the radial aspect of the arms. It faces the south and the light. It connects with the west, the autumn, heaven that withdraws, and the harvesting of the fruit that falls from the tree. *Yang ming* is about breaking up and discontinuity. For me it is about the human adventure, from the moment of conception to the end of our path. It has a dialogue with the *shao yin* Heart and Kidneys, with nature (*xing*) and with destiny (*ming*). In this discontinuity, this human adventure, the person needs to be protected. This is the function of the points ST-14, ST-15, and ST-16.

❖ Case History

A 25-year-old woman consulted me for a case of eczema along with allergies that affected her eyes and nose. She was highly vulnerable and said that she had never been protected. Small things were enough to either injure or please her; she felt uneasy when others looked at her. Her skin was very sensitive to pain. ST-14 provided a noticeable improvement.

The point located just above, ST-15, is indicated for people who tend to readily feel themselves to be under attack and are insecure. Both are connected to the protective function of *yang ming*, as are ST-13 (sweating) and ST-16 (diarrhea).

Rule and law; regulation, mediation, and freedom of movement; protection and nutrition in relationship to the outside world, connection, gathering-in and wholeness of the self: these are the basic mechanisms conveyed by the three yangs.

These six *jing mai* are further subdivided into twelve primary channels, twelve divergent channels, and twelve channel sinews. The pathways of all these channels are reproduced in the illustrations at the end of the book.

Twelve Primary Channels

The twelve primary channels *(zheng jing* 正經*)* are created from the division of each *jing mai* into two channels, the upper, linked to the arm *(shou)*, and the lower, related to the leg *(zu)*. They are called arm *tai yang*, leg *tai yang*, arm *shao yang*, leg *shao yang*, arm *tai yin*, leg *tai yin*, etc.

The primary channels connect us, first, to the exterior, to the cosmic qi that paces and influences our lives. Note that the five phases (五行 *wu xing*) need to be differentiated from the five movements (五運 *wu yun)*, which, coupled with the six energies (六氣 *liu qi)*, govern the evolution of rhythmic energy on earth. This set (*see* Fig. 1) governs a large part of our biological rhythms.

The five phases are normally laid out in the following order:

water → fire → wood → metal → earth

They are described in the following fundamental manner:

- Water moistens and flows downward.
- Fire burns and reaches upward.
- Wood bends and straightens.
- Metal is malleable and changes shape.
- Earth at the center has the paired movements of receiving and distributing, accepting and disseminating; this is particularly true on the nutritional level (*see* Fig. 2).

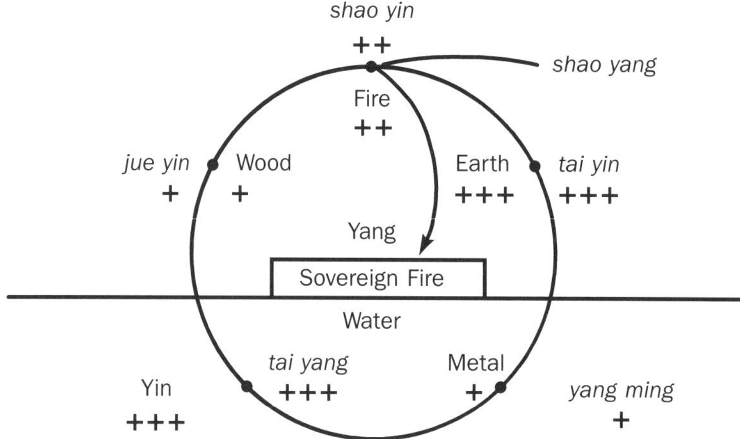

Fig. 1: Five Phases and Six Channels

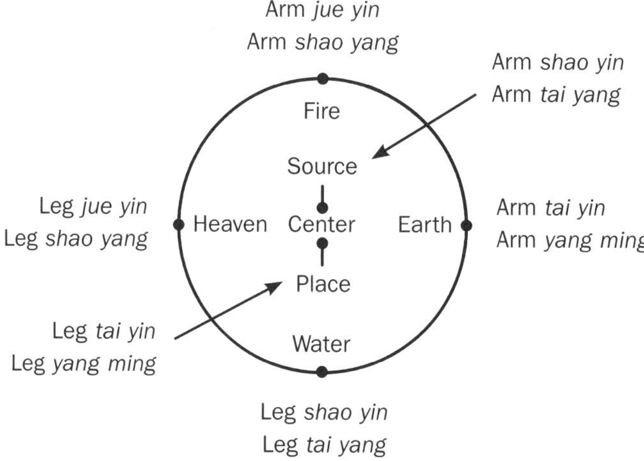

Fig. 2: Paired Movements of the Channels

Usage of the Five Movements

Our physiological activities vary in synchronicity with those of the cosmos at the level of the five movements. For example, our Liver organ and the corresponding channel display greater or lesser activity during certain days, months or years, independently of the four seasons; if this does not occur normally, it can result in 'desynchronization' syndromes: these are acute, usually painful, and characterized by spontaneous appearance and disappearance. They are treated with the transport points (well, spring, stream, river, and sea—*jing, ying, shu, jing, he*) along with the connecting *(luo)* and source *(yuan)* points.

The system of the five movements and six qi uses the traditional Chinese calendar concepts of the ten heavenly stems (天干 *tian gan)* and the twelve earthly branches (地支 *di zhi)*. Together, these set up interlocking cycles of 60 periods. By this method, every hour, day, month, year and age (of 60 years) is defined at the cosmic level and by turn at the human level, by a stem and by a branch, and therefore by a combination of a movement and a qi. Each moment is energetically defined by the conjunction of movements and qi of the hour, day, month, year and age. It is to this complex system that we now refer.

❖ Case History

A gentleman, age 62, who had been retired for two years, consulted me for a right-sided temporoparietal headache (which relates to the Gallbladder and *shao yang*) that had begun eight months before, getting worse at times, and at other times improving, but never disappearing completely. This headache was usually intense, unaffected by local application of cold or heat, not improved by pressure, often nocturnal and resulting in insomnia, but not occurring at a specific hour.

Therefore, this right-sided *shao yang* headache does not correspond to the eight parameters: it is not due to a local deficiency, excess or stagnation of yin or yang. The examination showed that it was also not mechanically related to dysfunctions of the cervical spine, teeth, or scars. It did not have an external climatic or dietary origin: it was neither modified nor triggered by climate changes or exposure to wind, cold or dampness.

Thus the etiology had to be internal. I immediately eliminated an extraordinary channel centered on *shao yang* because there was no sign of Yang Linking or of Girdle vessel involvement. The patient's normal digestion allowed me to dismiss a problem in the Gallbladder affecting *shao yang*, especially since he had no difficulty making decisions. Pain along a channel related to spring or to the wood phase (corresponding to the leg *shao yang* channel) seemed the most likely explanation.

The spontaneity of the beginning and development of the condition favored this hypothesis. The man before me was very alert, reacting to the slightest stimulus, ready to get up and move, doing everything quickly and therefore demonstrating an excess of the wood phase that is in motion. This excess had been compensated for by intensive activity, which was no longer the case since he retired. A macrocosmic excess of wood aggravated this movement and triggered the appearance of this pain.

We treated it using the techniques specified for desynchronization syndromes:

• dispersion of the wood phase at LR-2, bilaterally
• source of the affected channel: GB-40 on the right
• paired interior connecting point: LR-5 on the right

- contralateral connecting points in a midday-midnight pair: HT-5 on the left. (We will return to the use of these pairs later).

After a severe reaction the day after the first treatment, this patient was completely cured in three sessions. We advised him to pursue a course of annual preventive treatments to disperse the wood phase with LR-2 and GB-38, which are dispersion points, bilaterally.

❖ Case History

Mr. S., age 50, came to see me about acute pains in the left shoulder that had started four days before, suddenly, without apparent cause, unchanged by analgesics or injection. This wrenching pain (often *tai yang*) was located in a yang zone, although it could not be exactly defined. It was unaffected by pressure, cold, heat or the weather, but was aggravated by even the slightest movement.

We begin by analyzing the shoulder pain. This local symptom did not respond to the eight parameters, so I could eliminate a case of deficiency, excess or stagnation. The pain did not have an external origin because it was not affected by the weather and did not seem to have a mechanical cause. The spontaneous appearance suggested a disease that expressed a desynchronization between the man and his macrocosm in one of the five movements.

The history of this somewhat rigid and incommunicative patient revealed:

- acute epicondylitis (tennis elbow) originally on the right side and then on the left (which provided the origin of the pains), located on arm *tai yang*, which had appeared and disappeared spontaneously, accompanied by a strange sensation of "perceiving his stomach and intestines"
- a tendency towards soft, unformed stools
- some precordial tingling
- olfactory hallucinations.

These symptoms suggested a disturbance in the fire phase (defined by expansion). So we had pain in the left shoulder localized on arm *tai yang*, secondary to a deficiency in the fire phase and triggered by a desynchronization between this man and his macrocosm. We should remember that the fire phase is expansive; thus, if this phase is deficient in a person they are not expansive, but if it is in excess, they are overly expansive. The person here was not expansive at all. His fire phase was deficient with symptoms along the fire channels. When the cosmic fire phase is in excess he was better, as the cosmic excess compensated for his deficiency. Similarly, when the cosmic fire phase was deficient, he was worse. This explains the spontaneous appearance and disappearance of the symptoms.

This was therefore a deficiency of the fire phase expressed in one of his channels, arm *tai yang*, in the left shoulder.

We should note that most severe or acute pains are often secondary to a desynchronization between man and macrocosm: in that case, they do not correspond to the eight parameters.

The treatment was simultaneously symptomatic and systemic:

• Based on the precepts in Chapter 63 of *Basic Questions,* we punctured the stream point of arm *shao yin* on the right, HT-7, and connecting point of arm *tai yang* on the left, SI-7. This is also a case for applying the midday/midnight rule, calling for a contralateral puncture of the connecting point on the opposite channel. Arm *tai yang* is paired with leg *jue yin,* so we needed to treat LR-5 on the right.

• The overall condition reflected a yang impairment of the fire phase; the yang correspondences were affected; the signs were not very clearly related to the yin or yang organs and the impaired channel was yang. We were dealing with the arm *tai yang* channel. In this case of deficiency, we had to treat the tonification point, according to the mother-son rule. The mother of fire is wood, and its qi is wind. So we needed to behave as the wind of the macrocosm acting on the yin well point (HT-9) and on the yang stream point (SI-3). In this case, as the shoulder pain was along the pathway of the Small Intestine channel, the point to puncture was SI-3.

But that was not enough. We also needed to take the preventive step in the coming years of puncturing the tonifying point on arm *tai yang.*

This case history perfectly illustrates the diagnosis and treatment of pains that are secondary to a disturbance in one of the five movements and revealed by a desynchronization between man and his macrocosm. The problems of synchronization of five movements in humans we believe are found in conjunction with disruption of the five movements in the universe. But as, to my knowledge, there is no way to accurately predict these cosmic movements (and the people I have met in both China and the West seem to disagree with each other), so it is through the nature of the fluctuating symptoms that we can see this mechanism at work.

At the beginning, the treatment must be done twice with an interval of 48 hours and, if the pain has not disappeared, a third time three or four days later. Next, all one needs to do is follow up with the basic treatment one month and then three months later. Then it should be followed up with the preventive treatment. The needles should only be left to work for a short time (10 minutes) for the symptomatic treatment because we are dealing with a yang manifestation, which reacts strongly and quickly. In contrast, they should be left longer (20 minutes) for the basic treatment, in order to achieve a deeper reaction.

The pain disappeared completely with the third treatment, as well as the other symptoms.

Next, the twelve primary channels correspond to the five phases, in relation to the center and the four directions. Paired in an *exterior-interior* relationship:

- leg *jue yin* Liver and leg *shao yang* Gallbladder channels pertain to wood and the east
- arm *jue yin* Heart Master and arm *shao yang* Triple Burner pertain to fire and the south
- arm *tai yin* Lung and arm *yang ming* Large Intestine pertain to metal and the west
- leg *shao yin* Kidney and leg *tai yang* Bladder pertain to water and the north
- leg *tai yin* Spleen and leg *yang ming* Stomach pertain to the center earth, the place of life
- arm *shao yin* Heart and arm *tai yang* Small Intestine pertain to the center, fire, source of life.

The seasonal pathologies of the organs are treated at the alarm points, as we will see below. For seasonal pathologies affecting the channels we strengthen the treatment by using the transport (*shu*) points and the connecting/source points, as described above and in the case history of the marathon runner below, with ST-40 and SP-3.

The primary channels make up a daily circulation cycle of the nourishing qi that begins in the arm *tai yin* Lung channel and returns to it, at a peak within each of the twelve channels for a period of two hours.

Any two channels that are on the opposite sides of this cycle (e.g., Lung at 3 a.m. to 5 a.m. and Bladder at 3 p.m. to 5 p.m.) are paired according to the "midday-midnight" rule. (*See* Table 2.) A disturbance in one can cause a disturbance in the other. This is important to know for both diagnosis and treatment. The pairs linked this way are Lung and Bladder, Large Intestine and Kidneys, Stomach and Heart Master, Spleen and Triple Burner, Heart and Gallbladder, Small Intestine and Liver. These treatments also use the transport points and connecting points. The previous case history is an example of this.

A diagnosis of impaired channels is based on coexisting signs of trajectory, organ symptoms (which are usually subtle), and some pathognomonic signs, discussed below.

Table 2: Midday-Midnight Pairs			
Lung	3–5 a.m.	Bladder	3–5 p.m.
Large Intestine	5–7 a.m.	Kidney	5–7 p.m.
Stomach	7–9 a.m.	Heart Master	7–9 p.m.
Spleen	9–11 a.m.	Triple Burner	9–11 p.m.
Heart	11 a.m.–1 p.m.	Gallbladder	11 p.m.–1 a.m.
Small Intestine	1–3 p.m.	Liver	1–3 a.m.

- arm *tai yin* Lung: pain in the shoulders and back, aversion to wind, spontaneous daytime sweating and urinary frequency, dry hair and skin

- arm *yang ming* Large Intestine: dental pain, pharyngitis, cold gums

- leg *yang ming* Stomach: sighs, yawning, fear of people, fear of noises made by striking wood, weak legs

- leg *tai yin* Spleen: stiff tongue, pain at the root of the tongue, pain in the chin, lower back pain, amenorrhea, weakness in all four limbs

- arm *shao yin* Heart: dry throat, thirst, somnolence or insomnia, sadness, paleness or intense anger, epigastric bloating, lower back pain

- arm *tai yang* Small Intestine: pharyngitis, swelling of the chin, torticollis, shoulder feels pulled or fractured (*tai yang* type pains)

- leg *tai yang* Bladder: a sensation of "something attacking the head," a sensation of the eyeballs being pulled out, hemorrhoids

- leg *shao yin* Kidney: quickly satiated when eating, dull complexion (especially affecting the chin), constantly moving, numb lower abdomen, edema on the face or body

- arm *jue yin* Heart Master: hot palms, swelling under the arm (with leg *shao yang*), hysterical laughter, red face, feeling of oppression

- arm *shao yang* Triple Burner: deafness, pharyngitis

- leg *shao yang* Gallbladder: bitter taste in the mouth (with the Heart), sighing, muddy, dull complexion, diminished eyesight, difficulty walking, dizziness, pain in the thorax, sides or lower back making it difficult to twist

- leg *jue yin* Liver: dry throat, pale, dull face, lower back pain with inability to lean forward or backward, inguinal hernia, diminished eyesight, choking sensations, insomnia, depression, reduced libido, dizzy spells, dizziness, tinnitus, heaviness in all four limbs, impotence or priapism.

The divergent channels (*jing bie*) will not be discussed in depth here. They describe the relationships of the channels with the senses, brain, and head. They do not have any associated points, but only emphasize the fundamental relationships between the primary channels.

Twelve Channel Sinews

The channel sinews (*jing jin*) emphasize movement. The sinews refer not to the muscular form or flesh, but to that which animates the muscles and underlies their movement. The radical of the character for sinews (筋 *jin*) is bamboo, which consists of alternating knots and segments, concentrations, stops, moments suspended in the void, and expansions. Apart from being the symbol of linear time, this concept of bamboo supports muscle movements, the memory, genealogical lineage. As has been emphasized before, it is clear that the channels are not qi conduits comparable to water pipes; they are the vectors of the rules, laws and archetypes that we incarnate. The channel *jing* are not vessels (*mai*) and so are not colored by our own nature; they tell us that motion is the basis of the fundamental universal laws that "found and reveal the world."[4]

The diagnosis of a channel sinew impairment is based on the idea of locating a pain, usually muscular, along the course of a channel sinew. While these can largely be super-imposed on those of the corresponding primary channels, it is indispensable to know the differences. For example, the arm *tai yin* Lung channel sinew goes to the ipsilateral sternoclavicular joint; that of leg *tai yang* Bladder channel goes around the shoulder. This makes it possible to link certain cases of painful shoulder (such as subdeltoid bursitis) to these two channel sinews, which cannot be done on the basis of the pathways of the primary channels. But it is important to remember that with any channel sinew impairment there is an underlying and preexisting muscular tension in the area, often of long duration, and that this must be treated to obtain a lasting result. Most cases of sub-deltoid bursitis occur where there is tension in the nape of the neck and the trapezius muscles, for example due to the need to control everything or to being constantly on the defensive. In such cases, the treatment has to be adapted to the person and guided by the channel sinews involved, which can show the affected circuit.

Here are the different courses and symptomatology specific to the twelve channel sinews, based on a reading of Chapter 13 of the *Divine Pivot*, entitled "Channel Sinews." The corresponding illustrations are included, together with those of the other channels, in Appendix Two of this book.

LEG *TAI YANG* CHANNEL SINEW

Where its course differs from that of main channel:

- one branch goes down the fibula on the outside of the leg

- from the lower thoracic area there are two branches: one that goes to the axilla, the supraclavicular fossa, and then the occipital zone of GB-12; the other goes to the ac-romial zone of LI-15

- from the lower cervical region, there is a branch that passes through the supraclavic-ular fossa and ends at the side of the nose

- from the back of the neck, there is a branch that goes to connect with the root of the tongue

- starting from the region of BL-2, there is a branch that extends to the upper eyelid.

Specific symptomatology:[5]
- swollen and painful heel
- pains on the outside of the leg

- inability to raise the arm
- pain in the axilla and in the supraclavicular fossa
- facial neuralgia

LEG *SHAO YANG* CHANNEL SINEW

Where its course differs from that of main channel:

- one branch starts at the anterior end of the 11th or 12th rib and goes to the breast and the supraclavicular fossa
- at the front end of the channel, one branch goes to the top of the head and connects to the contralateral branch

Specific symptomatology:

- inability to flex and extend the knee
- lateral thoracic pain radiating to the breast and to the supraclavicular fossa

LEG *YANG MING* CHANNEL SINEW

Where its course differs from that of main channel:

- one branch starts at the ankle, rises along the fibula to the hip, and then to the lateral aspect of lower ribs, which it follows posteriorly to the spinal column where it goes into the posterior aspect
- a small branch from the nose spreads out on the lower eyelid like a net

Specific symptomatology:

- facial paralysis with deformation of the mouth: this is yang type if it is slack and there is inability to open the eyes, or yin type if there are spasms and inability to close the eyes

LEG *TAI YIN* CHANNEL SINEW

Where its course differs from that of main channel:

- from the pubis, the channel rises to the umbilicus
- it then goes deep down along the walls of the abdomen and thorax, entering the body of vertebrae on the anterior side of the spinal column

Specific symptomatology:

- wrenching pain in the genitals, radiating to the navel and the sides
- pain deep in the chest and in the spinal column

LEG *SHAO YIN* CHANNEL SINEW

Where its course differs from that of main channel:

- it reaches the genital area, where the three leg yin channels meet
- goes to the side of the spine, which it follows to the back of the neck, where it enters the occipital bone

Specific symptomatology:

- heavy sensation in the lumbar area (posterior yang side) and difficulty bending forward, toward the yin
- heavy sensation in the anterior part of the body (yin in relation to the lumbar region) and difficulty bending backwards, towards the yang

We think that these exchanges and disturbances in them are described here because it involves setting in motion the qi in the pelvic region, which is the most yin region of the body, and therefore corresponds to leg *shao yin.*

LEG *JUE YIN* CHANNEL SINEW

Where its course differs from that of main channel:

- it stops at the genitals

Specific symptomatology:

- lack of erection with retraction of the penis if yin type (cold) or with slackening if yang type (heat)

ARM *TAI YANG* CHANNEL SINEW

Where its course differs from that of main channel:

- on the face, starting in the zone of GB-12 leg *shao yang*
- a small branch goes into the ear
- a branch goes up the corner of the jaw, in front of the ear, comes to the outside corner of the eye and ends at the corner of the forehead
- a branch goes around the ear down to the lower jaw and back up to the outside corner of the eye

Specific symptomatology:

- ear pain radiating to the lower jaw
- if the pain in the ear radiates to the eye, the eye is kept constantly closed

ARM *SHAO YANG* CHANNEL SINEW

Where the course differs from that of main channel:

- one branch begins at the corner of the jaw and goes into the root of the tongue

Specific symptomatology:

- contractions of the tongue (the tongue's movements relate to arm *shao yin* and arm *shao yang*)

ARM *YANG MING* CHANNEL SINEW

Where its course differs from that of main channel:

- a crossing, mentioned before, with the channel sinew of leg *shao yang*: a branch starts in the cheek, goes up to the forehead and then to the top of the head, crosses to the opposite side and goes down to the corner of the contralateral jaw

Specific symptomatology:

- inability to raise the shoulder
- inability to turn the neck to either side

ARM *TAI YIN* CHANNEL SINEW

Where its course differs from that of main channel:

- a periclavicular branch that runs in an oval from the areas of LI-15 to ST-12
- a branch travels out on the inside walls of the thorax and diaphragm

Specific symptomatology:

- rapid breathing
- spasms of the chest
- spitting up blood

Note that the two *tai yin* channel sinews run along the inside face of the abdominal and thoracic walls: *tai yin* is the opening of yin toward the exterior.

ARM *SHAO YIN* CHANNEL SINEW

Where the course differs from that of main channel:

- enters the thorax at the axilla, runs along the inner side of the thoracic wall at the height of the nipple, and goes to the cardia; from there, it goes down the midline to the umbilicus

Specific symptomatology:

- qi build-up syndrome in the area of the navel along with a tumescent area the size of a fist[6]

- the two channel sinews corresponding to the two centers, arm *shao yin* (the Heart center) and leg *tai yin* (the Spleen center), are related to the umbilicus at the center of the body; the courses described are both energetic and symbolic

- a syndrome like that described for leg *shao yin*, located in the back rather than in the lumbar area; if the problems are yin, the body is bent forward, if they are yang, it is bent backwards, towards yang

ARM *JUE YIN* CHANNEL SINEW

Where the course differs from that of main channel:

- a small branch starts in the axilla and branches out on the anterior lateral aspect of the rib cage

- one branch penetrates below the surface in the axilla area and spreads out inside of the chest

Specific symptomatology:

- chest pain

- rapid breathing

Treatment

The treatment of a channel sinew impairment calls for puncturing the distal well points (at the tips of the fingers) along with the more proximal river *(jing)* point if the impairment has been present for a long time. It is also useful to puncture a meeting point:

- three leg yang: SI-18

- three leg yin: CV-3

- three arm yang: GB-13

- three arm yin: GB-22

The following two case histories illustrate the importance of knowing the details of the pathways of the channel sinews.

❖ Case History

Mrs. M., age 74, consulted me for a left-sided intercostal case of shingles (at the 3rd intercostal space) that had appeared six days before and was very painful. This robust, energetic woman was astonished by this case of shingles because she said she had never really been sick. Indeed, she did not report any medical history, other than an appendectomy at the age of 27. One important factor was the death of her husband three years earlier. Since that time, she complained of a lack of drive, without anxiety or insomnia, which she attributed to sorrow and the difficulty of living alone. Her pulses were strong, but the left distal Heart pulse was relatively weak. The shingles, already at the end of the eruption stage, were very painful: internal burning aggravated by the slightest contact and not fully relieved by application of cold. This indicated an excess of superficial yang, in this case, of fire. She did not report any recent contact with a carrier of shingles, chickenpox or herpes.

Considering the recent appearance of the condition, I began to clear this superficial pathogenic qi with a sweating technique from Nguyen Van Nghi using SP-1, SP-2, LU-9, and LU-10 on the left. Due to the intensity of the pain, she was given two treatments 48 hours apart, but they did not bring about any improvement.

I started asking more questions about this case of shingles and found there was a slight radiation of pain to the inside of the left upper arm and to the outside of the left forearm. It seemed to concern the arm *jue yin* and *shao yang* channels. The pain first appeared on arm *jue yin*. So, this was an excess of external fire in the arm *jue yin* channel sinew (located in the channel sinew because of the thoracic course followed), probably subsequent to deficiency of protective qi in this channel after the death of her husband and the resulting solitude. I punctured the distal well point, the starting point of the channel sinew, HM-9 on the left, and added the meeting point of the three channel sinews of the upper limb, GB-22. I also tonified the contralateral connecting point (HM-6 on the right) to bring the normal qi to the left arm *jue yin* channel, to the stream point HM-7 on the left. After three treatments within a ten-day period, the pain disappeared. She also recovered part of her drive. Her Heart pulse was improved, though not yet perfect. So I punctured the spirit point, GV-24.

There are three noteworthy items in this case. First, the possible implication of one of the three arm *yin* in case of intercostal shingles, which can only be explained by the courses of the channel sinews. Here, the arm *jue yin* had been previously made vulnerable by a Heart deficiency and so was particularly sensitive to pathogenic heat. Second, that although the pain in the upper limb was slight, it was important in making the diagnosis. And finally, the secondary manifestation located on the internal-external paired channel, arm *shao yang*.

❖ Case History

We have already seen the case of this young woman (*see* p. 40) when discussing the use of ST-28 in connection with the Bladder organ. Six months prior to that treatment she had asked for an urgent appointment for an acute, sudden pain in the right shoulder. In fact, this pain had been mild but continuous for several months, but had suddenly increased in the last three days. Localized in the shoulder, with no radiation to the upper limb or the neck, it was aggravated by any movement. Like a band, it covered the posterior, external and anterior sides of the joint. It was not influenced by local application of cold or heat, but it got worse toward the end of a particularly severe case of cystitis.

Considering the fact that any movement made it worse along with the suddenness of this aggravation, as well as the absence of a path indicating a primary channel, a channel sinew impairment seemed highly probable. The Bladder leg *tai yang* channel sinew, with a course that starts at the broadest back muscles and runs up to the shoulder before reaching the neck and the head, seemed to be the most likely one, especially in view of the history. So I punctured the distal well point, BL-67, and the yang channel sinew meeting point of the lower limb, SI-18, to which I added ST-28 as a booster. Puncturing these points resulted in relief from the pain for 48 hours, followed by a severe reaction for two days before the pain disappeared completely.

Eight Extraordinary Vessels

In Chinese these are called the 奇經八脈 *qi jing ba mai.* We have discussed the terms *jing* (channel) and *mai* (vessel) above. The word 奇 *qi* means extraordinary, rare, surprising, strange, irregular, marvelous, or curious. Larre proposed that this word can be seen as the opposite of the 正 *zheng* of *zheng jing* (the twelve primary channels), which means principal, right, regular, or normal. He once told me that *zheng* speaks of life as it unfolds, perceptible or not, measurable or not, understandable or not, while *qi* speaks of it as it is conceived and created. This concept is reinforced by the number eight (*ba*) which, in addition to representing diffusion into space with the eight winds, governs the multiplication and transmission of life, as in the eight trigrams of the *Book of Changes.* The combination of *qi* and eight communicates the functions of this group of channels: directing the mechanisms of our creation, at conception and at every breath.

For these extraordinary vessels I distinguish two types of functions. First and foremost, they are creative and in this way participate in all of our creations and plans, whether the conception of a being, our recreation with each breath, or even our artistic and spiritual creations. The second set of functions, which are better known, are regulatory.

Different points will be selected for each vessel, depending on which functions are desired.

From the creative perspective, the points for these vessels are:
• Penetrating: CV-4, ST-30

- Conception: CV-2
- Governing: GV-1
- Girdle: GB-26
- Yang Heel: BL-59, BL-62
- Yin Heel: KI-6, KI-8
- Yang Linking: GB-35
- Yin Linking: KI-9

From the regulatory perspective, the key points are:

- Penetrating: SP-4
- Conception: LU-7
- Governing: SI-3
- Girdle: GB-41
- Yang Heel: BL-62
- Yin Heel: KI-6
- Yang Linking: TB-5
- Yin Linking: HM-6

Personally, I use these vessels primarily in their creative capacity and have not studied their regulatory functions, which are well described in many acupuncture textbooks from China.

These eight channels constitute *four pairs*. Depending on the function envisaged, one may count them beginning with the Governing (*du*) vessel for their regulatory functions, or starting with the Penetrating (*chong*) vessel for their creative functions, as discussed below. They are paired as follows:

- Governing (*du*) and Conception (*ren*) vessels
- Girdle (*dai*) and Penetrating (*chong*) vessels
- Yin and Yang Linking (*wei*) vessels
- Yin and Yang Heel (*qiao*) vessels

Only the Governing and Conception vessels have their own points, like the primary channels.

Four of these vessels are related to the Kidneys. The Governing, Conception, and Penetrating vessels are generated from a common trunk that originates in the area of the Kidneys and emerges at CV-1. The fourth, the Girdle vessel, originates at the second lumbar vertebra and connects at that level with the divergent channel of the Kidneys. The other four vessels have their origin in the feet or the legs (the Yin Linking vessel). We should note that both the feet and kidneys have the form of seeds.

The Creative Functions of the Extraordinary Vessels

PENETRATING VESSEL

First of all, it is the crossroads at which the Penetrating vessel is linked to the primal qi (元氣 *yuan qi*) by its main point, CV-4 (*guan yuan* 關元, "Barrier of the Primal") and where it bursts in impetuously.[7] Originating, in connection with the primal, at the beginning of a creation (recalling that we are recreated at each breath), the Penetrating vessel is marked by the eruption of source qi, the source of life, at this crossroads. We can see how a disturbance in the Penetrating vessel could occur in the first moments of intra-uterine life when the mother is unwillingly pregnant and desires an abortion. It leads to great difficulty with emerging into life.

The symptoms are genital (in both men and women), sexual, digestive, lumbar, and pelvic, with unpleasant sensations of heaviness and pain, and in general, a sensation of burning within the body with fatigue. It may be the reason for some cases of infertility or miscarriage.

❖ Case History

Mrs. A., an elegant press agent, had experienced a substantial aggravation of her depressive syndrome since a vacuum aspiration was performed because of a false positive result on a pregnancy test. She had no more drive, desires, or impulses in any area of her life, including her sexuality. She slept poorly, awakening every two hours. She had no other physical symptoms. She had been in psychoanalysis for two years. The pulses were deep and hidden. Her tongue appeared normal. The preexisting Penetrating vessel deficiency was aggravated by the vacuum aspiration. CV-4, punctured and treated with moxa each week, healed this acute episode in five treatments. We advised her to follow up with treatments every two months during her psychoanalysis.

Further on, I recount a case history involving the Penetrating vessel in which I used SP-4, the opening point for this channel (*see* p. 108).

The Penetrating vessel, the origin, is also a future, a plan, a goal to be achieved: the human being, standing up, between heaven and earth.

❖ Case History

Ms. H., a reserved 37-year-old, came to see me one month after the death of her mother, with whom she had been very close, "too close." All of her symptoms had grown worse since then: intense, generalized muscle tension, low back pain on the left side, pain in the left side of the groin, intense vulvar itching, itching on the left big toe. She had been in menopause for the last six months, although she had had normal periods before that. She spoke quickly and also complained of intense anxiety that she had some problem with her throat. She could not stand to be alone. She was fragile and believed she was "in danger of dying." She lacked solid foundations: "I am walking through mud, I cannot lay down." In her expression, I could see extreme rage, which she did not deny. Her tongue appeared normal. The pulses were more tense in the proximal position. I punctured CV-5 to reinforce her foundations.

Two months later, because of her significant burning vulvar sensations, I punctured CV-1, since our trust-based relations made this acceptable. This point was used not only because of its local implications, but because it is the meeting point of the Governing, Conception, and Penetrating vessels. After two treatments, the symptoms had decreased noticeably. She managed to talk about her father, was able to envisage being a mother and felt the timid emergence of her femininity. By the sixth treatment, she said to me, "I can feel the life in myself and at the same time a lot of anger, sometimes even the urge to kill." Three months later, she said that she knew that she no longer wanted to be alone. Six months later, all of her symptoms had disappeared: "Life is in me and flowing; I am in love with a man who is available." CV-1, punctured a final time, had incited this woman to stand up straight, between heaven and earth.

GIRDLE VESSEL

This is the only horizontal channel; located at the waist, it encircles and orients. It is connected with the polar star: its role is to guide the lost traveler. To belt, to gird the waist to make it stronger, and then to orient and guide, these are the roles of the Girdle vessel.

If it is not functioning properly, the person is scattered and dispersed, because they are not girded. They are lacking in clear goals because they are not oriented, and often have low back pain and abdominal discomfort along with pelvic spasms, leukorrhea, and menstrual disturbances.

❖ Case History

Mrs. V., age 26, consulted me for a severe case of asthma that had appeared when she was 18, shortly after witnessing her uncle's death. This was the first time she had been confronted with death. She was never sick and did not have any other symptoms. She had a lot of qi but did not know how to manage it: she was too scattered and dispersed; she always needed the support of others (as compensation). Puncturing GB-26, which is named "Girdle Vessel" and controls the channel of the same name, cured this asthma in three treatments.

❖ Case History

Mrs. A., age 30, consulted me for severe, persistent insomnia that had lasted for nine years, although it did not tire her because she was very energetic. She had no profession, lacked discipline, and was incapable of settling down. Scattered and dispersed, she had embarked on many studies but never finished any of them. Puncturing GB-26 cured her insomnia in four treatments.

We note that dysfunction of the Girdle vessel, which then fails to gird and orient, prevents exhaling and sinking into sleep. In order to exhale, to confront death, or to let go into sleep, one must "gird one's loins," as God says to Job in the Bible. To gird one's loins is to be able to use one's physical and mental strength.

GOVERNING AND CONCEPTION VESSELS

The word 督 *du* means to control and govern. A deficiency in the Governing vessel, located on the midline and posterior aspect of the spinal column and skull, is characterized by a hunched posture, vertebral pains, a feeling of the head being empty, and depression.

The word 任 *ren* means to take charge. Here it refers to assuming responsibility for all aspects of our lives, while it also governs the formal boundaries, beginning with the skin. The Conception vessel, on the anterior midline of the trunk and face, contains and supports; it is often involved in infertility, urinary problems, leukorrhea, hernias, low back pain, and hydrocele or varicocele in men.

❖ Case History

Mr. X., age 45, was suffering from intense psychological distress. For the past six months he "felt at the end of his rope and had suicidal urges." He had a long history of alternating periods of feeling fine and of being depressed. While for years this type of breakdown had been preceded by periods of depression with feelings of failure and inferiority in all areas of his life, this latest period of distress was the worst he had ever experienced. He had difficulty expressing himself. The year before this crisis, he had endured a severe upheaval in his family and his working life and was unable to take on a new career opportunity that had arisen.

I did not find many symptoms: a few headaches, upper and lower back pains, hypersomnia and especially a hunched posture with his head pulled down into his shoulders, which strongly suggested a Governing vessel deficiency. Lastly, he had suffered from a lack of affection from his mother and the absence of his father, who he barely remembered. One very important factor was that he had never been addressed by his first name: his peers, parents, spouse and children all called him by a childhood nickname. Puncturing GV-1 led to substantial improvement after six monthly treatments, along with his choice after the third treatment to stop accepting this nickname and reclaim his true name.

One of the important aspects of the Governing vessel is that it reflects and resonates with the limits that come with names. This connects with the fact that to take any action in life necessarily means becoming limited, as every living being has its own nature and no being can be everything. The yang side of this limitation is reflected in giving it a name while the yin side is its taking a particular form. We know the importance of the name in relation to the specific cosmic nature, place and function of each being. The form, limited by the skin, is connected with the Conception vessel. This is demonstrated by the ability of CV-2 to treat skin diseases.

❖ Case History

This 36-year-old lady was tall, neat, cheerful and pleasant, full of *joie de vivre* and kindness. For three months she had been afflicted with a marked facial paralysis on the left side which, of course, depressed her a lot. It was obviously impossible for her to whistle or to blow into a tube; her left eye was wide open and did not close. The left side of the face was painful, especially when it was cold. Local heat improved it. This paralysis occurred after she had contracted Lyme's disease and especially, according to her, after her second child was born. Both her pregnancy, which was desired, and the childbirth were normal. The fact that the eye was open pointed to deficiency and cold. The treatment goal was to bring back yang heat to the face.

In 1986 she had undergone an operation for a T5-L1 scoliosis. Two metal rods were fitted into her back. She no longer suffered from it. This period of her life had taught her to put things in perspective and prioritize problems and finally to become somewhat wiser. She also complained of long-term bilateral frontal headaches around BL-2 that affected the eyeballs and occurred with menstruation or with pain in the nape of the neck. The parasagittal neck pains, also bilateral, would sometimes radiate to the left little finger. They appeared in a quite unpredictable way, and not apparently because of stress. She was not stressed by any particular worries; moreover, stressful situations tended to manifest as diarrhea rather than as pain in the neck.

She also reported an occasional paroxysmal supraventricular tachycardia. Her hands and feet were cold. Her pulses showed much energy and were normal. Her childhood was painfully marked by the alcoholism of an absent father.

The channels involved in her scoliosis and her headaches—*tai yang* and Governing vessel—were both related to the suffering she felt because of this alcoholic and absent father. The paroxysmal supraventricular tachycardia and the stress-induced diarrhea made me think of the Small Intestine and Heart channels.

All of these mechanisms converge toward SI-3, a point of the arm *tai yang* and a confluent point of the Governing vessel.

Further analysis of the paralysis showed deficiency cold in the face. The Yang Heel vessel, governed by BL-62, which is related to SI-3, makes yang ascend to the face. I needled it during the second session, after having tried SI-3 alone on the first occasion.

I added a symptomatic point on the head as the paralysis was severe and greatly handicapped this young woman, choosing among GV-23 on the Governing vessel, BL-1 on the *tai yang* channel, and ST-1, ST-3, or ST-4 on the Yang Heel vessel.

I only needled SI-3 on the left during the first session. During the following 48 hours this patient developed fatigue, pruritus, nightmares and a short episode of paroxysmal tachycardia, but her face was already better. On the fourth day, the onset of her period brought about the usual headaches. This confirmed that SI-3 was a good choice. In the second session, a week later, I added BL-62 on the left and GV-23, as I thought it would have an effect on the face and the headaches. The improvement was noteworthy except for the headaches.

One month later, at the third session, the symptoms had continued to improve, including the cold feet and hands, but not the headaches. I replaced GV-23 with BL-2.

The following month, the Institut Pasteur declared that her Lyme's disease had been cured. The improvement was remarkable; there only remained a slight 'curve' of the eye (which did not close completely) and the left part of the face. For her final two monthly sessions, I then replaced BL-2 with BL-1, which links leg *tai yang,* arm *tai yang,* leg *yang ming,* and the Yang Heel vessel. After the final session, her face had become completely normal.

This lady came back to me five months later because she wanted to stop smoking. In such cases, I always needle one of the connecting points, which govern the relationships with the exterior. In this specific case, it was obvious that SI-7, the connecting point of the arm *tai yang,* should be needled. I also chose a point on the head located on the same channel and related to the nose and the mouth, SI-18. Within two sessions, the treatment was a full success, which she confirmed when I happened to meet her in a shop.

❖ Case History

A 65-year-old man, intellectually brilliant and highly cultivated, held a subordinate administrative position for lack of ambition. He said that he was incapable of handling many of the practical aspects of life, accounting, his share of housekeeping, etc. He was married and had a 30-year-old son. He consulted me for a case of very itchy, generalized eczema that had appeared 18 months before. All biomedical test results were normal. He had been operated on for an inguinal hernia on the right side, and had suffered a heart attack at the age of 57. Treating the Conception vessel with CV-2 permanently eliminated this eczema in two sessions. I arrived at the diagnosis of Conception vessel because of his inability to take charge of his professional ambitions and many practical aspects of his daily life together with his skin problems and the hernia.

❖ Case History

A 60-year-old man who was vigorous and perfectly healthy suddenly experienced, for no apparent reason, acute pains in the lower lumbar region of the back around the midline. The pains were incapacitating and only relieved by assuming a fetal position. This athletic patient did not report any other symptoms or history of other such incidents. During the visit, he said he had been incapable of taking charge of his family, to the point where, although he was married and had four children, he still lived with his parents. Puncturing CV-2 cleared up the pain in two hours.

LINKING AND HEEL VESSELS

The Linking vessels are celestial and differentiate the yin and yang; the Heel vessels are earthly and marry them together. The Linking vessels are heavenly and govern space; the Heel vessels are earthly and govern time. The Linking vessels harmonize spaces separately, yang spaces for Yang Linking vessels and yin spaces for Yin Linking vessels. The Heel vessels govern our temporal changes, beginning with sleeping and awakening, in the daytime for the Yang Heel vessel and at night for the Yin Heel vessel.

The relation to basic heavenly principles, distinction between yin and yang, and the government of spaces all pertain to the Linking vessels. Rooting into the earth, marriage, beginning with that of the feminine and masculine in each person, and control of temporal changes are all within the sphere of the Heel vessels.

The Yang Linking vessel is responsible for pain caused by changes in atmospheric pressure: these patients are full of qi, even excited, and are able to predict the weather by their pains. Moreover, they are sensitive to all types of atmosphere, including human, as if there were no boundaries between themselves and others.

The Yin Linking vessel is defined by substantial headaches, jabbing or cutting precordial pains, and cyclothymic alternation between depression and excitation.

The Yin Heel vessel suggests pelvic problems (constipation, or painful menstruation), joint pains that are worse at night, and sleep disturbances.

The Yang Heel vessel can be recognized by pains that tend to appear in the daytime, difficulty falling asleep, and symptoms of excessive heat in the skin (acne, furuncles, eczema, psoriasis).

❖ Case History

Mrs. X., age 33, shed many tears as she listed her numerous problems. Renal colic alternating with soreness over the kidney, both on the right side. Acute lower back pain and sciatica that led to surgery for a herniated disc at L5-S1, which did not relieve the pain. Pains in the right ovary, independent of the menstrual cycle, but no organic lesion could be found. Excessive menstrual bleeding that led to the removal of a fibroma along with premenstrual headaches. She also had episodes of high blood pressure as well as Hashimoto's thyroiditis with hypothyroidism, treated with hormone supplementation. She also had stabbing precordial pains and tachycardia although the results of cardiovascular checkups were normal.

She had plenty of qi, was unaware of her limits, had no sense of emotional distance, experienced everything intensely, and had attempted suicide at the age of 16. The impairment of the Yin Linking vessel was obvious, with her lack of emotional detachment. Considering her substantial problems and their progressive nature, we recommended, in addition to in-patient supervision, acupuncture and psychoanalysis. There was a noticeable, gradual improvement and the progressing conditions were brought under control. KI-9, which I see as the main point for the creative aspects of the Yin Linking vessel, was the basis of my treatment.

❖ Case History

Mrs. K., who was rigid, self-effacing, small and dry, came to see me for two types of symptoms. There were problems that dated far into the past: multiple joint pains that moved around and were unaffected by the environment; constipation; slight urinary incontinence; and significant premenstrual syndrome. There were also more recent problems that had arisen five years previously, with a high level of inner tension that developed after the death of her husband: insomnia, tachycardia, eczema on her face with a burning sensation on the skin. The tip of her tongue was red; the proximal pulses were weak; the Heart pulse was tense. She had little self-confidence, was oppressed by her father, her brothers and her husband, and rarely expressed herself: "It isn't that I do not have anything to say." She had rejected her femininity and took a long time before agreeing to marry her husband.

The first symptoms were obviously due to a deficiency of the Yin Heel vessel with an inability to embrace her femininity, to marry the yin and the yang. The second set of symptoms was connected with a constraint of the Heart fire following the death of her husband, which was reinforced by a failure of the Kidney qi to rise to the Heart, due to the Yin Heel vessel deficiency. Puncturing KI-6 (the master point of Yin Heel vessel) and KI-6 (to release the Heart constraint) brought about a spectacular improvement in all of her symptoms.

❖ Case History

Mr. N., age 49 and an actor, consulted for left-sided cluster headaches that had worsened during the previous three-and-a-half months. The pain started behind the eye, extended to the temple, and then to the occipitoatlantal area. During an attack, his nose ran, his eye watered, and his upper eyelid on the same side of the face drooped. He could not think of any factors that triggered or aggravated the problem. This pain emerged at the base of the skull and involved the two orifices of the skull, the nose and the eye. Energetically speaking, the runny nose, the weeping eye, and the drooping eyelid showed it was linked to the *tai yang.*

The base of the skull separates and unites the skull and face, heaven and earth, intellect and sensations (with the seven orifices), reason and affect, spirit and emotions. Symbolically, it is like the diaphragm that separates the chest and abdomen. They are often simultaneously disturbed. The base of the skull is primarily governed by the *tai yang* and GV-16 on the midline and by BL-1 and BL-10 on the sides. One could also add the appropriate barrier points: BL-2, GB-14, GB-3, or ST-7 (see pages 127–133 for a discussion of barrier points).

The patient's history included ophthalmic migraines and eczema recurring from time to time. The principal etiology of ophthalmic migraines is, above all, endocranial phlegm (often accompanied by numbness of the tongue), an excess of cephalic blood, or a disturbance in the heel vessels.

In addition, he had disturbed sleep patterns with difficulty in falling asleep before two or three in the morning, and fatigue in the lower limbs when standing for prolonged periods, which caused him problems at work.

In view of the lateral nature of the pain, I first thought of an impairment of BL-1 (primarily signaled by the symptoms in the eye, nostril and eyelid), linked to a disturbance of the Yang Heel vessel (difficulty falling asleep, eczema, fatigue in the lower limbs, and ophthalmic migraines). However, this laterality did not exclude a mechanism involving the midline, especially as the pain, of the yang type, was located above (yang) and to the left (also yang). Considering the location of the pain, M-HN-3 (*yin tang*) seemed more likely.

When I asked this man about his life, he said that he was going through a melancholy period of transition and wavering. He said he knew intuitively that it was time to break up with a girlfriend for whom he cared a lot: "It is a serious step to take, and I do not know exactly where I am in the process; fortunately, I have something solid to lean on—my vocation as an actor." This torn feeling, this transition, and this wavering was manifested at an intermediary level, at the base of the skull, serving to separate and unite the reasoning and affective aspects. Needling BL-1 and BL-62 on the left cleared up this neuralgia in one treatment. Seven months later, it had not returned. He subsequently told me that this visit calmed him, helped him serenely to decide on the separation and to rediscover his "wholeness."

SIXTEEN CONNECTING VESSELS

The connecting vessels (絡脈 *luo mai*) are vessels but not proper channels (經 *jing*). Why? Because they do not transmit essential truths, they do not reveal the laws of the world, and they are not the foundation of the world, as the main channels are. The connecting vessels are literally 絡 *luo*, which originally referred to the weft of a fabric against an existing warp (經 *jing*), the word used for the main channels. It weaves the fabric of relations that make up our everyday life by relying on the channels.

Let's begin by looking at their functions and dysfunctions:

- Inside of our bodies, the connecting vessels link the yin and yang channels in an exterior-interior relationship (*biao-li*), and all aspects of the body, from the largest to the smallest, from the most coarse to the most subtle, to the qi, blood and fluids.

A pathology of the yang connecting vessels leads to a difficulty in linking the yang to the yin, which then stagnates on the surface, in the exterior. This will result in patients who are agitated, angry, irritable, overly sensitive—all signs of exterior yang excess. By contrast, a pathology of the yin connecting vessels leads to a blockage of yin deep down inside. Such patients are introverted and rarely show their feelings and emotions, even if they are boiling with anger inside.

Here are four possible uses of the connecting points:

- In case of an imbalance between two paired exterior-interior channels, by puncturing the connecting point of the channel that is in excess and the source point of the paired channel

- To regulate the functions and circulation within a given channel, especially at the pivots like *jue yin* and *shao yang*, by stimulating the connecting and associated points of the same channel

- To link symptoms from different parts of the body by puncturing the connecting point alone, depending on the symptomatology

- To connect two channels that are in excess when they are related by the midday-midnight connection of the traditional Chinese clock (*see* p. 80). When there are symptoms on two channels that have this type of relationship, one should puncture a point on one of the affected channels and the contralateral connecting point on the related midday-midnight channel. This can enhance the therapeutic action. An example of this was seen earlier in the pathologies of desynchronization between man and the universe with the main channels (*see* p. 76).

- The connecting points are also involved in all of our communications and relations with the outside world, through the sense organs, the skin, and orifices, that is, all of our means of contact with the world.

The symptomatology[8] of the connecting points is important and not widely known. (*See* Table 3.) They contribute to the diagnosis and indications of these points.

Certain connecting points complement their connecting functions (linking yin and yang) with those of the opening points of the extraordinary channels, also known as confluent points (交會穴 *jiao hui xue*). These are LU-7, HM-6, SP-4 and TB-5. Clearly, these two properties are not independent: the first, of connecting, is the basis for the second, of opening. An acupuncture point is actually a convergence of mechanisms that are different but related. The choice of the point to which one associates it, or the mere fact of puncturing it, orients its effect. For example, while I use HM-6 alone for a diaphragm problem, I would add KI-6 to also treat the Yin Linking vessel, or TB-4 to treat the connection between the arm *shao yang* and the arm *jue yin*, or ST-40 if there was a midday-midnight issue, and so on.

I have already mentioned TB-5 along with TB-16 in the windows-of-heaven case study (*see* p. 50). I also utilized HM-6 for a case of shingles, to use the connecting-

Table 3: Symptomatology of the Connecting Points	
LU-7	• Heat in the thenar eminence or palms • Yawning, coughing, dyspnea, frequent urination • Sadness, grief
LI-6	• Painful gums, grinding of teeth, cavities and toothaches; deafness • Painful obstruction of the diaphragm, sensation of cold in the teeth and gums • Mental problems, excessive talking
SP-4	• Acute intestinal pains, vomiting, profuse and watery diarrhea • Abdominal swelling, large stools • Sighing and complaining, melancholy, schizophrenia
ST-40	• Mental disturbances, epilepsy, madness • Feeble, emaciated, weak legs; inability to flex the knees; cramps in leg muscles • Hysterics, overexcitement, hallucination, actions such as dancing on tables or throwing off one's clothes
HT-5	• Fullness in the area of the diaphragm • Inability to speak due to emotion • Emotional lability, tightness in the heart, lack of self-confidence, agoraphobia, inexpressive face
SI-7	• Loose joints, difficulty moving elbows • Sties and excrescences on the neck and face, warts • Mental illness, apprehension and overexcited speech

KI-4	• Anuria with anxiety, constipation
	• Back pains (T5-T6) radiating anteriorly to CV-17; low back pain
	• Inferiority and failure complex, lack of authority, joylessness, timidity, nervousness, seeks solitude, a "desire to shut out the world and close the door," apprehension
BL-58	• Stuffy nose, runny nose, pains on the top of the head and in the back
	• Nosebleeds, runny nose
	• Depression, hysteria, madness
HM-6	• Pains in solar plexus, heartburn
	• Stiff neck, mental fatigue
	• Forgetting words, indecision, anxiety due to yin deficiency, an absence of willpower with anxiety, laziness
TB-5	• Spasms in the elbow
	• Limp elbow
	• Excitation, tremors
LR-5	• Extreme and painful erection
	• Sudden itching of genitals
	• Lack of joy, melancholy, frequent sighing, worry
GB-37	• Cold hands and feet: qi disturbances
	• Powerless, flaccid legs; cannot rise unassisted from a seated position
	• Epilepsy, palpitations

associated system to link the two right and left branches of the arm *jue yin* Heart Master channel. I will now use a case history to illustrate the use of connecting points in their capacity for controlling the internal relations of a person, in this case in a connecting-source pair.

❖ Case History

A 32-year-old filmmaker with a Bohemian look came to see me for headaches, usually on the left side, very intense, pulsatile, located on *tai yang* from BL-2 to BL-8, causing a sensation of the ipsilateral eye being pushed forward. The headaches were aggravated by pressure on the eyeball and relieved by local application of cold; they were sometimes accompanied by dizziness and vomiting. They often occurred following a period of tension and overwork, while he was decompressing. Alcohol had no impact. The responses to cold and to pressure suggested a yang excess, and the lack of impact from alcohol implied that it was not a blood problem. Because of the localization on the *tai yang* channel, I thought of BL-5, BL-7 and BL-8. BL-10 was not involved, as the pain did not concern the occipital area or the nape of the neck.

In addition, I noted *tai yang* pains in the mid and lower back, more often on the left, and intermittent pains on the posterior aspects of the legs along the pathway of the leg *tai yang*, making it impossible to bend the knees. The evident impairment of leg *tai yang* could be due to a problem with that channel, or it could be secondary to a problem with leg *shao yin* (by the external-internal pairing), arm *tai yin* (by the midday-midnight pairing), or leg *tai yin* (by the ascending-descending rule). We have seen these pairings with the primary channels.

I saw that there was a history of pharyngitis and a case of epididymitis that lasted for a year. He reported frequent soft stools, especially when he was tense; bouts of a dry, hacking cough, although he did not smoke; some precordial pains that were neither stabbing nor cutting in nature; and that he felt satiated quickly when eating. His urine was normal. He slept well and often dreamed that he was taking flight. The proximal radial pulses were deep but the pulses at KI-3 were full. These signs evoked a disturbance in leg *shao yin,* especially because of the pharyngitis and the fact that he was quickly satiated. The absence of stabbing or cutting precordial pains eliminated the implication of the Yin Linking vessel, for which he did not display the associated behavior in any case, particularly the alternating periods of depression and excitement. A recurring dream of taking flight suggested that the qi was blocked above. This could be the qi from the Lung, the Heart, or one of the three yang channels, in this case most probably *tai yang.*

The man was often physically very tired; he had little endurance. He was irritable, extremely sensitive, and easily discouraged. He was engaged in a profession that was insecure, dependent on the television channels, which might or might not buy his highly original films. He had been married for five years and had a two-year-old son. He described himself as an "outlaw" who lived outside the rules and without a clearly defined place in society. A history of an absent father who treated him like a child could be one explanation for these problems.

Remember that *tai yang* is associated with the law, rules, and the father. The dreams and sensitivity suggested that leg *tai yang* was not connecting with leg *shao yin*. The lack of rules seemed to indicate that the origin was in *tai yang* for this "outlaw."

The connecting point, BL-58, the name of which (*fei yang*) means "flying yang," connecting the leg *tai yang* to the leg *shao yin*, was strongly indicated. So I started by puncturing BL-5 and BL-58. I hesitated between using KI-11, the root of production of the five organs, in consideration of the fatigue and the epididymitis; KI-18, because of the soft stools, cough, and epididymitis; and KI-3, the source point that makes an effective pair with the connecting point BL-58. At the first two sessions, I chose KI-18, which is, in my experience, a point for draining the Spleen, perhaps in order to cleanse it, to eliminate toxins, etc. The results were spectacular. A third treatment consolidated these results.

I saw him again eight months later for a recurrence of the headaches, a pain in the right shoulder on *yang ming* that was interfering with abduction, and intense fatigue. He was unsuccessfully trying to sell an ethnographic film on Indonesia at the time. Two treatments with BL-58 and KI-3 relieved these problems, including the shoulder pains (remember that the leg t*ai yang* channel sinew moves in a belt around the shoulder). This case history seems to be a particularly good illustration of the pathology of a connecting point in an external-internal pairing.

I will add another case history to illustrate the diagnostic and therapeutic procedures of using the connecting points.

❖ Case History

A 56-year-old woman who worked as a bookseller and practiced yoga came to me for a long-term problem with insomnia. She had difficulty falling asleep, awoke frequently and could only fall back asleep after a long time. She did not have nightmares. She reported some episodes of sleepwalking in childhood, did not cry out or speak during her sleep, did not grind her teeth and did not suffer from sleep apnea. She did not have recurring dreams. Since she had a lot of qi, she was not very tired, considering her lack of sleep. Her tongue appeared normal. Her pulses were full; there were no deficient sectors.

There was little to report in physical terms. She had had four abortions because circumstances did not permit her to keep the children. She digested her food well and did not have any particular pains. Her periods had been normal, she had no children, her menopause was not being treated except with food supplements and was progressing without problems.

She had undergone psychoanalysis for ten years for a depression connected to her childhood and this was now cured. She was touchy, quick to react, easily carried away, highly emotional, sensitive and impulsive. She had been severely bullied and was very unhappy during her childhood. In fact, she had only begun to feel truly happy since her marriage, twelve years before. She could not understand why she continued to have trouble sleeping.

Which mechanisms could be involved?

Considering her sleepwalking, qi levels, normal pulses, and absence of other symptoms, one could suppose pathology of the ethereal soul, the Girdle vessel, or of a yang connecting point. Nothing suggested any organ, or the Governing vessel.

Could the ethereal soul be the cause? No, because there were no Liver signs. And the Girdle vessel? She was neither dispersed nor scattered, had neither low back pain nor white discharges, did not easily twist her ankles, etc.

Could the cause be a yang connecting point? Probably.

- We could eliminate GV-15 because she did not have an overly extended posture, did not stutter in childhood, and her spine was normal.
- She was not nervous and did not have the cutaneous symptoms of SI-7. There was no sign that suggested *tai yang* (BL-58) or *yang ming* (LI-6 or ST-40).
- Her impulsive behavior, her sensitivity, and her emotional lability went with *shao yang*. She did not have cold hands and feet, cramps, weak legs, gallbladder problems or epilepsy in her history (GB-37).
- This left us with TB-5, even though there were no other signs of the Heart Master in an external-internal pair, elbow pains or tremors.

I therefore punctured this point bilaterally. She started improving from the first treatment. After the second treatment a week later, she slept six hours straight and then fell asleep again fairly quickly. She arrived for her third treatment six weeks later with a torticollis on the right side, which was relieved 48 hours after a puncture of TB-16, also a point on the arm *shao yang*. At the fourth and final treatment, two months later, she said that she was sleeping well but had been suffering for six days from a pain in the left shoulder along the arm *shao yang*, which I treated with TB-14 in addition to the usual point.

We should note the emergence of pains, unusual for her, along the channel being treated: was this an elimination reaction?

I also want to describe a case that required puncturing the connecting and associated points of the same channel.

❖ Case History

Mrs. M., a 46-year-old teacher, small and slender, and energetic if not outright nervous, came to see me for the first time in 1979 for headaches that were either on the right or left, often severe, non-pulsatile, localized along the *shao yang* channel, and did not respond to cold, heat or pressure. I could not find any triggering or predisposing factors, including climate, nor any signs that would suggest either Yin Linking or Yang Linking vessel dysfunction.

What could I deduce? That the headaches did not correspond to the eight parameters, that they did not concern the blood (they were not pulsatile nor influenced by alcohol or by the menstrual cycle) and that I would have to find out to which *shao yang* mechanism they corresponded.

She also complained that she had frequent feelings of instability, that she was bothered by noise and often experienced spontaneous blockage in her left ear. Which *shao yang* point could this be? Above all, GB-2, which is responsible for ear blockages and for headaches.

I also noted that she sometimes had slow digestion, alternating between constipation and yellow stools, flatulence, and sensitivity to chocolate and coffee. Otherwise, all was well: there were no other pains, no gynecological, urinary, pulmonary, cardiac or other problems.

Which mechanism could be the cause? The Gallbladder, although I could not say whether it was the origin of the problem or the secondary result of a disturbance in another *shao yang* mechanism.

This woman was energetic and decisive, divorced, with one son, and a spiritual seeker. But she was very scattered and had always been going in all directions at once, in all areas of her life. She needed "psychological help and support." Her tongue looked normal. So I chose GB-2 and GB-26, since the proximal pulses were deeper.

What could be the *shao yang* mechanism in question? She had neither the typology nor the symptomatology of a Yang Linking vessel problem. A *shao yang* axis? There were no signs of arm *shao yang* and other leg *shao yang* symptoms. She was not impulsive. It is true that she had a wandering nature, but her dispersion suggested the Girdle vessel, as did her tongue and her pulses. The Gallbladder appeared to be secondary rather than the original cause.

So I needled the points. She was well after three treatments.

I saw her again in 1981 for a relapse of the same symptoms. She had found a spiritual master, through his writings, but she had not yet decided to meet him. Two treatments restored her equilibrium.

She returned in 1995 for frequent dizzy spells with blockage in the left ear and breathing difficulties. She could not fully exhale. "It's blocked before it gets to my neck," she said. She was out of breath and her nose was stuffy. She had met her spiritual master and was now living in an ashram. But as she progressed with her purification, her fears of death and of her mother increased or emerged. "I have lived in fear all my life." Naturally, she linked this fear of death with the breathing difficulties.

Was there a relationship between the Girdle vessel and this difficulty with exhaling? Yes. A person needs strong loins (Kidneys) for support, to be able to exhale. See the case above (p. 91) concerning the Girdle vessel in connection with shortness of breath on exhalation and a confrontation with death. To die is to expire and the Lung door of the corporeal soul is an "exit into life and entry into death".

I punctured GB-26 and LU-2 because it was "blocked before the neck."

She returned again in 1998. This time she had serious digestive problems as well as vulvar and anal itching, nausea and strong-smelling urine. She was out of balance and had pains in her left ear, no headaches, a surprisingly marked hallux valgus, pain in the right sacroiliac joint and a highly sensitive GB-29. "My childhood fears have returned with a vengeance, along with their ghosts. At the same time, I am learning to detach from my body and its somatic and psychic pains; I am unstable, not dispersed, but unstable. I wake at 5 a.m.. My qi is on the surface and up high."

Why was GB-29 sensitive? Because it corresponds to the adolescence that she was reliving at this time.

Was the Girdle vessel still involved? If not, which mechanism should be addressed? I understood that her problems had shifted from the Girdle vessel to *shao yang* blocked at the surface, without connection to *jue yin* (sensitive hallux valgus, anal and vulvar itching). What should be treated? The connecting point of leg *shao yang,* which links this channel to leg *jue yin* in an exterior-interior pairing. I punctured GB-37 and GB-41, as GB-41 is the opening point of the Girdle vessel and the combination of the associated and connecting points of the same channel is a regulating technique. The signs cleared up quickly. After the third treatment she was much more peaceful.

I saw her again in 2001. She had undergone a cholecystectomy for gall stones. Now she was suffering from serious vertigo; her left ear was blocked and oversensitive to high-pitched sounds; her head felt hot. She had mild headaches and digestive problems. Her breathing was better than before. Her mother had died. "We were able to see one another again before she died; it was a gift of the goodness of life." Moreover, she often felt a presence around her saying, "I am arriving at my destination." "But what is causing this imbalance? Can acupuncture help me find the right place, and stop fearing my fear?" I gathered that she wanted to find the right middle ground of the Gallbladder.

Which central point could help her? I felt that this point was GV-7, located on the midline at the level of BL-19. Its name is 中樞 *zhong shu,* or "Center Pivot." In the next three weeks, she accidentally fell on her knees four times. After the second session, the dizzy spells stopped and she felt better.

She returned in August 2003 and January 2004 to have this point punctured and to have its meaning and importance explained.

What do these three treatments have in common? The need for centering, first, at the level of the Girdle vessel, which is of the order of man between the Linking vessels, which are heavenly, and the Heel vessels, which are earthly; and next, by the pivots *shao yang* and *jue yin* to communicate and free internal circulation and the Heart Master (Pericardium), the servant of the Heart, as well as the Liver, general of the armies. This is done to achieve the justice and middle ground of the Gallbladder. This aspect of the organ often makes me think of the internal master, that which is in the center of us and knows what is right.

The following example illustrates the use of a connecting point in its role of governing our relations with the external world.

❖ Case History

A little girl, age 10, was overeating, defensive, and complained of multiple allergies: nasal, some asthma-like bronchitis, eczema, urticaria, and several bouts of angioedema. She was sensitive and felt everything, even if she did not show it. She was fearful, but showed off to hide it. There was some sleepwalking (which often implies TB-5 or BL-47) but she slept well. Her pulses were superficial, showing that she had blocked everything at the surface in order to protect herself: this explained the allergies, the hyperdefensive reactions, and the obesity. I decided to puncture the points ST-15 (seen above with *yang ming*) and TB-5, the connecting point of arm *shao yang*. After six monthly treatments, her allergies had improved and she could stop all treatments. I recommended psychotherapy and quarterly acupuncture as follow-up. Her weight did not change, showing that she still had major problems with hypersensitivity and insecurity.

I now want to make two remarks concerning SP-21, on the great connecting channel of the Spleen, and SP-7, on the *tai yin* connecting vessel.

❖ Case History

Mr. A., 53, was a solicitor. He was overweight, hyperactive, and tough in business. He had been suffering from insulin-dependent diabetes since the age of 19 and sought help for the neuropathy that was affecting his extremities. The lower part of his legs and his hands were very cold and presented chilblains; most of all, they were very painful, as if squeezed and crushed. The pain was severe enough that the prescription of an NSAID and morphine analgesics was justified.

The rest of the history added very little. He suffered from insomnia partly because of the pain in his feet that was aggravated when he was in bed. His blood pressure was slightly high but well controlled. His pulses were wiry and deep, his tongue was normal, neither purple nor trembling.

This married man had two children he loved dearly; he liked amassing estates and money, and admitted that he was not very generous. He was not really prone to giving. Considering the symptoms of cold, which pointed to qi and blood not reaching the extremities, and his weight and personality, it occurred to me that this man kept everything to himself and lacked centrifugal movement. I thought of the two central organs, the Heart and the Spleen, and of the middle burner. Actually, as far as the yin organs are concerned, the center has two sides: the Heart belongs to the subtle side, the side of the spirit, and the Spleen belongs to the sensitive side, the side of the flavors and the intention.

The pulses, the tongue, which was neither pale (deficiency) nor purple (stagnation) nor trembling (wind), his friendliness (when not at work), and the absence of other symptoms did not suggest a Heart disorder. On the other hand, his diabetes, weight, and toughness in business could signal a central obstruction of the Spleen, even though he did not have digestive disorders. The pulses and the absence of digestive disorders ruled out qi and blood constraint in the middle burner.

The Spleen could be treated with the following points: LR-13 (alarm point) associated with SP-6, which has a central action on blood; or KI-17, which, to my mind, regulates the transportation function of the Spleen.

But the paresthesias led me to think of a connecting channel implication. Considering the responsibility held by the Spleen, the choice was between one of the three following connecting points: SP-4, SP-7 and SP-21. I considered that his obesity was in part due to using his extra weight to protect himself from psychological aggressions as well as using food as compensation for other things that are lacking in his life. I preferred to use SP-21.

As soon as I had needled SP-21, the extremities improved by 50 percent. Unfortunately, 48 hours later, he developed a very painful orchiepididymitis on the right side that was successfully treated by antibiotics. While the pain had improved during the week, he noticed that the improvement was better before he ate, which confirmed the role played by the Spleen. The orchiepididymitis can be seen as a reaction to the treatment of the *yang ming*, coupled with the *tai yin* in an exterior-interior relationship. Needling ST-29 relieved the orchiepididymitis within 72 hours.

After the second treatment, a fortnight later, the pain was still largely improved over eight days but a particularly violent attack occurred on the ninth day and required the administration of morphine. On the tenth day, the pain gradually receded again. The patient reported hypoglycemic episodes secondary to this session. I needled SP-21 accompanied by ST-40, a connecting point, to reinforce the effect of the leg *tai yin* point. His touchy nature and irascible temper were indications for the latter point.

After the third treatment, 20 days later, he had much less pain during the day but still experienced a severe attack between 5 and 8 a.m. The hypoglycemic episodes had disappeared. I do not think ST-40 was of much use. I punctured SP-21 alone for this fourth treatment. A month later, the patient had improved by 60 percent with a relapse around the time of the Heart channel (11 a.m. to 1 p.m.). The patient told me he was very worried about his daughter who he feared might have osteosarcoma. They had not yet received the results of the tests.

When I saw him a month later, he said the improvement had been steady (60 percent) for three weeks in spite of the confirmed diagnosis of his daughter's osteosarcoma and of the still present insomnia. He suffered from pain attacks from time to time but they were less severe. His extremities were less cold. He did not return for treatment.

❖ Case History

Mrs. T., age 38, was an administrator. She was tall, thin, reserved if not uncommunicative, and rarely smiled. She complained of pains that were all located along the leg *tai yang*, on the left side. She reported intense menstrual headaches around BL-2, neck pains which started at BL-10 and radiated down the back, occasional sciatica without low back pain, and rare occurrences of torticollis secondary to colds. Only one of her relatively constant pains was on the right side, under the right big toe; it was intermittent and aggravated by prolonged standing. She reported scoliosis since adolescence, but no history of low back pain. She had very straight posture, almost rigid, and reported that she was very tense, especially at night.

Apart from these pains, she complained of alternating diarrhea and constipation, rare pains in the right iliac fossa (also on the right side), a feeling of abdominal distention and slow digestion. Her periods were late and scanty, for which she took the hormonal drug dydrogesterone. Her tongue appeared normal, and her pulses were deep (which mirrored her closed attitude).

On her second visit, she told me that she frequently suffered from dyspareunia.

She was married, with no children "for the time being," and described herself as being tied up in knots, and sometimes tending to overreact but not "boiling inside." She had few friends and did not confide much in anyone; she could remember no major traumas either in childhood or later. This patient seemed to be defined by being closed, or rather as failing to open up. She did not feel welcome herself and also did not welcome others; she was closed to them, as well as to her own sexuality.

The symptoms of this patient made me think of the two main channels linked with openness in Chapter 6 of *Basic Questions*, namely the *tai yang* and *tai yin*, primarily the leg channels, as the *yang* pains were on the left and the *yin* pains on the right. Was the origin of the disease *tai yin* or *tai yang*? It was difficult to say *a priori*. The importance of the pain spoke in favor of *tai yang*, but her attitude, her digestive problems, and the dyspareunia suggested *tai yin*. Moreover, *tai yang* and *tai yin* are coupled as far as ascent-descent is concerned: while *tai yin* ascends, *tai yang* descends.

Which points should be needled? To begin with, at least a connecting point responsible for the exterior-interior exchanges. BL-58 and BL-39 are connecting points of the leg *tai yang*. The two connecting points on the leg *tai yin* are SP-4 and SP-7. Why are leg *tai yang* and leg *tai yin* the only channels to have two connecting points? I cannot say. Has it something to do with their opening function?

Two treatments using BL-2 and BL-58, then BL-5 and BL-58, completely failed. It is true that the symptomatology of BL-58 is more reactive, more "skin deep" than this patient presented. I did not needle BL-39, which requires more signs of heat in the pelvis.

I then considered *tai yin*. I needled SP-4, also a key point of the Penetrating vessel, because of the dyspareunia. There was a slight improvement, barely enhanced by the so-called "regulating" pair of SP-3 and SP-4. For lack of a better solution, I decided to treat the other connecting point, SP-7.

From then on, the improvement was evident in both the pains on her left side (headaches, neck and back pains) and in the big toe on the right foot, the digestive problems, and, after the third treatment, the dyspareunia. After four monthly treatments of SP-7, she was basically cured. We pursued maintenance treatments every quarter and then every half year.

CHAPTER SIX

ACUPUNCTURE POINTS

T HE MOST COMMON WORD used to define an acupuncture point is *xue* (穴): a cavern, a dwelling dug in the earth, or a cave. In a mountain, a cavern is the empty space where exterior winds and underground airstreams gather, where the qi of heaven and the qi of earth join and transform themselves; this is where man naturally goes into retreat. As we know, emptiness is the guarantor of a good functioning of the different sorts of qi, of their movements, condensations and transformations. It is most probable that the specific anatomic structure of an acupuncture point will never be revealed for it embodies emptiness. Needling it must be painless. The point is a well. The acupuncture needle goes into it through its hole and goes straight down to the bottom without deviation or going further down. The practitioner, like the calligrapher or the jade engraver, foresees what will come out of the needle and knows when to stop to avoid obstacles, to avoid touching sinews, veins, nerves. The acupuncturist's void matches the emptiness of the point.

Symbolically enough, traditionally (but not completely accurately) there are said to be 365 main acupuncture points, as many as the days in a year. In fact, most books describe 361 points: 218 on the six main yang channels, 91 on the six main yin channels, and 52 on the Governing and Conception vessels. All the regular points are located on either the 12 main bilateral channels or the two median vessels.

Traditionally, each point has one or more names, a location, symptoms, and specific functions.

What Do Acupuncture Points Do?

We do not yet know how acupuncture works. Surely, it can only be neuroendocrinological; but we cannot explain the diversity of effects of the thousands of different possible combinations. All we can do is turn to Chinese tradition and to the notion of qi: linked to form, to manifestation, to the appearance of a form, qi is perhaps in-*form*-ation. Puncturing a point may also enable the body to recall information that it has forgotten or no longer uses for its general functioning because it has become obstructed. Clearly, one should not place too many needles in a patient: the body can understand and perceive what I want to tell it if I provide only a small amount of information that is also coherent; it cannot do so if I inundate it with information in the form of needles. Moreover, these pieces of local, regional or general information must be complementary rather than conflicting. It will be geared to answering the question that is always posed before any enduring pain or symptom: What are the regional and general disturbances that maintain the body and prevent it from being healed? This forces us to try to understand the being as a whole, to look past symptoms and focus on the person, a concept that we will expand upon in our conclusion.

Puncturing (with a needle), heating (with a moxa stick or cone), or massaging (especially for small children) all stimulate a point and its functions. Before puncturing, I massage to familiarize myself with the point, sense the surface opening and the underlying direction. I choose the needle (the diameter and length) according to the depth of the point. With the needle in hand, I clear my mind and center my weight in my pelvis so that the needling motion can occur spontaneously; it is during that suspended moment that I allow needling at the end of exhalation.

To conclude this section, I want to stress the importance of teamwork between the patient and practitioner. The former observes and is precisely aware of the symptoms that have arisen between two sessions; the latter interprets and translates these; it is the soundness of this relationship that makes it possible to find the effective point. Because it is often a 'minor' initial symptom that provides the key, patients must therefore feel they are in a relationship of trust, so that they can say anything without fear of causing trouble or of appearing ridiculous.

Points: Names, Locations, Functions and Symptoms

By tradition, each point has one or more names, a location, symptoms, and functions.

NAMES

The names are significant, even if it is sometimes difficult to understand the reasoning behind them. Certain points even have secondary names that explain their function. The name of CV-5 is Stone Door (*shi men*), and as a foundation stone, it is indicated in breakdowns, when, under certain life circumstances, a person has the feeling that everything is crumbling; in this case, the pulses in both of the proximal positions are deep and broken down as well. GV-3, or Yang Barrier *(yang guan)*, enables the yang qi and the Lung qi to descend to the pelvis, sacrum and lower limbs. LU-2, or Cloud Door *(yun men)*, at the top of the thorax, governs the exit of qi from the Lung upward toward the clouds. BL-58, or Flying Yang *(fei yang)*, makes it possible to keep the qi of leg *tai yang* from 'flying' off the surface, bringing it deeper, toward the leg *shao yin* with which it is paired. In my experience, patients with a dysfunction affecting this point often dream that they are flying away.

Points with the same Chinese character in their names have similar functions. Some examples are points with the characters for spirit *(shen* 神*)*, wind *(feng* 風*)*, pivot *(shu* 樞*)*, and vitals *(huang* 肓 *)* in their names. Thus, the "wind" *(feng* 風*)* points are readily attacked by external wind, and, in the interior (like the wind), facilitate the flow of the different forms of qi in the corresponding areas. These are GV-16, BL-12, SI-12, TB-17, GB-20, and GB-31.

This idea can lead us to research the related functions of groups of points. Not only do points whose names use the word spirit *(shen)* often have psychiatric indications, but so do those with the word divine *(ling* 靈*)*. The *ling* points are HT-2, HT-4, GB-18, KI-24, and GV-10.

The names of the points can help us to understand when they should be needled.

❖ Case History

Mr. N., a smiling, squat, medium-sized 51-year-old man was an Argentinean writer who came to see me in 1993. He left his country in 1981 soon after his father had gone into exile, persecuted by the dictatorial government. His father was a tolerant, human, kind and generous man who died soon after moving to France; he was simply unable to deal with what had happened to his country.

Mr. N. consulted me for pains that were all located on the right side of the body: in the nape of the neck, the trunk, the upper and lower limbs, the hip and the groin. They had been aggravated by a fall ten years previously. He complained of a constant tension in the pelvis. These pains, aggravated by cold, were clearly linked to the weather. The soreness along the pathway of the Yang Linking vessel implied that he should react acutely to all climatic and human environments; this in fact was the case.

He did not complain of other symptoms. He slept well, had a lot of energy, but could not tolerate heat as well as he previously could.

Moreover, he mentioned a huge grief "there, in the chest" since his father's death and exile.

He divorced his wife and had chosen not to have any children, even though it had been a difficult choice to make. This type of issue often involves the Gallbladder, *shao yang*, or Kidneys, *jue yin*.

The first obvious point to needle was TB-5 as the opening point for the Yang Linking vessel. It seemed wise to needle another point in connection with Argentina, for TB-5 did not take into account the depression and the grief constrained in the interior. I then chose CV-18, a point linked to the arm *jue yin* because of its pairing with the arm *shao yang* in an exterior-interior relationship. This is a major point linked to the *jue yin* as a node (based on Chapter 5 of *Divine Pivot*), especially in connection with family lineage; it also connects with a compression of the energy in the chest. After two monthly treatments using TB-5 and CV-18, the improvement was quite noticeable. The pains nearly disappeared and the psychological state of the patient was gradually improving.

The patient came back six months later, complaining of frontal headaches; in addition, "grief and tears are buried; I cry silent tears." Two points have "close to tears" or "cries silently" in their names: GB-15 and GB-41. I chose GB-41, the opening point of the Girdle vessel, coupled with TB-5. The headaches disappeared within 48 hours.

Three months later he came back with a severe urticaria that had started eight days before. Had he eaten some kind of fish that triggers urticaria? In fact, he already suffered from this condition as a child but could not think of a triggering factor. To be coherent, I chose another point of the *shao yang*, GB-31, very much indicated in cases of pruritus. The effect was immediate.

He consulted again eight months later. On a physical level, he was well, apart from a frequent sensation of closure in the chest. But fear had not left him and "the ancestors are present." First his grandfather had "died, lost in the forest, wandering, and was never buried," and then his father had died a long way from home. Which points refer to the ancestors? TB-7 and SI-11. Of course, I chose TB-7, located on the arm *shao yang*. Two months later, he could feel that his chest was opening and fear was going away. I needled this point once more three months later, after which he said, "Now, our journey is over." Note how, in his evolution and personal journey, I always followed the course of the *shao yang* as the main thread of my choices.

LOCATION

Each point located on one of the primary channels, or the Governing or Conception vessel, is defined by a location with points of reference found on the skin, bones, muscles, etc. For example, CV-6 is on the abdomen, 1.5 units below the navel, along the midline. BL-25 is in the loins, or lower back, vertically located between the 4th and 5th lumbar vertebrae and horizontally at 2 units from GV-3. TB-10 is at the elbow, 1 unit above the olecranon. ST-41 is at the center of the anterior ankle crease. ST-4 is on the face, at the height of the mouth's labial commissures, directly underneath the pupil when the patient is looking straight ahead. Once the area has been defined, we have to locate each point precisely, by massaging the depression in which it is located to determine the corresponding special skin texture, the opening, its direction and depth, and, in a manner of speaking, to ask for permission to puncture it.

Here I report a case that shows how the anatomic or energetic location of a point can be a useful guide.

❖ Case History

Mrs. G., age 56, was a midwife who consulted for "a lack of drive and enthusiasm." "I'm sinking," she said. She complained of a sensation of epigastric heaviness and oppression radiating to the back, between the shoulder blades. Her back and her shoulders felt heavy. Her chest felt closed. The onset of these symptoms coincided with the menopause. She had few other symptoms apart from occasional bouts of hypertension, but her underlying blood pressure, checked three times a day, was normal (135/75 mmHg). Her sleep was satisfactory. The first time she came, her proximal pulses, as well as the KI-3 pulses, were deep. Her married life was difficult: "the situation is not ideal but bearable; we each live our own life; we share the same views on the children's education." Her father died young in Poland, and her mother had left this country when she was a teenager, and, as a Jew, had to live hidden for several years. "Maybe it can explain why I do not like to be seen?" she asked … and also why her chest and shoulders were closed.

On her first visit, I needled CV-5 to treat the fact she felt she was "sinking." Why did I not choose CV-3 or CV-4 or CV-7? She had no urinary problems or constipation requiring the use of CV-3; there were no signs linked to the Penetrating vessel, no fatigue or cold requiring CV-4; and there were no symptoms related to the lower burner that could justify needling CV-7.

After I had needled CV-5, she felt tired for three days, but then felt a bit more lively. Maybe she was "sinking" a bit less. The KI-3 pulses were back to normal.

I still had to open the closed chest, which can be done with some points on the *tai yin*, *yang ming*, Conception and Governing vessels. Nothing in this pattern called for the *tai yin* or the *yang ming*. When I asked her, "Do you feel that you always want to control everything?" she answered, "Yes, very much so," which stressed the role of the Governing vessel, the function of which is to control. I chose to needle the Governing vessel point which opens the chest, GV-10, located between T6 and T7. The improvement was remarkable, including a marked decrease in the sinking sensation and the feeling of heaviness in the epigastrium, the back and the shoulders. The patient was obviously much more cheerful. Two other treatments using this point reinforced this result. The origin of the disorder could be linked both to the absence of the deceased father (because of the relationship between *tai yang,* the Governing vessel and the father) and to the fact that her mother did her best to stay hidden, especially during the war.

SYMPTOMS

Symptoms of various types are attributed to each point. For example, for LU-1 there is chronic impairment of the nose, throat, lungs and bronchi; anorexia, vomiting, particularly during coughing fits, coldness in the diaphragm, edema on the face or the four limbs; shoulder and back pains; and insomnia with awakening around 3 a.m.

Certain points are connected with psychological or behavioral signs, such as "insanity, raving, seeing the devil, spasmodic laughter, logorrhea, confabulation, convulsions combined with fear"[1] for LI-5. Others are associated with dreams: apart from the usual intestinal, urinary, gynecological, and lumbar signs, GV-5 is also associated with "snake dreams."[2] All of this information is useful in clinical examinations.

❖ Case History

In a case that was previously presented (see p. 34), a young woman presented with uterine bleeding that had continued for 18 months. Surgical intervention was envisaged. After an initial session where I punctured a thoracic point she dreamed of "two wooden snakes fighting a duel," which led me to realize that her combined symptoms corresponded to GV-5, Suspension [and] Pivot (*xuan shu*), which causes the qi to rise from the pelvis to the upper body, thus releasing certain excesses from the true pelvis. The bleeding (which was due to the fact that the qi in excesses can push the blood out of its normal paths of circulation) ceased within 12 hours and did not recur.

The lists of signs attributed to each point by Chinese tradition are not restrictive. Furthermore, in the West we have found indications and symptoms that are not, to our knowledge, described in the Chinese literature. For example, LR-11 is remarkably effective for certain sacroiliac and sciatica pains although, as far as I know, these symptoms are not included in the Chinese repertory for this point. KI-27 is one of the most effective points for pain on the front side of the shoulder and of the upper limbs, as well as in allergic rhinitis (hay fever). In my experience, a dysfunction in BL-58 often results in dreams of flying.

WHICH POINT FOR WHICH FUNCTION

Functions are attributed to certain points. These include the actions of the alarm points of the Gallbladder for GB-23 and GB-24; treating yang deficiency in the lower parts of the body for GV-3 ; treating the origins of Conception vessel qi for CV-20 and Governing vessel qi for GV-7; and the intersection of the Kidney, Spleen and Heart for CV-23.

Other points belong to groups that define their properties. There are general command points at the extremities of the limbs, from the elbows to the hands and from the knees to the feet. Each yin channel has five transport points (*wu shu xue*)—well, spring, stream, river, sea—that regulate all activities of the channel and synchronizes them, at each moment, with the cosmic energies. Each yang channel also has, in addition to these five points, a sixth source *(yuan)* point that refers to the origin of the channel's qi. All have points for tonification and draining and dispersion.

As I have so far mainly focused my attention on specific points instead of point groupings, I tend to use transport points less often than most of my colleagues. That having been said, these are the cases in which I do choose them: first, relying on their specific properties, I can turn to one of these five points to reinforce the action of a particular point. For example, the well point is located where the channel starts: "The well point is responsible for all that begins" (*Classic of Difficulties*, No. 16). I needle it when I want to 'sweep' the channel, that is, to act on the entire channel. I also needle well points so that afterwards new symptoms will appear to guide me toward the points to needle next.

❖ Case History

Mrs. M., age 39, was a Spanish teacher and a tango singer. She was small, thin and lively, and one day, at 1 p.m., she asked for an emergency appointment, as she had to sing at 9 that evening and had been suffering from a hoarse voice since the previous evening. She had no fever, her nose was not running, and she did not cough. This is something that happened fairly frequently to her, although no triggering cause, infectious or not, could be identified. In any case, she was prone to frequent nasopharyngitis and hoarseness. Her tonsils had been removed when she was a child.

She reported a long-term intestinal frailty with painful attacks of diarrhea three times a year, and intolerance to cow's milk.She was nervous, quick-tempered, sensitive, impatient, suffered from bruxism and felt very tense, experiencing at that time a frequent sensation of cold in the nape of the neck and the back. Her sleep was also fragile as she had difficulties falling asleep or frequently woke up during the night at the slightest noise. She had no recurring dreams or nightmares.

Her pulses were normal. Her tongue had a white coating at the root.

The implication of the arm *yang ming* seemed likely with both nasopharyngeal and intestinal problems. The main point responsible for sudden hoarseness on this channel is LI-18. Which other points of the arm *yang ming* have acute hoarseness in their indications? LI-4, LI-10, and LI-17, but LI-10 was not implicated in patients with all of these neurological, painful dental and intestinal signs; and LI-17 was a possibility but the hoarseness of the voice linked to this point usually appears in a context of inflammation, of laryngitis and of a painful sore throat making drinking and eating difficult, which was not the case here. I then needled LI-18 and added, because of the urgent need, LI-4 to reinforce its action. She was able to sing that night as usual.

Sometimes I use the correspondences with the five phases. As mentioned above in the discussion of the main channels, in desynchronization syndromes, I first use the tonification or draining points. Then, in acute cases due to external pathogenic qi, like a common cold, I use the correspondences between these five points and the external pathogenic qi, like the spring point corresponding to heat in the yin channels and to cold in the yang channels. I then tonify the spring point to bring heat to a yin channel invaded by cold.

Following the *Classic of Difficulties*, No. 74, as a preventive treatment I will sometimes regulate an organ by needling the well point in spring, the spring point in summer, the river point in autumn and the sea point in winter, adding the stream point at the end of each season.

It also happens, when I want a more global effect on the organs, that I treat the yin organs using the spring and stream points of its channel, and the sea point on the corresponding yang organ channel.

But most of the time, as often as possible, I needle the specific points that are discussed below, as I consider them to be more precise and more efficient.

❖ Case History

Mrs. J., age 40, consulted me for hyperthyroidism diagnosed two years before. Her daily prescriptions were avlocardyl (a beta blocker), tranxene (a benzodiazepine), and neomercazole (an antihyperthyroid medication). Her symptoms were classic ones: a small goiter, bilateral exophthalmia, slight tremors, tachycardia, weight loss, and aggravation of an old diarrhea pattern. The history revealed a pronounced weakness after physical effort, some hypersomnia, a frequent stifling sensation in the throat, significant hair loss, long-term diarrhea with loose stools but no pain or distention and no special food intolerance, and an inability to vent her anger. Her tongue was slightly trembling. Her pulses were rapid and moderately empty at both right and left proximal positions.

I diagnosed a Yin Heel pattern, as it is responsible for some types of hypersomnia where the yang cannot communicate with yin, here secondary to the fact that yin cannot ascend. The empty proximal pulses were in favor of this diagnosis.

Moreover, the exophthalmia, tremors, loose stools, trembling tongue and the inability to express anger manifested a constraint of the Liver organ or of the leg *jue yin* channel. This channel corresponds to wind and anger, goes through the eyeballs and guides to the head the yin coming from the lower part of the body, from the feet and the pelvis, with the help of a window-of-heaven point, SI-17, which, like all the points belonging to this category, governs the neck area.

Three factors were then involved: the Yin Heel, which could not anchor the pelvis; an obstruction of the *jue yin,* with the inability to vent anger; and a dysfunction of the window-of-heaven point SI-17, with the goiter. Consequently, the treatment was a bilateral needling of KI-6, a key point and the starting point of the Yin Heel; LR-6, an accumulation point favoring the 'dis-obstruction' of the leg *jue yin*; and SI-17.

This patient was given three treatments one week apart, three treatments two weeks apart, and then three sessions once a month, followed by one treatment every three months. After the fourth session, the fatigue, diarrhea, and hypersomnia had disappeared so she could stop taking the tranxene. After the sixth session, she stopped the avlocardyl, as her tachycardia had disappeared and did not return. After the eighth session (three months of treatment), she noticed a deep improvement and began to cut down the neomercazole. She still could not express her anger. The exophthalmia had receded on the left, although her hyperthyroidism was better.

Other points are said to be specific. They have special functions: the associated and alarm points govern certain aspects of the yin organs; the eight meeting points open the eight extraordinary vessels; the barrier points control the circulation of qi to the joints; the window-of-heaven points link the head to the trunk; the four connecting points in the group cause yin qi to rise from the four limbs and bring down yang from the body. There are eight meeting points described: for qi (CV-17), blood (BL-17), vessels (LU-9), sinews (GB-34), yin organs (LR-13), yang organs (CV-12), bones (BL-11), and marrow (GB-39). Thanks to this function, the action of GB-39 in improving tolerance to chemotherapy has been understood. There are other groups of specific points that I myself do not use, such as the four seas (*Divine Pivot,* Chapter 33).

Let's take the example of the Lung. In addition to being the master of qi, Chinese medicine endows it with several functions including directing downward and clarifying the qi and fluids, as well as autumnal gathering and spreading. To me, the Lung as master of the qi is related to the back points, which are associated with the corporal soul made alive, that is, BL-42, BL-13 (the Lung back associated point) and GV-12 on the midline. Its downward-directing function is devoted to KI-27, and the function of clearing to KI-26. The autumnal gathering is governed by LU-1, an alarm point. The spreading is governed by LU-2, Cloud Gate, a door that opens onto the exterior, the skin, the clouds, etc.

It is the same on a symbolic level. The Lung is the roof of the organs and is related to the order of heaven, as we shall see more precisely in the chapter on symbolism. I see the Lung as being endowed with the qualities of heaven: purity, justice, and both dissociation from the One and reunification, or return, to the One. Purification and the clarifying of qi and fluids correspond to KI-26. Justice and, pathologically, an oversensitivity to injustice[3] correspond to KI-22. Reunification and relationship with unity is linked to a median point, CV-20 *(hua gai)*—or Splendid Canopy, where canopy *(gai* 蓋*)* refers to a covering like a roof where the two sides join together.

❖ Case History

Mrs. C., age 39, slightly plump, who was smiling but looked tense, with an apparent ease for expressing herself, consulted for anxiety attacks accompanied by a sensation of oppression in the chest, a feeling of cold, and tremors. The symptoms started when she was 20 and were much worse when she was driving. She said she was irritable and prone to fits of tears. She could not think of any disturbing events that had occurred when she was 20, but reported that she had been left with her grandmother from birth until she was two. When she consulted, she was a married woman with two daughters; she was happy and did not understand the reason behind these anxiety attacks.

On a physical level, she reported a weakness of the lungs, mainly of allergic origin, a pain in the right thumb along the arm *tai yin*, a pain in the right shoulder along the arm *tai yin* and arm *yang ming*, and frequent rashes affecting the face and the neck. Her body was often swollen and she used to wake up at three in the morning, but there were no other significant symptoms.

Her history included two instances of pneumonia. One of them, a year earlier, had been triggered by "a huge" injustice. No doubt the Lung was involved, maybe because of the separation she experienced when she was born. Which Lung points should we choose?

LU-1, an alarm point, is related to mourning, to grief, and could treat the irritability and the rashes of the face and neck, the edemas and the waking at 3 a.m. It is the emblematic point of the autumnal harvest. It seemed well suited here.

The back associated point, BL-13, is more focused on acute patterns. LU-2 deals with a sensation of fullness in the chest, frequent sighing, repressed anger and peripheral heat signs. It did not seem to fit in this picture. KI-27 directs Lung qi downward, and when dysfunctional, there is fullness above with such symptoms as allergic rhinitis, asthma, pains in the anterior part of the shoulder and severe insomnia. It did not seem to be indicated in this case either.

As far as the aspect of the Lung as the roof of the organs is concerned, CV-20 is used when separations that should have happened do not occur, for example, to cut all ties with the energy of the mother.

BL-42 stores up the essence of the Lung and links it to the corporeal soul, to the "entering and exiting," and, to begin with, to "exiting from life and entering death." It was a possible choice.

GV-12 is related to the desire to kill people, to madness, to hallucinations and raving. There are no signs suggesting that it could be applied here. To me, KI-26 is the point that clarifies the qi and fluids of the Lung, but this patient had no phlegm or turbidity.

I started by needling LU-1, but it did not bring any improvement other than a little less irritability and her sensation of oppression was very slightly reduced.

On her second visit, the patient told me about her enormous dread of madness, of the "intense fear she might become mad." Yet nothing either in her family history or in her own life could justify this fear and she had always refused to seek a psychotherapist's help. I then needled BL-42, which did not bring any modification in her symptoms.

On her third visit, she told me of the utmost fear she had when her husband was not with her. She would sometimes imagine that she would be prostrated, feel suffocated, sweat all over, and have a tremendous fear she might want to harm her children and would be unable to stop herself. GV-12 then became the obvious point to needle (its indications include the fear of not being able to control oneself). A trust-based relationship had to be established before she could confess to this "shameful" symptom. From then on, the improvement was noticeable. Three other sessions allowed for reinforcing the results, after which she was well enough to decide she did not need more treatments. She still comes back with her daughters from time to time.

❖ Case History

Mrs. P., age 39, was a receptionist. She was full of energy, active, friendly, impulsive, quick-tempered, and fairly plump. She came to me for significant alopecia on the temporal and frontal areas that had started four-and-a-half years previously. It had not responded to any treatment and compelled her to wear a wig. Together with the alopecia, she had sweating of the hands together with solar plexus anxiety attacks which stifled her, made her agitated and besides herself, and with which she could not cope. From time to time she also had palpitations.

Moreover, her skin had been very sensitive ever since she was 22, when she had suffered from patches of itchy eczema that had never completely cleared; they were mainly located on the elbows, knees, hands and feet. The history showed everything else was normal, including her sleep. She was happily married and had two children, ages 9 and 3.

The alopecia started after she had undergone two stressful events: first the death of her best friend's daughter, who died of a brain tumor at the age of 8; and then an important disagreement at work with her boss and some colleagues. After this, she had had less drive.

Her tongue looked normal. Her distal pulses were deeper on the left side than on the right.

What are the mechanisms ruling the skin in Chinese medicine? The *tai yang* governs the exterior and points on its arm (e.g., the connecting point SI-7) and leg (BL-40 among others) channels. Heat from the *yang ming*, Lung and Heart can also reach the skin. I first thought of the Heart because of the anxiety, the palpitations and the pulses, because of its exterior-interior connection with the

Small Intestine (arm *tai yang*), and because this highly reactive woman who could become beside herself with anxiety suggested a disharmony between the Heart and the Small Intestine, together with a disrupted communication between the two channels. I needled the connecting point of the arm *tai yang*, SI-7 (which also governs the skin), and HT-4, a *ling* point well suited to her lack of drive and her anxiety. The eczema improved but then came back, as did the anxiety and the lack of drive; the alopecia and the moist hands remained unchanged after the first two sessions. In addition, a big quarrel at work did not help.

On her third visit, I considered treating the leg *tai yang*, particularly BL-58, a connecting point that is indicated for very edgy people who are very quick-tempered. After doing so the eczema disappeared, as did the sweating; she was less touchy, but the alopecia and the anxiety were still unchanged, even with the addition of BL-40 during the fourth session.

I then came to think that I might have misunderstood the distal pulses, especially as the alopecia was accompanied by a sensation of oppression and not by palpitations and tachycardia; I realized that the deepest pulse was not the Heart pulse, but the Lung pulse, which was more wiry. I then asked myself: Which feeling or sensation has been the strongest when she had to face these traumas? The answer was immediate: injustice. KI-22 regulates the expression and dissemination function of the Lung and responds very specifically to injustice. After I had needled it for the first time, the patient noticed that her hair had started growing again and that she felt much more relaxed. I then added BL-58, a connecting point on the leg *tai yang*, which had already been needled during the third and fourth sessions, for the leg *tai yang* and the leg *shao yin* are coupled in an exterior-interior relationship. It was thought that facilitating the communication between the leg *tai yang* and the leg *shao yin* in this reactive and edgy patient would reinforce the action of KI-22. Each time she came afterward, once every two weeks, she confirmed that she was improving at all levels. After a fifth treatment using KI-22 and BL-58, she was nearly cured.

WHICH POINT FOR EACH PATIENT

The functions and indications of the point or points should cover most of the patient's symptoms, match their typology, behavior, history and life, as well as their self-perceptions. Rarely, in acute cases, this may be a symptomatic point for the purpose of providing relief, although experience shows that the point that treats the person is always, even in acute cases, more effective than a predetermined formula. It may be a point that restores the qi that has been lost or expended or else a deficiency of blood or insufficient fluids, because nothing can be regulated if there is a general state of deficiency. It may also be a general point that corrects all of the disrupted mechanisms or, even better, a point that translates the practitioner's perception of the patient at this given moment.

This depends on what the patient is seeking, the knowledge and orientation of the acupuncturist and the relations established between the patient and the practitioner.

One principle seems fundamental to me. The practitioner should not anticipate; his task is to respond to the body's needs, because the body, with its given symptoms, asks for treatment of the points needed at this particular moment. This is true for each and every session.

To conclude this section, I want to stress the importance of teamwork between the patient and practitioner: the former observes and is precisely aware of the symptoms that have arisen between two sessions; the latter interprets and translates these into a point. It is the soundness of this relationship that makes it possible to find the effective point, because it is often a "minor" initial symptom that provides the key. Patients must therefore feel they are in a relationship of trust such that they can say anything without fear of causing trouble or of appearing ridiculous.

Stimulating Selected Points

❖ Case History

Mr. C., age 50, a civil servant and weekend marathon runner, came to see me for a pain in the right foot that had appeared fourteen months before without apparent cause, located on the leg *tai yin* Spleen channel between SP-3 and SP-5 and, at the height of the attacks, radiating along the leg *yang ming* Stomach channel from ST-36 to ST-45. Climate, cold, heat, and change of shoes had no effect. This pain usually appeared at the 15th kilometer of his weekly long run, forcing him to quit. A rheumatologist, physiotherapist, osteopath, and podiatrist were all unable to obtain any improvement. Given the absence of local factors, I investigated the possible causes of this pain in acupuncture terms: Stomach and Spleen and the leg *yang ming* and leg *tai yin* channels. There was no digestive pain or other symptom that would permit me to implicate one of these mechanisms.

For the moment, I was perplexed and moved on to the general examination. The history did not turn up any other symptoms. This married man, a father of three girls, and sometimes jazz musician, claimed to be perfectly happy. The tongue was unremarkable and had no coating.

But when I took his pulse, I was surprised. The pulse was impalpable, which showed that he had 'broken down' at some point in his life. The man was astonished, and confirmed this diagnosis. Eleven years before, he "went through hell" with his second girl, who experienced a terrible anxiety neurosis (still unresolved) and he was smoking hashish to escape his malaise. The family was taken completely by surprise and was unable to understand this crisis. In such a case, the pelvic point indicated is CV-5, "Stone Door," which, when punctured, helps rebuild the individual's grounding—a psychological and energetic foundation.

How does this explain the pain in the foot? The feet, like the pelvis, are a foundation, a support. A pelvic deficiency is often the cause of pain in the feet. And what explains the location on the *yang ming* and *tai yin* channels? The dissociation between the outward appearance—the happy marathon runner, jazz musician, father and husband—and the inward suffering that he repressed and could not explore. It so happens that *yang ming* and *tai yin* link the external to the internal, such as the outward appearance and the inner experience.

I punctured, on the right, the points that connect these two channels, SP-3 and ST-40. The first session, after 48 hours of intense fatigue, resulted in a clear improvement in the foot; according to the patient's estimate, about a 40 percent improvement. The second session completely eradicated the pain, which still had not returned fifteen months later. His overall condition was better too; he feels "much more relaxed."

One of the conclusions that may be drawn from this case history is that we need to remember to ignore the symptom and pay attention to the person.

Note: A brief description of the categories and indications for all the points discussed in any depth in this book can be found in Appendix One.

Weave of Points

I would like to call attention to the immense weaving that is created by the acupuncture points. We have seen examples of this throughout the book: they constantly interact with one another. This hints at the architecture of the human body described by Chinese medicine that emerges through the points, with each point representing a convergence of information and the sum of this information assuming control of the functioning of our lives.

An example is CV-5 (*shi men,* "Stone Door"), a foundation (concerned in cases of breakdown), the alarm point of the Triple Burner and therefore of our nutrition; it also controls the gestational envelopes that take part in our perpetuation. In fact, it is responsible for maintaining life.

It also mediates between the original qi of the Kidneys (*yuan qi*) that emerges at CV-4 *guan yuan*; it is also a main point of the Penetrating vessel (opened by SP-4), and of the body qi produced under the control of CV-6, the "Sea of Qi."

We should note that there are two points of the leg *shao yin* Kidney channel at the same level as CV-4 and CV-5—these are KI-13 and KI-14—and that SP-14 is at the level of CV-6. All of these take part in the dialogue between Kidneys-origin and Spleen-life. CV-5 interacts with GV-5 and shares with it the role of a mediator. Above GV-4 (*ming men,* literally "Life Gate" or "Gate of Vitality"), which is the gate to our own *ming men* and prenatal energy, GV-5 brings up the qi from the Kidneys, the root of production of the five organs, from the level of the prenatal origin toward the other viscera, beginning with the Spleen, the minister of the granary, which is the level of the post-natal qi at

GV-6. Here again, the dialogue between the Kidneys and Spleen is at work. Furthermore, at the same level of GV-5 on the back, we find the back associated point of the Triple Burner, BL-22, which, as explained before, has a mediatory function; and also BL-51, a *huang* point that helps govern lactation. Below GV-4 is GV-3, which pertains to the Large Intestine, the Kidneys and the pelvic envelope, and it receives the qi sent down by the Lung via CV-20.

Thus, a point should not be viewed in isolation. We have to create a dialogue with one or several other points to understand it better. Let's consider, for example, GV-26 and CV-9.

GV-26

Its name is 水溝 *shui gou,* which means "Water Ditch." Its other standard name is 人中 *ren zhong,* meaning human being and middle, the "Middle of Man." Both of these terms relate to its anatomical position in the philtrum. It also has three less common names, all of which include the character 鬼 *gui,* meaning ghost, this being the earthly dialectic to the heavenly spirit.

Its indication is as a resuscitation point; it brings the soul back into the body, it reestablishes the relationship between yin and yang when their separation has induced a loss of consciousness. It is indicated for epileptic seizures; it treats delusions, madness with agitation, mania, fright or hysteria. According to its functional indications, it revives consciousness and sedates the mind. Among the other problems it treats are eye disorders, loss of taste, glossitis, intense thirst, diabetes, jaundice, pain and stiffness of the spine, and low back pain.

Located at the junction of the upper third and lower two thirds of the philtrum, it is between the nose, which welcomes the heavenly qi, and the mouth, which welcomes the fruits of the earth. It therefore relates to man.

In *taijiquan* and Daoist meditation, it is the great circle, the end of the Governing vessel and its junction with the Conception vessel. This allows it to be seen as the junction of heaven and earth, or anterior and posterior heaven.

It relates to both Intestines: it is located along the arm *yang ming* channel, at the contralateral meeting point, between LI-18 and LI-19. The *Systematic Classic of Acupuncture and Moxibustion* says that it is on the arm *yang ming* channel, and not on the Governing vessel. In the same book it is said that one can judge the state of the Small Intestine "by the length of the philtrum and the thickness of the lips."

CV-9

Located on the midline, 1 unit above the navel, CV-9 is called *shui fen* 水分; *shui* means "water" and *fen* means "to divide, to separate, to spread, to distinguish," and most importantly, "a share, the share that falls to each of us."

The *Classic of Difficulties*, No. 44, states: "The Large and Small Intestines meet at the screened gate, (*lan men* 闌門)," which I take to be level with CV-9.

It is said that this point corresponds to the separation of food into fluids (going to the Bladder) and solids (going to the bowels) and, in the case of the Large Intestine, the separation into pure and impure fluids.

Its indications comprise:

- a sunken fontanel or a fontanel that does not close properly

- abdominal disorders with diarrhea

- ascites and edema

- stiffness and contraction of the spine or of the lumbar area
  (similar to GV-26)

In the case of edema, the efficacy of this point, whether needled or treated with moxa, is unclear to me; in any case, any effects are short-lived.

Common Characteristics

Both GV-26 and CV-9 are related to the Large Intestine and Small Intestine.

Both are points with the word "water" in their names.

They share the same topology, as both are close to some sort of navel, as are all the others points in this section. Indeed, if we consider the head and the trunk as representing heaven-man-earth, the navel is in the middle, separating the epigastrium (man) and the pelvis (earth); the thorax being celestial. In the same way, the philtrum, where GV-26 lies, is between the upper part of the face, together with the eyes, the nose and the ears (man), and the lower part of the mouth and chin (earth), with the skull being celestial.

Differences

It seems to me that CV-9 separates, puts everything back in the right place as always, when the pure and the impure are mentioned.

GV-26 unites: soul and body, yin and yang, the Governing and Conception vessels, and beyond this, the resonances of heaven and earth.

❖ Case History

Miss P., age 32, was small, plump, and apparently quiet, and she did not speak much when she first came, although this changed on subsequent visits. She sought help for tobacco addiction, but the history revealed she had been suffering from severe anxiety attacks since the age of 15. She felt knots in the solar plexus and was chilled, often had loose stools and constantly experienced embarrassment. She could not say what triggered the attacks, but she knew for sure that it all began after a distressing and prolonged series of maxillofacial treatments for dental problems. She took half a Déroxat (paroxetine, an antidepressant) tablet every evening and had been seeing a psychotherapist for 18 months. She stated that her childhood, while "by no means joyful," had not been painful or difficult. She slept well and did not lack drive.

On the whole, she was in good health except for recurring back pains; she did not suffer from scoliosis, lower back pains or neck pains. These thoracic pains, in the absence of scoliosis or other vertebral aches and pains, were due to solar plexus anxiety attacks. I find that this etiology of back pains is a frequent one.

The examination did not show anything special. Her proximal pulses were deep but the KI-3 pulses were full, which suggested that some type of qi could not descend. The maxillofacial treatments that had taken place just before the anxiety attacks started, even though these went on for 17 years, had blocked the descent of qi in the face in the area of GV-26, which, as seen before, governs the descent of the energy.

I therefore needled this point. During the following 48 hours her anxiety attacks intensified and she was so disconnected from the world that she "did not touch the ground." But on the next day, both her anxiety attacks and her back pains had disappeared. They did not come back, even after she discontinued Déroxat. She felt "more firmly on the ground than before."

She returned some weeks later for her tobacco addiction treatment, which I had decided to postpone when she first came. We know the relationship between GV-26 and the arm *yang ming*. To be consistent, I chose the arm *yang ming* channel point at the level of GV-26, which is LI-19, and added a connecting point, LI-6, governing the relationships with the exterior. She quit smoking easily after two sessions.

Remember that, for every patient, we need to determine the two or three points indicated at the time of their visit, that is, the two or three pieces of information that are no longer circulating in the body's economy.

Barrier Points

INTRODUCTION

These are of great practical importance, especially in cases of pain. In my book *Acupuncture*, I defined the barrier points as those that encouraged the circulation of qi, in three stages, throughout the body: in the limbs, the head, and the trunk. This idea has proven very useful to many practitioners over the years.

These barrier points are often located near the joints where they allow the yin and yang qi to come out of the trunk and into the roots of the limbs, reaching the extremities, and then return. They also control the exchanges between the face and skull, in both directions. Likewise, they control the ascent and descent of the yin and yang qi in the trunk, between the thorax and the pelvis. The same is true throughout the body. I will provide a few typical examples here.

Obstruction of these points results in a blockage of the flow of qi, with excesses upstream, deficiencies downstream, and repercussions on the channel where the concerned point is located.

The diagnosis of deficiency or excess of yin or yang qi is made on the basis of three characteristics:

1. type of pain
2. response to local pressure
3. response to local application of heat or cold

So we can see that:

- Pain caused by an excess of yin is of the yin type, aggravated by local pressure (because it is an excess) and improved by local heat (yang).
- Pain caused by a deficiency of yin is of the yang type, improved by pressure and by cold.
- Pain caused by an excess of yang is of the yang type, aggravated by local pressure and improved by local cold.
- Pain caused by a yang deficiency is of the yin type, improved by pressure and heat.

All types of excesses are aggravated by rest (during which the qi accumulates) and are improved by activity (during which the qi is dispersed). The opposite is true of problems due to deficiency (*see* Table 4).

Pain can be due in some cases simply to qi not moving in a particular part of the body. For these cases we use the term stagnation. The diagnosis of stagnation is made on the basis of improvement with movement, massage and heat. There can be yin stagnation (with yin-type pain) or yang stagnation (with yang-type pain). This is the only case where a yang pain is improved by heat.

BARRIER CONCEPT

This problem has never been thoroughly studied and we have only found three references to it in classical Chinese texts. The most important is in Chapter 71 of the *Divine Pivot*, which states, "If there is a pathogen in the Lung and Heart, its qi lingers in the two elbows. If there is a pathogen in the Liver, its qi flows into the two axillae. If there is a pathogen in the Spleen, its qi lingers in the two hips. If there is a pathogen in the Kidneys, its qi lingers in the two popliteal fossae." We have based our schema on this passage, with some modifications.

The barrier concept implies that there is a physiological stagnation of qi at the joints. We need to apply a qualitative dialectic to the joint barriers where qi is stagnat-

Table 4: Barrier Point Diagnosis	
PARAMETER	CHARACTERISTIC
Yin-Yang	**Yin** · dull, continuous, deep pain
	Yang · sharp, intense, superficial pain
Cold-Hot	**Cold** · better with heat, worse with cold
	Hot · better with cold, worse with heat
Deficiency-Excess	**Deficiency** · better with pressure
	Excess · worse with pressure
Stagnation	Better with movement, local massage, heat

ing, that is, we need to relate this dialectic to three terms (*tai, shao, jue/ming*) at the three articulations of the limbs: shoulder, elbow and wrist for the arm; hip, knee and ankle for the leg.

Of course, we must apply this to each limb at the yin and yang exits from the trunk to the extremities and at the yin and yang entrance points from the extremities into the trunk.

Thus, yang qi emerging is one of the following:

- *tai yang*, the most characteristic (greatest)—supreme at the shoulder and at the hip, the joints that are closest to the trunk
- *shao yang*, intermediate—at the middle joints, elbow and knee
- *yang ming*, least characteristic—at the joints of the extremities, the wrist and ankle

Incoming yang qi is one of these:

- *tai yang*, because it is highly characteristic, at the distal joints, wrist and ankle
- *shao yang* at the intermediate joints, elbow and knee
- *yang ming* in the proximal joints, shoulder and hip

Likewise, the yin qi that goes out is:

- *tai yin* in the shoulders and hips
- *shao yin* in the elbows and knees
- *jue yin* in the wrists and ankles

Incoming yin qi is:

- *tai yin* in the wrists and ankles

- *shao yin* in the elbows and knees
- *jue yin* in the shoulders and hips

It is understood that Chapter 71 of the *Divine Pivot* is referring to the quality of the incoming or outgoing qi, and not to the corresponding organ.

This text associates:

- the Spleen (leg *tai yin* channel) with the hip, where the qi that exits is more characteristic, and therefore *tai yin*
- the Kidney (leg *shao yin* channel) with the knee, where the qi that exits is *shao yin*
- the Lung (arm *tai yin* channel) with the shoulder, where the exiting qi is the most characteristic and therefore *tai yin*
- the Heart (arm *shao yin* channel) with the elbow, where the qi becomes *shao yin*

We have moved successively from a dialectical quality of qi to a channel with the same name, and then to the corresponding organs.

As we have already said, these phenomena impact the primary channels of the same names, on the upper or lower extremities, depending on the specific channel involved. So, for example, the yin exit at the hip, *tai yin*, affects leg *tai yin*; the yang entrance at the shoulder, *yang ming*, affects arm *yang ming*, and so forth, and this is both physiological and pathological. In this way, a blockage in the yin exit at the hip, for example, can lead to an accumulation of yin upstream, a deficiency of yin downstream, and a painful impact on leg *tai yin*. Likewise, an obstruction of the incoming yang at the shoulder triggers a buildup of yang upstream, a deficiency below, and a painful impact on arm *yang ming*. One can easily see the diagnostic usefulness of these concepts and they also have considerable therapeutic significance.

The diagnosis of an excess is not based solely on manual pressure. The pressure may be broader, such as a bra, belt, or collar, but also coughing or the pushing required for a bowel movement. Likewise for deficiencies: an abdominal deficiency due to a yin deficiency may, for example, be improved by pressure on the stomach, but also by coughing, during sexual intercourse, or before a menstrual period. It will be aggravated during and after the period, as in the case of defecation. For headaches, pressure on the eyes will reveal whether there is a deficiency or excess.

We will define the points that govern the passage of these joint barriers using the fundamental concept that a phenomenon impacts the channel to which it is dialectically linked, and emerges at some point along this channel.

Taking a careful history is the primary way of understanding whether or not the barrier concept should be used and which points are most appropriate. Range of motion exams contribute little here while palpation is primarily concerned with whether the area is hot (yang) or cold (yin). The history can tell us where the pain is, which channel or channels it radiates along, whether it is improved by the local application of cold, heat and pressure, and finally how the pain is affected by movement or the lack thereof. This allows us to diagnose empty, fullness or stagnation of yin or yang and to deduce the relevant point barrier. If cold, heat, pressure or movement do not affect the pain, the barrier approach will not be helpful.

BARRIER COMMAND POINTS

These points command the entry and exit of yin and yang qi at the level of the joints that serve as barriers to the flow of qi. From this perspective, we can look at each of the four limbs and their subsets of joints with the more superior in every context being yang and the more inferior yin.

Altogether there are seven joints, divided into two groups of four and three. The legs and arms each have four basic sets of joints and they are preceded by three major joint areas:

• proximal: shoulders and hips

• intermediate: elbows and knees

• distal: wrists and ankles

The limbs must connect with the trunk: the qi goes from the trunk to the extremities and, inversely, returns from the hands and feet to the trunk. Obviously, this qi flowing back and forth must have both yin and yang aspects, so the yin and yang qi comes and goes between the extremities and the trunk in each of the four limbs.

Qualities of qi are defined according to the source of the qi, depending on whether it is found in the extremities or in the trunk. The qi is most highly characteristic *(tai* or "greater")* at the outset; it becomes gradually less so and more attenuated as it moves through the body.

The qi that comes from the periphery, hands and feet, as well as the distal joints, the wrists and ankles, is strongly characteristic in the extremities.

The qi that comes from the trunk, shoulders, and hips is strongly characteristic in the roots of the limbs.

Dialectically, I would qualify these energies as *tai*, supreme, highly characteristic, at their origin; *shao*, lesser, at the intermediate joints; and *ming* or *jue*, exhausted, at the end of the circuit, according to a qualitative dialectical order.

Note that I only list below those barrier points that we have developed ourselves. Nothing is noted when we have used cleft points or any of the five transport points in the barrier point scheme.

TRUNK EXITS

The command points, which conduct the qi to the extremities, are always on the proximal side of the articulation *(see* Table 5).

Yin Qi Exit from the Trunk to the Limbs

The barrier points at the shoulder and hip are located on the *tai yin* channels, as the qi is *tai yin* here. They are LU-2 *yun men* ("Cloud Door"), located on the arm *tai yin* primary channel, and SP-12 *chong men* ("Rushing Door") on the leg *tai yin* primary channel. Both of these points have the word *men* 門 (door) in their names, reflecting their ability to open and close the flow of qi.

Yang Qi Exit from the Trunk to the Limbs

At the upper limbs, the outgoing qi is controlled by *tai yang,*[4] at the shoulder, specifically SI-11 (天宗 *tian zong,* "Heavenly Ancestor"), one of the points with *tian* ("heaven") in its name, which connects the trunk to the heaven of man. Remember that traditionally in China, humans are represented with uplifted arms. This is why the qi that arrives at the shoulder is *jue yin.* It is not the qi "from the Liver, stopping at the underarms," as some authors claim, but *jue yin* qi. That is to say, although the Liver is *jue yin*, not all *jue yin* is Liver.

The exiting qi is controlled by *shao yang* at the elbow, and by TB-13 arm *shao yang*. It is controlled by *yang ming* at the wrist, and LI-9 arm *yang ming*.

At the lower limb, the outgoing energies are controlled by:

- *tai yang* at the hip, and BL-29 leg *tai yang*

- *shao yang* at the knee, and GB-33 leg *shao yang*

- *yang ming* at the ankle, and ST-37 leg *yang ming*

TRUNK ENTRANCES

Yin Qi Entrance from the Limbs to the Trunk

The qi that comes into the roots of the limbs is *jue yin* and the command points are therefore located on the *jue yin* channels. These are HM-2 (天泉 *tian quan,* "Heavenly Spring") in the upper limb, a "heaven" point (like the arm *tai yang* point SI-11) that facilitates the entry of yin at the shoulder, and LR-11 (陰廉 *yin lian*), which activates the entry of yin qi at the hip.

Yang Qi Entrance from the Limbs to the Trunk

The end of yang qi circulation that arrives at the trunk is *yang ming*. At the shoulder, LI-15 (肩髃 *jian yu)* commands the entry of yang qi; at the hip, ST-31 (髀關 *bi guan,* "Hip Barrier") plays the same role. These points activate the entry of yang and yin at the shoulders and hips.

A number of articular barriers do not have their own specific points (such as the yang entering the wrist or the knee). In such cases you must use one of the command points of the corresponding channel, since these points have the property of sweeping all the activities that affect their channel. The best approach in such cases is to puncture the cleft unblocking point, which unblocks the qi of the corresponding channel, including the barriers.

Table 5: Barrier Command Points

	EXITING		ENTERING	
	YIN	YANG	YIN	YANG
Shoulder	LU-2	SI-11	HM-2	LI-15
Elbow	HT-6	TB-13	HT-6	TB-7
Wrist	HM-4	LI-9	LU-6	SI-6
Hip	SP-12	BL-29	LR-11	ST-31
Knee	KI-5	GB-33	KI-5	GB-36
Ankle	LR-6	ST-37	SP-8	BL-63

APPLICATION TO PATHOLOGY

In practice, the barrier points are highly effective; we use them in articular or periarticular pathologies, primarily in a case of diffuse, general impairment, which strongly suggests a "barrier" blockage that is not allowing yin or yang qi to flow through in one direction or another. In that case, there are local symptoms of yin or yang deficiency or excess, returning to the basic eight parameters for diagnosis as discussed above in the beginning of this section.

Alternatively, they can be used in the case of pain localized on one segment of a channel that suggests a barrier problem. If, for example, the yang does not exit the trunk to go into the shoulder or hip, which is therefore *tai yang*, a pain appears, on the one hand, of a yang-deficiency type downstream in the extremity located on the *tai yang* channel on the arm or thigh, because of this the qi cannot come out since it is the most characteristic. Normally, there will be a sign of congestion or excess in the part of the trunk nearest the limb (i.e., the upper chest or pelvis). If, in addition, the yang is not coming out at the elbow or knee, meaning at the intermediate level of *shao yang*, the pain produced by the blockage is localized on the *shao yang* channel of the forearm or leg. If, once again, the terminal yang is not coming out at the wrist or ankle, the pain is localized on the *yang ming* channels. Another example: if the terminal yang, *yang ming*, cannot enter the shoulder or the hip, the pain is localized on the *yang ming* channels of the shoulder or hip; in this case, there is an excess of this qi that accumulates upstream.

We will review all of this material with the pathology, but I want to draw special attention to two points. First, the therapeutic precision of these points. In the last example in the paragraph above, where the terminal yang does not enter the hip, only ST-31 on the leg *yang ming* can relieve this pain. Second, with these barrier points we can achieve an immediate, substantial improvement, so they are also a therapeutic test.

❖ Case History

Mrs. S., age 42, came to see me for acute left-sided lower back pain that appeared two days before for no apparent reason and without any other accompanying symptoms. This intense pain was very circumscribed and located just lateral to the left sacroiliac joint. It made any movement difficult, did not radiate, and was only very slightly relieved by heat. It did not appear to be influenced by environmental factors. The pain was unchanged after four treatments on the left with BL-57, BL-67, BL-29, and finally BL-36.

At this point Mrs. S. told me that there was a little radiation of the pain into the left groin. This could be seen as a blockage of ST-31 *(bi guan,* "hip barrier"). This point affects, on the one hand, the movements of the hip, and on the other, the return of the yang of the lower limbs into the pelvis. An obstruction with hip pain here is with or without radiation to the lumbar area.

On examination, I then found a painful spot deep and on the left, directly below the outer edge of the paravertebral musculature, above L1, approximately in the area of BL-50 (the back associated point of the Stomach). I decided to puncture only ST-31 on the left. The pain disappeared within 48 hours. The stiffness that remained disappeared after a second treatment of the same points.

The pain may be localized on the channel of the same name as the blocked qi, when the corresponding organs are normal. For example, the yin qi, *jue yin,* or terminal yin cannot enter the hip when the pain is localized on the channel of the same name in the thigh, leg *jue yin,* and the Liver, Gallbladder, and wood phase are all normal. This means that if there is pain along these channel pathways that does not match the eight parameters described above, the treatment must use something other than a barrier point.

Here again we see that the channel is indeed a privileged place where all the physiological and pathological phenomena that are linked to it both resonate and manifest, regardless of their origin or localization.

❖ Case History

Mr. M., age 50, suddenly experienced a flash of heat along with a cracking sensation in the lumbar region, vomiting and very severe pain on the back of his leg as he was trying to lift a heavy car.

Let's analyze this pain according to the eight parameters. The type of pain was yang, severe, deep, relieved slightly and temporarily by heat, aggravated by movements; pressure had no effect. Remember that movement improves cases of stagnation because it causes qi to circulate, and also improves excesses by expending the qi. This pain, which was aggravated by movement and improved by heat, either corresponded to a deficiency or else did not fit in with the eight parameters. The pain was deep, severe, and located along the pathway of the foot *tai yang* channel. This pain was aggravated by coughing (which increased the pressure in the abdomen). This means that there was an excess in the abdomen and a deficiency below the cutoff that was preventing the qi from flowing from the abdomen to the leg along the leg *tai yang* channel.

Vomiting and hot flashes also correspond to this qi cutoff: the yang from the trunk, which could not descend, rose up in the wrong direction, bringing up the food and triggering a flash of heat. The qi that comes from the trunk to flow into the leg is, qualitatively, *tai yang* and comes out at BL-29. Since it could not reach *shao yang*, it spread out from here to the *tai yang* channel, which explains the trajectory and the type of pain.

For treatment, we tonified BL-29, the barrier point, reinforced by needling both the cleft point, BL-63, and river point, BL-60, which transmit qi to the areas that depend on this channel. I punctured BL-29 first, then BL-60: it is a rule of thumb to always puncture in sequence going from yang to yin, except in the special case of GV-20, which can cause fainting if punctured first. In other words, one should always puncture from top to bottom, and from left to right, etc.

As the goal of the treatment was to bring the qi out at BL-29 and make it circulate through to BL-60, we had to tonify those points. We left the needles in for just ten minutes to avoid an excessive treatment reaction, and repeated this the next day. If there was no improvement after the second session, it means that this pain is not treatable by acupuncture because it is structural. The pain diminished by 50 percent after the first session and disappeared two days after the second one.

❖ Case History

Mr. A., age 32, an athlete, had been lifting heavy boxes of books and, after the third box, felt a very sharp pain in the right lumbar area, which immobilized him. This acute pain, located in the right sacroiliac joint, extended into the buttock and thigh along the *tai yang* channel. It was not affected by coughing. All movements were painful, but this pain became even worse after long periods of sitting. Pressure had no effect on it. Heat improved it, while cold had no effect. The big toe on his right side was also numb. Otherwise, this man was in excellent health and had no previous lumbar, vertebral or joint problems.

What are the first diagnoses that come to mind? A qi barrier (in this case BL-29) or a sinew problem. If the problem involves BL-29, the pain would be aggravated by coughing (pressure). Since this was not the case, a sinew problem seemed likely, considering the circumstances of the occurrence, which eliminated the intrusion of a pathogenic climatic effect.

The sacroiliac joint is controlled by the sinews[5] of the leg *tai yang*, leg *shao yang* and LR-11. The extension of the pain to the buttock and thigh suggested *tai yang*. The absence of lateral pain (*shao yang*) and radiation to the big toe (*jue yin*) does not suggest the other two mechanisms. So I punctured the well and river points of the leg *tai yang*, BL-67 and BL-60, along with the local painful (although not tender) points, located along the inside line of leg *tai yang* on the back, about 5cm above the sacroiliac joint. This had no effect.

I then applied a principle that I consider fundamental: if the treatment of the painful area is ineffective, this means that the origin of the pain is somewhere else. I did not find anything in the area of the two right thoracic and lumbar leg *tai yang* channels or in the knee. Searching in front of the area, I found on the right side of the groin a very painful LR-11 (one should always also test the contralateral point for comparison) and punctured it, along with LR-4, the distal river point of the channel. The pain increased during the evening and then disappeared during the night.

Which symptom might have led me to make this diagnosis from the outset? The aggravation after prolonged sitting, which cuts off the qi circulation in the hips and in the groin. Also, the tingling in the large toe of the ipsilateral foot draws attention to this diagnosis. Radiation of the pain to the foot is an important indicator that one of the three leg *yin* is responsible.

The general history-taking revealed that this highly energetic man had occasional insomnia, poor sleep quality and had experienced somnambulism in childhood, suggesting the command point for all the Liver functions, BL-47. Can we establish a link between this disturbance of BL-47 and this painful location on leg *jue yin*? Yes, because when a function is defective, the muscles, tendons and other structures that depend on it are not as well supplied and therefore more vulnerable and do not recover as well. Since the pain disappeared after I punctured LR-11, I punctured BL-47 at the second session. The improvement in the quality of sleep was so remarkable that this man asked for a third visit to complete the correction of his sleeping problems.

ON THE HEAD AND NECK

The energies concerned in this case are especially yang, because we are dealing with the upper, heavenly part of the body. (*See* Table 6.)

Between the head and the trunk: the energies (which are yang in this area) descend from the head to the thorax via the sequence BL-10 to GB-21 to ST-11; and the energies rise from the thorax to the head via the points SI-14 to TB-15 to ST-3 (still along the *tai yang* → *shao yang* → *yang ming* progression).

Between the top of skull and face: the qi descends from the top of the skull to the face via BL-6 to GB-3 to ST-7 and rises from the face to the top of the skull via BL-2 to GB-14 to ST-8. A case history involving GB-3 follows.

Table 6: Barrier Points of the Head and Neck

	BETWEEN HEAD AND THORAX		
Rising	SI-14	TB-15	ST-3
Descending	BL-10	GB-21	ST-11
	BETWEEN TOP OF SKULL AND FACE		
Rising	BL-2	GB-14	ST-8
Descending	BL-6	GB-3	ST-7

DIFFERENTIAL BETWEEN DIFFERENT TYPES OF BARRIER POINTS

❖ Case History

A woman, age 30 and four months pregnant, consulted me for severe headaches that had begun during the third month of her pregnancy. The pregnancy was desired, and had proceeded normally. The headaches were severe, frontal, helmet headaches accompanied by a feeling of weight and of heaviness in the head. Noise and light had no influence. This patient had nothing to say about any effect on the pain of a local application of cold or heat (to help differentiate yin and yang), nor whether pressure on the eyes made any difference (to help differentiate deficiency and excess). What can be concluded? Very little. The headaches seemed to be intense and due to an excess, because of the sensation of weight and of heaviness in the head. An excess of yang? More we cannot say. Note the frontal location and the non-pulsatile type of pain (meaning that the blood was not involved).

The history revealed that this young woman had suffered from premenstrual headaches since puberty. They were sometimes unilateral, right or left, located in the temple and the eye, sometimes bilateral, frontal and band-like. They sometimes radiated to the back of the neck at GB-20 and sometimes to the ipsilateral ear. The weather did not have any influence (a sign of Yang Linking vessel dysfunctions). Above all, I noted the radiation along the lines of *shao yang* (see the illustrations of the primary channels on the head in Appendix Two, p. 249) and to the ear. The qi problem therefore seemed to be on *shao yang* bilaterally, sometimes unilaterally. Considering the frontal location, one may surmise there was a blockage of GB-14, GB-5, GB-3, GB-1 or TB-23 with the latter tending to cause pain in the eyes and eyebrows. GB-14 has significant ocular symptomatology. GB-5 corresponds more to radiation to the outside corner of the eyes, to the nose and to the teeth, because of its connection to the arm and leg *yang ming* channels. GB-3 is indicated by the temporal location of the pain and its auricular effect.

In the history, there was little of note except for migraines on the maternal side, which spoke for a hereditary type of blockage in GB-3. Her tongue appeared normal. I successfully tonified this point bilaterally.

CHAPTER SEVEN

HUMANS IN THE COSMOS: THE FOUR SEASONS AND THE HUMAN BODY

Seasons in Chinese Medicine

The four seasons make up the rules and the mesh of the net.[1] They tell of the evolution of the energies of heaven and earth, the concerted actions of heaven and of earth, and how man, according to Chinese medicine, must harmonize his own energies with those of each season to avoid dysfunction.

The four seasons refer not just to the changes of seasons as seen throughout a year, but also symbolize four characteristic periods of a day, or even of a life, because these same cyclical variations are reproduced in the course of a day, a year, or a lifetime (*see* Fig. 3).

It should be noted that in the Chinese tradition, the equinoxes and solstices mark the middle of a season, its apex. Therefore, according to Chinese time, summer begins on May 5th, autumn on August 5th, winter on November 5th and spring on February 5th. It is easy to see that the air and the light at that time become somewhat different; it is a small yet perceptible change.

How is each season defined? First by two specific functions, second by its relationships with heaven and earth, then by man's resolve (his spontaneous, instinctive, animal will) which naturally springs at each season and in each being, and finally by the Dao, the way that one must follow during this period.

SPRING

- Spring is "bursting off and unfolding."[2]

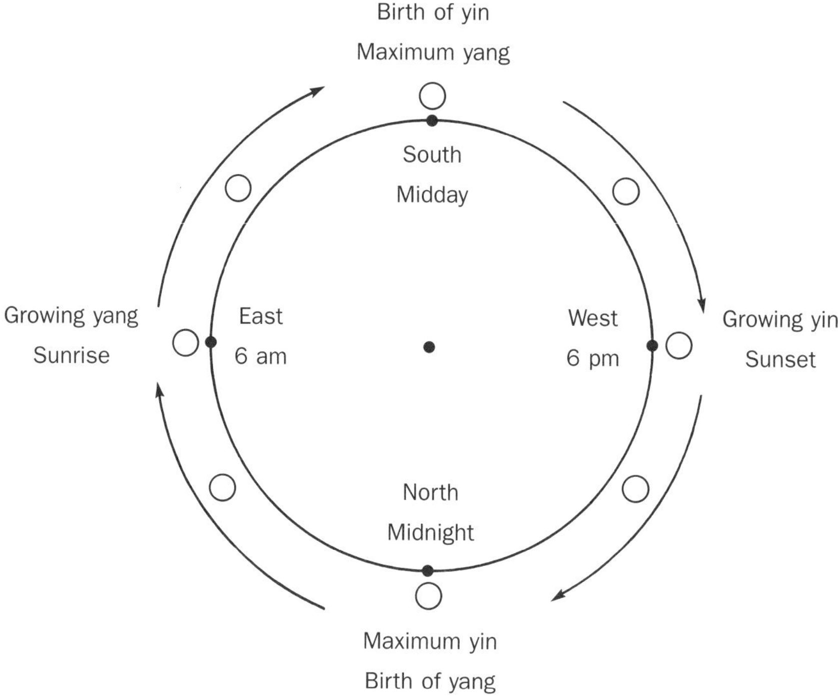

Fig. 3: The Four Seasons

- Heaven and earth "act together to produce life."

All creation is then brought into life: the 10,000 beings are flourishing, vegetation comes to life and emerges from the earth. The character 生 *sheng*, etymologically speaking, is "a plant which springs from the earth, which goes higher and higher."[3] This very well illustrates the movement of spring, which bursts out, unfolds, displays and grows.

- "Man's resolve favors the upsurge of life." It then lets energy emerge and spread outside. "The body feels well; it gets up at dawn and goes to bed at night." It paces the courtyard with a free heart. Its task is "to reward and avoid punishing, to favor life and avoid killing, to give and avoid taking." Convicts were therefore not supposed to be executed in the springtime, but in autumn, in accordance with the season.

- In spring, the energies express themselves, and the deepest types of qi emerge. At six in the morning, night and yin disappear and the day, sun and yang appear. It is important to understand that these phases occur within us at all times, but that they are magnified during spring and at six in the morning.

- The spring movement of wood is easy, supple and free; it is a continuous movement, similar to the sap of the tree, going from the roots to the extremities of the branches.

- There is an acupuncture point, LR-14, which corresponds to the end of the night, to the cyclical end of yin. Its name is *qi men* 期門. *Qi* here means time, period, phase, expiration date, and immobility while *men* means an exterior door. It governs the end of the menses, the end of pregnancy (postpartum difficulties, expulsion problems), and the end of the procreative phase of life, at the time of menopause. It is then a favorite point when something has to come to an end but does not, or does not end properly, as if night (yin) would never end and be replaced by day. A difficult separation? For the transition from the end of a phase to the beginning of another phase involves a separation, a sacrifice which has nothing to do with a moral or mystic law but is an archetypal law of life.

It should be noted that, on an intuitive level, I would not put the point that governs menopause in the springtime, when life is bursting forth and expanding. To explain this position, I mention the traditional Chinese rules for the life of a couple. Up to the time of menopause, the man and woman must keep everything separate: bed, sheets, towels, and tableware … everything, down to the smallest details. They only join in sexual intercourse. When the wife reaches the age of 49 (7 x 7), symbolic of menopause, they put everything together. It is as if this man and this woman, as individuals, until now confined to their masculine or feminine spheres, acceded to a state of androgyny, blending in them and between them the masculine and the feminine. In Africa also, women are often only allowed to join the tribal councils after menopause; prior to that, they are excluded. This is why menopause, which marks the beginning of this time of unity, can be seen as the dawn of a new life. It is also the spring and not the autumn of life. It does not have to be thought of as a pathology, except in cases of disorders.

SUMMER

- It implies "to proliferate, to multiply, to be luxuriant" as well as "to flower, to cause to flourish." The function of summer is to make perfect. While spring is birth, summer is the apogee of vitality.

- The energies of heaven "thrive" and the energies of the earth "bring out the flower." Heaven and earth blend their energies, as in a sexual intercourse. Creation "makes flourishing perfect." The 10,000 beings "flower and fructify" *(shi* 實*)*.

- Man follows this movement in getting up early and going to bed late, in tempering his vital forces that tend to be overly exuberant. "Without violence, he favors the brilliance of beauty and strength," easing "the outward expression and the evacuation of the energies." It is worth noting that at the very moment when the energies, the desires, the ambitions reach their climax, when sun and fire (light and warmth) reach their peak, man humbly controls, assists without any violence, and discharges all excess.

- The Dao of summer is to maintain the development of life.

- When the sun reaches its highest point, when yang too reaches its highest point, something of the order of night, of yin, is born, because it is when a phase is at its peak that its contrary begins to peep through, to sprout and to be born. Here the movements of qi are: reaching a peak, bringing out, bringing yang to the surface and giving birth to yin.

- The summer movement of Fire expresses luxuriance, fructification, flowering, the peak of life.

AUTUMN

- It is both "overabundance and harmony." The function of autumn is then to gather, to pick up, and to harvest.

- "Heaven withdraws and hurries, the earth is shining and beaming." The same brilliance can be seen in the complexion and the eyes of a person: when someone is anxious, his complexion and his eyes are dull: "the brilliance of the spirit radiance is hidden." "Autumn is the season of peace and of quietness."

- Man is then on his own, peaceful, in harmony. Heaven, the father, has withdrawn and man quietly "displays his radiance," mature, adult, self-sufficient. Man "harvests" and "gathers all types of qi" without letting the energies be spread and lost outside. Autumn is the time when man has to turn towards himself again. He then harvests the fruits of spring and summer. To be in harmony with the energy of the season, he has to go to bed early and get up late.

- The Dao is to "maintain the harvest of life."

- Here, the qi movements are internalization, disappearance of day, yang, sun, and appearance of night and yin.

- The autumnal movement, related to metal, marks a discontinuity, a separation, similar to the ripe fruit that falls from the tree and will never return to that tree.

WINTER

- Winter means "to shut inside and to store up."

- In winter, the relationship with heaven is disrupted, "no stimulation ever comes from the yang," the earth cracks, water freezes; earth yields no more fruit, it "hides and stores up, preparing through this retreat the root of a new upsurge."

- The role of man is to be "buried, hidden, turned towards his own self, busy taking possession of himself."

- The Dao is to maintain "the storing up of life."

- Night (yin) has reached its peak. Day (yang) begins to be born, like the sprout in the earth that contains all the future, like the seed or the first cell of a human being that contains the entire being. The qi goes into retreat, recedes to the inner reaches.

- The winter movement of water marks the transition from the invisible to the visible, from the non-differentiated to the differentiated, the first moment of each creation.

Seasons of Man

Four seasons in a year, four periods in a day, four ages in a life, four seasons for a man.

- Childhood is the spring of man, with the "upsurge of life."
- Adolescence and early adulthood are his summer. He prospers and fructifies, accompanied by all the related desires, lusts and ambitions. It is necessary to know how to "facilitate the radiance of strength and beauty."
- In autumn heaven withdraws: it is the age of mature adulthood. Man, who till then was subjected to the order, to the rule, to the law, to the father, now finds his own rule, his own way of life; he displays the radiance of the spirit and renounces his desires and ambitions with a peaceful and quiet mind.
- Winter, old age, the fourth period of life, sees him go into retreat to prepare the seed for a new upsurge. "Storing up, exclusively turned towards his own self, busy taking possession of himself," he now turns towards the underground sprouting of a new life.

These four permanent phases, magnified at certain times of year, day or life, cohabit and balance each other. For example, the passionate luxuriance of summer is echoed by the necessary burying and retreat of winter. Everything has to be lived at the right time, everything has to be balanced.

ALARM POINTS

Each organ has one alarm point, except for the Gallbladder, which has two. These alarm points are linked to the five phases (五行 *wu xing*). The *wu xing* are made up of four phases that correspond to the four seasons and directions and one central phase. Each alarm point corresponds to one of the five phases and, in particular, to the corresponding organ and season: in a way, it is the seasonal alarm point of the organ (*see* Fig. 4).

FIVE PHASES

The five phases are named in order: water $\rightarrow$ fire $\rightarrow$ wood $\rightarrow$ metal $\rightarrow$ earth. All natural, cosmic and human phenomena are correlated to these five phases, four of them peripheral and one central. For example:

- Water, of the winter and the north, corresponds to the Kidneys and to cold.
- Fire, of the summer and the south, corresponds to the Heart Master[4] and to fire.
- Wood, of the spring and the east, corresponds to the Liver and to wind.
- Metal, of the autumn and the west, is in a continuum with the Lung and dryness.
- Earth, at the center, governs the Spleen and dampness.

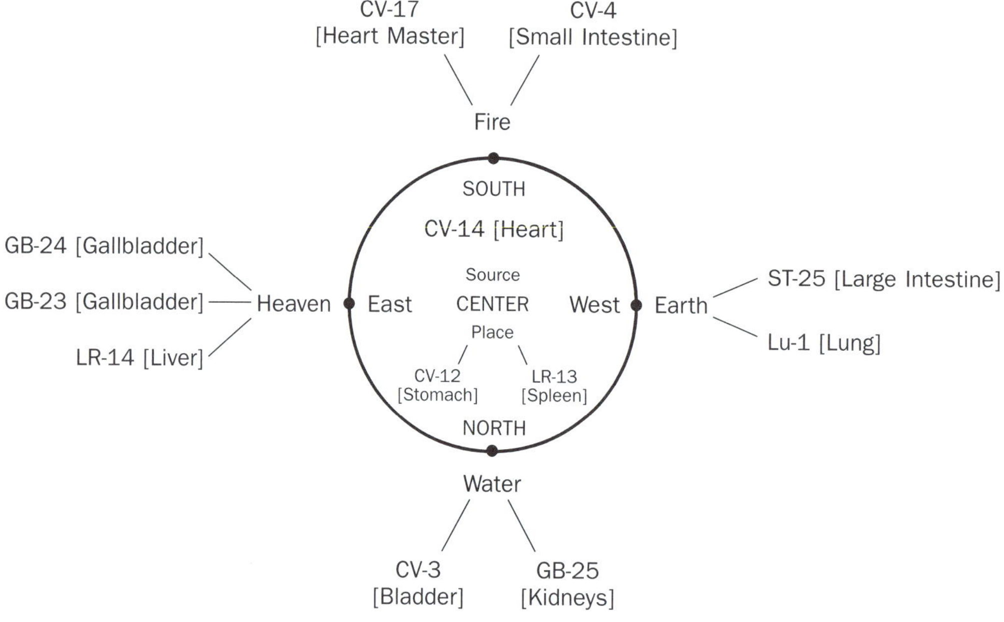

Fig. 4: Alarm Point Correspondences

Functions of the Center

There is duality in the center. "At the center (of the empire), next to the sovereign who must have virtue from heaven, there will be a hero who tends to the earth."[5] In man, it is the same: the center is dual: the Heart (sovereign) on the heaven side and the Spleen, in charge of tending to the earth. This is like the solar system: the sun is the source of life and the earth is the place of life. This corresponds to both heliocentric and geocentric views of the universe.

The sovereign Heart is controlled by CV-14, along the midline, at the tip of the xiphoid process.

The alarm point of the Spleen is LR-13 at the end of the 11th rib.

The Stomach, which is paired with it, corresponds to CV-12, which is in the epigastric area and along the midline.

In the following case histories, pay attention, in passing, to the apparent subtlety of the organ signs at these points. This shows once again that these organs have functions that are much broader than those acknowledged in the West.

❖ Case History

A young woman, age 38, slim, stooped and tired-looking, came to see me for frequent anxiety attacks and insomnia. The anxiety attacks were severe. They caused symptoms including tightness in the throat, thorax and abdomen, with sensations of coldness in the bones, diarrhea, tachycardia and tremors in the lower limbs. During these attacks, she was prostrate and frozen. The attacks correspond to a freeze, a massive invasion of the qi by cold, usually internal, due to a general deficiency of fire (e.g., related to CV-6), affecting the Gallbladder and the sovereign Heart. They may be compared and contrasted, schematically, with anxiety attacks that are fueled by excesses of fire, either, for example, in the Heart where the fire is either compressed at the center (related to CV-15) or where it cannot return to its home in the Heart (related to CV-16).

She slept poorly, waking at four in the morning and unable to fall asleep again for two hours. She said that she had little drive. We found little in terms of somatic disturbances, apart from an episode of hypothyroidism, with fatigue, chills, constipation and weight gain, which subsided after a short allopathic treatment. The hypothyroidism reinforced the suggestion of internal cold caused by a deficiency of fire, which is of major importance in this case.

All of this had begun after the sudden death of a close friend, which had reminded her of the deaths of her brother and her father, five and seven years previously. Her tongue looked slightly pale.

The deep pulses in both proximal positions and the weak pulses in the Heart area suggested a breakdown (in the feet) and a Heart origin for the fire deficiency. Her stooped posture reflected this breakdown: she could not hold herself up straight, feeling unable to get any bearing on a solid floor. This type of breakdown should be treated with CV-5. CV-6 could also be considered if there was no deficiency of fire in the Heart, which manifests with the coldness and the somatic symptoms.

Which points should I choose to treat the deficiency of fire in the Heart, considering her sensation of being "chilled to the bone"? This sign is connected to the points CV-14, the alarm point of the Heart, along with HT-4, HT-5 and BL-43. HT-4 is for cases of depression, sadness, fear, excitability, muteness or aphonia, which did not correspond to this patient, especially since her short, thick hands did not seem to indicate points on the upper limbs. HT-5 suggests an emotional intensity, frequent nervousness, a lack of self-confidence, distance from others ('misanthropy'), loss of speech and blockage in the diaphragm: this did not appear to fit this case either. BL-43 suggests greater physical and mental exhaustion, and loss of memory, even though it is indicated for cases of separation or the loss of loved ones. CV-14, which governs the Heart fire center, closely matches this patient, with her anxiety and occasional panic attacks, even though she did not have pulmonary or gastric signs. It was especially apt as it is located on the same channel as CV-5. So I punctured CV-5 and CV-14. There was rapid improvement after the very first session. After the third session, she was sleeping much better and had far less anxiety. She returned six months later. A conflict with her 18-year-old son had caused a relapse. Her equilibrium was restored in two sessions.

❖ Case History

Mr. C., age 43, was a teacher who came to see me for a syndrome that had been progressing for five years, consisting of sensations of knots in the stomach accompanied by nausea, weakness in the limbs, an empty feeling in the head, dizziness and tingling all over the body. Against this background of a permanent moderate state there were occasional acute attacks that left him powerless. His hands and feet were not cold; they did not change color. His blood pressure was normal. There was no lightheadedness. He could not tolerate being touched in the stomach area and asked not to be punctured on the solar plexus. This suggested a qi blockage in the center with a peripheral deficiency, especially of yin; there was no sign of blockage of the yang or of blood.

Otherwise, he was well and there were no other symptoms. His history included acne during his adolescence, a very painful romantic breakup at the age of 27, the death of his twin sons when they were six months old and he was 32, the death of his father when he was 39, and the removal of a leiomyoma from his stomach when he was 40. His tongue appeared normal. The proximal and distal pulses were deficient, suggesting a blockage at the center and confirming the symptomatology. So I punctured LR-13.

Following a worsening of symptoms for 48 hours, he was well for seven days. I repeated the same treatment at the second session two weeks later. He was better after another 48-hour reaction accompanied by "morbid thoughts and apathy." At the third visit, a month later, we punctured the same point plus SP-8, an unblocking cleft point, to reinforce the effects of LR-13. He continued to show visible improvement. Two months later, he was no longer having attacks and the background symptoms had practically disappeared. He reported a period of three days during the seventh week when his limbs felt weak again. Two sessions at three-month intervals practically eliminated the syndrome.

From our point of view, LR-13 governs the center/earth/Spleen, like the center Hall of Enlightenment to which the emperor returned after visiting each of the four cardinal directions, and like the last 18-day segment of each of the four seasons that enables the seasonal qi to return to the center so as to be transformed for the next season. The important point about LR-13 is the possibility—or impossibility in a case of pathology—of returning to the center, the imperial place of transformations. The leiomyoma in the stomach was probably evidence of that impossibility in this man. The failure of the middle qi (中氣 *zhong qi*) to be distributed to the periphery is only the apparent consequence of this non-centered condition.

Phases and the Four Seasons

These symbolize four characteristic periods. They can apply not only to a year, but to many time periods because the same cyclical variations are reproduced in the course of a day, a year or a lifetime.

■ SPRING

Spring corresponds to wood and the easterly direction. In the spring, vegetation comes to life and emerges from the earth; deep qi is exteriorized; the yang qi appears, like the sun that rises at six in the morning. At the same time, the yin qi declines, like the night that fades at the same hour. It is important to understand that these phases occur within us at all times, but that they are magnified in the spring, at six a.m., and in adolescence. The spring corresponds to the wood phase, the easterly direction, and the Liver and Gallbladder. The alarm point of the Liver is LR-14, while the Gallbladder has two alarm points, GB-23 and GB-24.

LR-14, located on the nipple line, in the sixth intercostal space, is the alarm point of spring and of the Liver. It corresponds to the end of night, the end of a yin phenomenon. In women, it governs the end of the menstrual period, the end of pregnancy ("postpartum difficulties, expulsion problems"[6]). It is effective at the time of menopause, the end of the procreative phase of life, to treat hot flashes, etc.[7] It governs the end of the qi movements that rise from below, from the depths of the yin zones to the upper areas of the thorax.[8] It is therefore indicated when something that must end does not end, or ends badly, whether it is a case of bronchitis, the qi rising to the chest, a menstrual period, a pregnancy, a procreative period, a separation, etc. It is as if the night (yin) does not end as a means of allowing the day to appear.

❖ Case History

Ms. S., age 25, was a tall, slender student who was rather reserved, blushed easily and was often indecisive, "always sitting on the fence," as she said. She came to see me in 1996 for various symptoms.

Her primary complaint was furuncles that were very disturbing and painful, located on her chin and forehead, which had been progressing for seven years. They had responded to autovaccines in 1995 but had returned, despite a long-term homeopathic treatment. They seemed sensitive to stress but were hardly influenced by menstrual periods or digestion. To which qi would these boils correspond? Fire due to either qi constraint or an accumulation of damp-heat, that is, toxins due to poor draining of the blood in particular.

She also suffered from painful localized muscle tension, especially in the back of the neck and in the trapezius muscles and on the lateral aspects of the lower limbs. The connection with *shao yang* is obvious here. This tension was not related to the weather. The young woman was not dispersed or scattered and had neither leukorrhea nor low back pain, which eliminated the Yang Linking vessel and the Girdle vessel.

She also complained of digestive problems with nausea, alternating constipation and diarrhea, and increased gas before her periods. She did not tolerate fats, coffee, chocolate or eggs, which pointed to the Liver or Gallbladder.

Her periods were often several days late but the premenstrual syndrome was constant. She frequently had chilblains in the winter and her hands and feet were usually cold.

Her tongue appeared normal. Her pulse was deep at the left middle position.

She was cheerful and had plenty of drive, had a history of somnambulism at the age of ten and awoke frequently. She did not report any recurring dreams. She said that she did not have her feet on the ground, so she readily took refuge in ideas. In 1997 she began to learn *taiji* and in 1998 she began psychotherapy.

Let's analyze all these factors.

Which qi are we dealing with here? Liver or Gallbladder, *jue yin* or *shao yang*.

What are the arguments in favor of these mechanisms? The fact that she is always sitting on the fence points to *shao yang*, her indecision to the Gallbladder, poor circulation to *jue yin*, poor drainage with a buildup of impurities ("bad blood") to the Liver, and most of the other signs could be attributed to one of these four etiologies.

Is there a defective relationship between *shao yang* and *jue yin*? Apparently not. An origin in GB-37 would result in greater irritability, reactivity, and yang manifestations on the surface. Poor communication from LR-5 (*jue yin* to *shao yang*) would indeed correspond to persons who are reserved but who are "joyless, and sigh frequently." Neither of these two points seems to match her.[9] I began by treating *shao yang* at GB-21. Located on the trapezius muscle, at the beginning of the trunk, and corresponding to the hinge-like quality of *shao yang*, it is the meeting point of the five organs and governs the female pelvis, including obstetrics. Two sessions at three-week intervals, adding the well point and the root, GB-44, at the second session, had no effect.

How should I work on the Gallbladder? I rejected the choice of GB-23, because this patient, although reserved, was open: she was not a misanthrope. I decided to adjust in two ways: treating the digestive, middle burner aspects of the Gallbladder by puncturing CV-11 and to purify the blood with SP-10. This was also unsuccessful.

At this point, I decided it would be better to approach another aspect of the Gallbladder, considering her periods, that is, treating the Gallbladder as an extraordinary organ. The corresponding point BL-48 is located at the level of BL-19 on the outside branch of the leg *tai yang* channel. This branch has points that store the organs' essence and spirit, including points for the spirit, corporeal soul, ethereal soul, intention and resolve. There are only two yang organs that have points on this branch, the central yang organs Stomach and Gallbladder. BL-48 seems to control the Gall Bladder as an extraordinary organ. Puncturing it twice had no effect.

My other choice was to treat the Liver. Considering the somnambulism, sleep disturbances, the coming and going that could not flow easily like tree sap flowing from the ends of the roots to the tips of the branches (explaining the cold feet and hands, the reserved expression, etc.), I thought of the point that corresponds to comings and goings in the Liver, the "Gate of the Ethereal Soul" (*hun men*), BL-47. Puncturing this point twice did not bring much of a change in her symptoms.

At the next visit, she told me that she was suffering from her indecisiveness and feeling of always being on the fence, which led her to "take refuge in ideas" because of her problems with living in the present. As an example, she described an emotional relationship that she knew had grown empty but that she could not manage to end: "I am still hanging onto a relationship that is over." So I used the Liver point that corresponds to the ending of night to permit the coming of day, the end of winter that allows spring to burst forth, the point that helps end one cycle in order to begin another (like, among others, the circulation of nutritive qi that ends with leg *jue yin* to begin with arm *tai yin*). This springtime point in the Liver is LR-14.

After three sessions, there was a considerable improvement all around, including in the furuncles. She has now begun a new life, is teaching in Switzerland, and is doing well with one treatment a year—in the spring, of course.

The Gallbladder has two alarm points, GB-23 and GB-24, which correspond to the sun rising in the morning, and to the springtime externalization of qi energies.

❖ Case History

An international lawyer, age 52, consulted me for tremors. He had little to report: some flatulence and insomnia. He was very austere and incommunicative, simply complaining of inner and outer tremors: "It feels all agitated inside, it's moving but it cannot come out." All of these signs evoked a blockage of GB-23, including the difficulty with interpersonal relationships. What was causing this constraint of qi inside? Why could It not express itself? "In some way, I am betraying myself. I am an international lawyer, I have my own plane, I travel the world, but every quarter, I need to take my camel and my tent and go off in nature to recover my peace and serenity and return to myself." Most of the time, his life was not his own; it did not match up with his inner nature. His true qi as a man of nature was repressed within; it was moving and causing him to tremble. Puncturing the corresponding point, GB-23, near the axilla, relieved his tremors and insomnia. GB-24 has similar symptoms, but with a yin blockage; in fact, it is connected with *tai yin*. This point treats Gallbladder pathologies marked by difficulty in making decisions or sadness; also, commonly these patients will have constipation.

■ SUMMER

The function of summer is to cause to flourish, bear fruit, and perfect. If spring is birth, then summer is fructification, the apogee of vitality. This is when the sun culminates, the yang qi culminates, and qi is externalized. At the same time, something is born that is of yin, of the night, because it is at the time when a phase is at its peak that the contrary agent begins to be born. This season corresponds to the fire phase, like the Heart Master and the Small Intestine. These alarm points are CV-4 and CV-17.

The midline pelvic point CV-4, alarm point of the Small Intestine, corresponds to this beginning, this birth of yin qi in the summer and to the south. This point has several summer-like functions. It sets the qi in the pelvis in motion, as is implied in its name 關元 *guan yuan* or "Pass Source."[10] It corresponds to the source qi, the yang and fire of the Kidneys, which put the yin of the Kidneys in motion. When it malfunctions, there is exhaustion with deficiency, with a deep sense of inner cold, premature aging, and genital and sexual problems: it is considered to be a point that tonifies the entire body.

As the alarm point of the Small Intestine it has the function of fructification (a function that corresponds to summer) of the products absorbed through eating food. This combination of two summer seasonal actions explains the symptoms of digestive and urinary problems connected with this yang organ.

❖ Case History

A woman, age 41, consulted me for headaches and excessive sweating. She could not pinpoint when the headaches had begun. With no apparent cause, they occurred in attacks that lasted for four days. Neither the weather nor her periods, digestion, or emotions had any effect on them. The pains were deep, endocranial, intense and tight. Local application of cold provided momentary relief. Pressure on the eyes did not change them, and they were accompanied by a marked sensation of fullness in the head. Of the yang type, alleviated by local cold, accompanied by a feeling of fullness, they corresponded to an excess of endocranial yang. The first point to consider was BL-8, which clears endocranial yang. In this case, it brought quick relief. BL-7 would be the next point to consider if BL-8 had failed, as it is difficult to make a clinical distinction between the two.

The sweating, which had begun four years earlier, was mainly at night. It also occurred during naps. In the daytime, it was localized in the armpit. The patient could not say whether it was hot or cold sweating. It was abundant at night and had increased during the past year. Examining the overall condition of the patient was necessary to get a more precise idea of the etiology.

She was a young woman, but said that she felt tired. She was rarely cheerful or energetic and reported that this horrible fatigue was worse in the morning and had increased over the years. She did not suffer from sudden exhaustion during the daytime. The main causes of morning fatigue are stagnation of the Gallbladder qi, general stagnation of yin or of yang (corresponding to CV-4 or GB-25, respectively), or an insufficiency of the "morning audience" of the Lung (related to LU-1). In this case, yin stagnation seemed likely.

She was very sensitive to cold and often felt chilled to the bone, but reported occasional heat sensations in her head. Her sleep had been poor for a long time; she had difficulty falling asleep, but did not have nightmares. Sensitivity to cold contributed to the stagnation. Any generalized yin stagnation is accompanied by a leakage of yang, which explained the feelings of heat, the headaches and the insomnia. The leakage of yang increased and revealed the blockage of cephalic yang at BL-8.

She was an accountant, an orderly person, who smoked sixty cigarettes a day and paid little attention to her diet; she did not like meat or fruit. In the past six months, she had experienced pain in the knee joints. She did not report any cardiac or pulmonary symptoms, coughing, spitting or shortness of breath despite her tobacco addiction. She digested all foods well. She often had gas and had been constipated for a long time. Urination was normal. Her periods occurred every 28 days. She constantly had a white vaginal discharge. The mother of an eighteen-year-old son, she had given birth eight months before to a second child, whom she had spent three years trying to conceive. She had been bedridden for the last six months of the pregnancy. Three-and-a-half years before, she had miscarried. Her sexual relations were satisfactory. Apart from an appendectomy and breast plastic surgery, she did not report any significant surgical history. As she digested well and her periods were normal, the possibility that the Penetrating vessel was implicated was discarded.

As a child she had been sent to a boarding school where she stayed until the age of ten, at which time her father had died. She tried to escape the material and emotional difficulties of her childhood by marrying at the age of 17. She quickly became pregnant and then found herself alone with her son; she stayed alone for ten years. For the last several years, things had been better. Her deep and short pulses, as well as the tooth marks on the sides of the tongue, justify CV-4, which brought a very important improvement after two sessions. (It must be stressed that CV-4 is the convergence of three functions: it sets the yin in motion, it is the alarm point of the Small Intestine, and the Penetrating vessel.) This improvement increased with the following sessions. The headaches disappeared once BL-8 had been needled three times.

CV-17, a thoracic midline point, controls the culmination of qi and its distribution to the exterior, at the surface.

❖ Case History

A woman, age 50, came to see me about fatigue that had persisted for the last four years, or rather, for a tendency to fatigue. She awakened readily in the mornings but her endurance was limited. She chilled easily, slept well and did not sweat. She reported difficulty concentrating, became easily fatigued mentally, and had a slight deterioration of her eyesight. She had occasional sore throats, feelings of oppression, some tachycardia during effort, and for the last year especially, could no longer tolerate wearing her bra. These symptoms indicated a case of excess in the chest: any excess is aggravated by local pressure, as in this case, with the bra compressing the thorax. Her digestion was good, stools were regular and urination was normal; she was menopausal. She had never had any problems with menstrual periods or with pregnancy. There was nothing else of significance in her history.

The diagnosis was clear. It was a qi deficiency with an excess in the chest. So why was the qi that comes into the chest to be distributed throughout the body failing to circulate? The history showed us that this woman had been pursuing spiritual growth but lived with a man who was very strong, active and materialistic and who was opposed to this pursuit. She felt confined. I punctured HM-6, which controls the upper burner, and CV-17, which, in addition to being the alarm point of this burner, controls the externalization and distribution throughout the body of the thoracic qi. By the third session, there was a vast improvement.

■ AUTUMN

Autumn is harvest time. Here, the qi movements are internalization, disappearance of day yang with sunset and the appearance of night yin. It is related to the metal phase, the Lung and the Large Intestine. The alarm points here are LU-1 and ST-25.

LU-1, a lateral thoracic point, on the second rib, is the alarm point of the Lung, and is in charge, in humans, of the autumn harvest. For humans, harvesting includes eating and breathing. If there is no harvest, one cannot swallow (resulting in nausea or vomiting) or breathe (resulting in coughing). If the surface energies cannot be harvested into the trunk, "the feet, hands and face are swollen."[11] These phenomena offer a concrete illustration of how the autumn phase is occurring in us at all times.

ST-25, located on either side of the navel, midway between the upper (heavenly) and lower (earthly) halves of the body, is the alarm point of the Large Intestine. The name of this point is 天樞 *tian shu* or "Heavenly Pivot." It connects heaven and earth and, in the *Great Compendium of Acupuncture and Moxibustion*, it is said to be the alarm point of the middle burner and as such connects the upper with the lower. More specifically, in the autumn it receives; it harvests from the earth the influences that have descended from heaven.

❖ Case History

Mrs. P., age 71, came to see me in December 1998 for intense pain in her right knee that had appeared after a sprain in her right ankle. In fact, the incident had only been a triggering factor, because she had already had the same pains twice, one year and four years before. The pain was deep, in the joint, and radiating from the popliteal fossa, and aggravated by certain movements and by going down stairs. The knee was swollen and hot. It had already been aspirated twice, but the condition had returned. In addition, she had stiffness in the pelvis; she was constipated and urinated very little. Her digestion was slow and she had gained considerable weight in recent months although she had not changed her eating habits. The proximal pulses were superficial and deficient.

I had been treating this woman occasionally since 1994. She was small, slim, elegant, stylish, sensitive and impassioned, although she had no self-confidence and pursued many activities. These were both earthly delights and "spiritual seeking," although she did not manage to bring these down-to-earth activities and heavenly aspirations into harmony. Moreover, I had noted during her first visit that "heaven and earth need to be joined." Her symptoms at the time had been as follows: heartburn (treated with omeprazole); colitis with alternating constipation and diarrhea, aggravated by dairy products and raw vegetables; a frequent cold sensation in the lower abdomen; a hallux valgus; erratic pains; hypertension that was being treated; and a history of asthma between the ages of 18 and 42. At the time, I concluded that the *yang ming* (Stomach, Intestines) and *tai yin* (Lung, hallux valgus) needed to be connected. The aggravation caused by cold foods, the feeling of cold in the lower abdomen, the hypertension and even the asthma all showed that heavenly yang qi was not descending to the abdomen.

In 1998 I began by treating her knee locally with ST-35 and GB-31, which is often effective in cases of knee joint effusion. There was only a slight improvement so I decided to set aside the symptom, or rather, to include it in an overall picture of the person: heaven and earth must be married within humans, at *yang ming* and *tai yin*. I therefore chose a point on the *yang ming* channel that serves to bring heaven down to earth, ST-25. After two sessions, the knee pain disappeared. The intestines were also markedly better. A relapse three months later was healed in one treatment of the same point.

■ WINTER

In winter the earth no longer produces; it hides and stores up. The qi recedes to the inner reaches. The night (yin) climaxes while day (yang) begins to be born, like the seed in the ground that contains the future plant, or the first cell of a human being that contains the entire being. It is related to water phase, the Kidneys. The alarm points here are CV-3 and GB-25.

CV-3, a pelvic midline point, is the alarm point of the Bladder, and corresponds to the retreat of qi to the depths, to storing up and to the seed that germinates underground.

❖ Case History

A young woman, age 30, suffered from infertility. After an operation to remove a cyst from her right ovary, she had malodorous menstrual periods, pruritic discharges, burning sensations after intercourse, and stabbing pelvic pains that increased after bowel movements (a sign of deficiency). In addition, she was constipated, had difficulty holding urine in, often had red hands and feet, slept poorly, was sensitive to noise and was very tense, both physically and psychologically. Her adolescence was difficult and marked by a sexual assault. Her problems started after this attempted rape. These symptoms told me that her qi was not returning to the deepest recesses, the most yin areas in the true pelvis in the lower part of the trunk, in winter and, for this reason, the pelvic blood was stagnant and was not being drained. Beginning with the second session, puncturing CV-3 considerably improved all of these symptoms and enabled her to become pregnant.

GB-25, the alarm point of the Kidneys, located at the ends of the twelfth ribs, governs the winter movements of yang qi at midnight. If this qi is not put into motion in the pelvis, the result is low back pain that makes it difficult to stand for long periods of time, spasms in the lumbar region and hips as well as in the shoulders and back, diarrhea, flatulence, and dysuria.

❖ Case History

A woman, age 47, a sculptor who was massively built and strong, came to see me for migraines and fatigue. Her incapacitating headaches had begun during adolescence, occurring monthly or bimonthly, and were unilateral, occurring on either side of the skull, along the *shao yang* channel. They were intense, without any connection to menstrual periods, climate, cold, heat, or diet. They usually lasted 36 hours and responded poorly to various therapies. The etiology was unknown.

Her fatigue was physical (reduced strength and endurance), psychological (reduced drive), sexual (reduced desire), and intellectual (reduced concentration and memory). This suggested involvement of the Kidneys. The fatigue was primarily in the mornings; it was so intense on awakening that she often wondered how she could face the day. The problem had arisen insidiously and grown steadily worse.

In the history, I noted two cases of renal colic without any stones being seen on imaging studies. The Kidney pulses were deep. She was dedicated to her art and regretted her inability to have children. One point seemed indicated to me: GB-25. Located on *shao yang* (the pathway for headaches) and corresponding to the Kidneys, it spurs the movement of yang energies through the body, particularly in the morning. Puncturing this point monthly brought a rapid improvement in her migraines and fatigue: "You have set the power of my kidneys in motion," she astutely observed. Interestingly enough, in French the word for kidneys, *reins,* is used in numerous expressions referring to both the lower back as well as to power and wealth.

CHAPTER EIGHT

SYMBOLIC LANGUAGE OF CHINESE MEDICINE

MY APPROACH TO CHINESE medicine requires that we attempt to deeply penetrate and decipher this symbolic language, while simultaneously not lose sight of the medical perspective and the grounding and practical applications that it brings. This is what is at the base of my own approach to this medicine. It has become increasingly clear to me that, in order to gain an in-depth understanding of Chinese medicine, including clinical practice, we must first pursue our understanding of its symbolic underpinnings as far as possible. I have briefly discussed this issue in the Introduction.

What is a Symbol?

The word symbol comes from Latin *symbolus,* meaning symbol or creed (as the mark of a Christian), a sign, which in turn comes from the Greek *sunbolein* 'mark, token' from *sun-* 'with' plus *ballein* 'to throw.' These were tokens that were broken in half and given to people of the same group so that later, if necessary, they could recognize each other by fitting the halves together to make the coin whole again. It was used in other circumstances as well, such as a tablet split in half and used to enable an envoy form another country to be recognized. Its usage implies a movement in which one engenders two (broken into two) and returns to one, and therefore a relationship between the one, founder, and the many, manifest.

A symbol is complementary with myths (writing tradition) and rites (acted tradition). In Chinese I have learned that there are two characters for that which have a similar meaning. The first is 符 *fu,* which refers to a talisman such as those used in Daoist religious ceremonies. The second is 象 *xiang,* which, according to Wieger, means a "symbol, to symbolize, represent, resemble, appearance, and elephant" with a commentary that states it refers to the elephant's footprints.[1] The elephant is no longer there; it is not visible. *But the footprints tell us it exists and has passed this way.* As stated in Chapter 7 of the early Han work the *Huainanzi* (淮南子), "Long ago, before there was either heaven or earth, there was only symbol *(xiang)* but no form (行 *xing).*" This shows that symbols and form constitute an inseparable pair. Symbols and essences *(jing)* are the origin of forms. So symbols are the foundation of the life of the many, and forms are their manifestations.

Symbols link the visible and invisible, perceptible and imperceptible, and the concrete mechanisms of life to its foundational archetypes and laws. The world of symbols is therefore one of a mediating intermediary. It connects the plane of archetypes and of the fundamental laws of life and the natural order of the living with that of forms and of materialized beings. It enables us to understand in which forms a symbol manifests, such as an anatomical form, and, conversely, which symbols manifest as which forms, parts or organs of the body. Symbolic vision therefore adds a vertical dimension to the horizontal inventory of forms, structures and mechanisms of life: in this case, the body is also the incarnation of the archetypes. So the importance of symbolism is evident. The human body is an incarnation of archetypes; symbolic, traditional Chinese medicine reveals the traces of the archetypes in the human body.

SYMBOL IN CHINESE MEDICINE

In order to further our comprehension of Chinese medicine, we need to understand that this medical system uses a language that is primarily symbolic. What does this mean? Chinese medicine assumes that all living beings, whether they belong to the animal, vegetable, mineral, or human kingdoms, are subject to the same laws. Their structures, in various forms, embody the same principles and archetypes. Their relationships are governed by the same rules and regulations. Symbols are the bridge, the intermediary, between these principles, rules, basic laws, archetypes, and the infinite number of living structures and forms, each one being both universal (since they embody the same principles) and specific, singular (because each being is unique).

Major Symbols of Chinese Medicine and Their Clinical Applications

THE CLINICAL USEFULNESS OF THIS SYMBOLIC VIEW

This symbolic view can be both diagnostic and therapeutic, since it permits the linking of mechanisms and structures that otherwise have no apparent relationship, such as, for example, when they both come under the same symbolic designation as earth. My purpose is to apply all these symbols to the human body, its functions, structures, mechanisms, areas, and so on, all on psychological, diagnostic and therapeutic levels.

This symbolic method allows for establishing physiological and pathological relationships between areas, organs, structures and mechanisms which otherwise have no other links. It then allows us to understand and treat patients who could not have been treated otherwise. Let me cite a few examples to make things clear before we go deeper in this explanation. As far as the body areas representing heaven/earth are concerned, the skull and the thorax are related to heaven because they are situated at the top of the head and trunk. The face and the abdomen are further down and pertain to earth. The base of the skull and the diaphragm, the in-between structures, separate heaven from earth. Other examples concern the organs. The Lung above, being the roof of the organs, corresponds to heaven; the Kidneys below, the base, correspond to earth. The Heart corresponds to fire, and the Kidneys to water. The Stomach is more of the water type and the Gallbladder of the fire type.

Where will all of this lead us? First to some correspondences of heaven and earth, water and fire, and so on, that do not entirely match the traditional ones and can appear to be contradictory. For instance, I see a symbolic and physiological correspondence between the Lung (heaven) and the Kidneys (earth): numerous pulmonary diseases have their origin in the Kidneys and vice versa. Or, the air inhaled by the Lung (heaven) must descend from the thorax (heaven) to the pelvis (earth) and the Kidneys (earth) and then go up again with exhalation. The Heart fire descends to control the Kidney water and conversely the Kidney water ascends to control the Heart fire.

But it is also possible to relate areas partaking of the same symbolism, like the skull and the thorax, which correspond to heaven, and the face and the abdomen, which correspond to earth, and the base of the skull and the diaphragm, which separate heaven and earth. We shall see that there are often simultaneous "celestial" disorders of the skull and thorax, or of the "in-between," the base of the skull and the diaphragm. This is true regardless of whether a problem in one area induces a problem in the other or if they are both disturbed by the same factor.

In succession, I will examine the most important pairings:

- heaven/earth,
- heaven/human/earth triad
- water and fire
- entrances and exits, and comings and goings
- clear and turbid

Heaven and Earth

I will use a common approach to studying a symbol—determining the qualities that are attributed to it in Chinese tradition—in order to understand the corresponding functions and define the mechanisms that embody them in human beings.

Heaven is 天 *tian*, "the sky, firmament, the principle of heaven animating the universe, yang, nature, that which is natural, day, time, imperial." Earth here is 地 *di*,[2] "the earth, the principle of earth quickening the universe and corresponding to yin, the region, country, terrain, soil, place, situation, disposition, substance."[3]

Corresponding Qualities, Functions and Mechanisms

What are the qualities attributed to heaven and earth? Which are the resulting Chinese medicine functions and mechanisms? And how is this useful in practice?

- Heaven is vitality, activity, strength, and power. Earth is rest, receptivity, and docility.

- The natural order of the living, rules and law, are of the order of heaven, symbolized by jade. The warp and weft, the weave of all that embodies and realizes this order, rule, and law belong to the order of earth. Anything that defines a rule or establishes a law should be placed under the symbol of heaven. That which embodies and realizes these rules or laws is under that of the earth.

- A passage in the *Lie Zi* states that "The function of heaven is to give life and to cover. That of the earth is to give shape and to carry."[4] This means that which covers and protects is of the order of heaven. That which carries, supports, receives, contains, and embraces is of the order of earth. The mechanisms that contain an element of initiative, momentum, origin, or beginning are of the order of heaven; those that contain a response, a realization, or a completion come under the symbol of earth. For example, the sperm that induces conception is of the order of heaven; the egg that receives it and carries it to term over the nine months of pregnancy is of the order of earth. The catalyst of a reaction is of the order of heaven, and the resulting reaction is of the order of earth, because it is heaven that takes the initiative and earth that carries it out to completion. Heaven is creation, the masculine principle, the father, that which causes existence. Earth is fertility, nutrition (the cauldron), the feminine principle, the mother, that which causes growth. Heaven is that which gives life, that which takes the initiative in life. Earth is that which gives shape, that which has the capacity to give shape.

- The order of heaven and earth comprises the father and mother, and the paternal and maternal aspects in each person, whether they are man or woman. The father proclaims the law, the rules, and the limits; the mother nurtures. The father covers and protects; he causes existence. The mother carries, bears, and receives; she causes growth. While the father gives both a name as well as rules and limits, as adults, it is up to us to find our own rules, thus becoming our own father. Because a just law is both universal and personal (always yin-yang, complementary and not mutually exclusive), our personal rules are a personal interpretation, according to our individual nature, of the universal law.

TAI YANG AND TAI YIN

A channel located on the back, upon which we lean, in a way, is called *tai yang*; it represents the father and the ruler on this channel, an acupuncture point called the "Window of Heaven," BL-10. This helps us institute, adopt and learn our own set of rules and laws, to learn our own personal interpretation of these universal laws.

❖ Case History

A young man, age 28, consulted me for psoriasis and migraines that alternated between right and left, starting from the occiput and rising to the top of the skull, with wrenching pain that radiated along the nape of the neck. These migraines were clearly caused by a dysfunction in point BL-10. As a way of rebelling against his father, he had no profession; he did not know his vocation or even his own wishes. In his skin and at the point BL-10, his body had stored the memory of this difficulty with finding and actualizing his law, his rules and his place. Puncturing this point cleared up the migraines and psoriasis, and an understanding of the point's function helped him become aware of the meaning of his symptoms.[5]

Opposite *tai yang*, *tai yin* is the mother, earthly, which receives and nurtures and to which we return. A case history mentioned earlier, in the section on connecting vessels, represents this (*see* p. 108).

HEAVEN AND EARTH IN OUR MORPHOLOGY

Navel

Above the navel is heaven, below it is earth, and parallel with it is ST-25, the "Heavenly Pivot," that we will come back to and which plays the role of linking our heaven and earth (*see* Fig. 5).

Diaphragm

In the trunk, the diaphragm separates and unites the thorax, which is found above and is heavenly, and the abdomen, which is below and earthly. It separates and unites the abdomen and thorax, and therefore also everything that is of the order of instinct and feelings. In addition, it permits that which is pure and heavenly to rise to the Lung, Heart and brain and prevents that which is impure and earthly from rising. The diaphragm separates in order to reunite, filters in order to blend, and keeps the pure and the impure in their proper places: it has the function of maintaining wholeness, that is, the harmonious relationship among all the structures of a being.

❖ Case History

A 54-year-old man was torn between his mother, an ascetic and very pious woman, and his sister, a beautiful young woman in distress who only felt alive through pleasure and sensuality. These two highly contrasting women both called forth his protective instincts. But he could not reconcile within himself their two as-

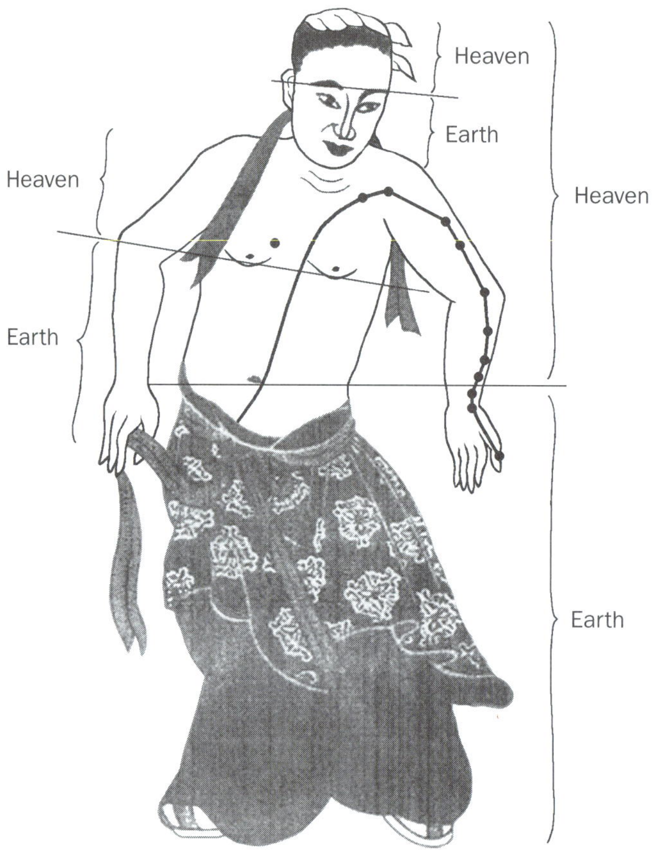

Fig. 5: Heaven & Earth in the Human Body

pects. The contraction in his diaphragm testified to this lack of communication within himself: he felt a tight band around the base of his thorax that made him feel like he was suffocating, prevented food from passing through the cardia of the stomach, and caused hiccups and aerophagy. Analytic psychotherapy and monthly or bimonthly acupuncture treatments with LI-6 to address the part of the body that had stored the memories of this pain helped him harmonize these two aspects of the feminine principle and liberated his diaphragm.

Base of the Skull

The base of the skull, between the top of skull and face, is of the same order as the diaphragm. It separates and unites the top of the skull and the face, heaven and earth, the intellect and feelings (through the seven orifices of the face), the rational and the affective, spiritual and emotional. Symbolically, it is analogous to the diaphragm, which separates and joins the thorax and abdomen. They are often disturbed at the same time. A case history from the previous section on the Yang Linking vessel demonstrates this (*see* p. 103).

Note the symbolic analogy between the diaphragm and the base of the skull, separating and uniting two areas of heaven and earth. The frequent symptomatic associations that can be explained by this analogy are clear. There is a perfect continuity, typical of acupuncture, between the archetype and the function, the symptoms that signal a disturbance and the corresponding points. Now we have a better understanding of the medical use of symbols. They allow us to link functions, zones and structures that have no apparent connection to one another, and to understand which archetypal disturbance, in this case either heavenly or earthly, is at the source of the imbalance.

LUNG AND ITS EARTHS

The Lung, which is the canopy of the yin organs, brings down the air that is inhaled, the qi and fluids; it is associated with the pure and the just. It purifies and clarifies the qi and fluids that come to it. It is also especially sensitive to injustice. These are all heavenly qualities.

The Lung, of the order of heaven, carries on a dialogue with various earths: those of the Large Intestine, Kidneys, and Spleen. Down below, the Large Intestine, which is paired with the Lung, receives the qi and information brought down by the Lung; it transmits and then sends them throughout the body (*Basic Questions,* Chapter 8). One point corresponds to this function, GV-3.

❖ Case History

A woman, age 31, who was bossy, rude in her speech and brusque in her manner, presented with skin allergies along with nasal and bronchial respiratory problems. Her symptoms seemed to be triggered by exposure to the sun. Her breathing was often shallow and superficial, especially at night. Her painfully tense neck, headache and red face evoked a circulatory and respiratory blockage of qi above the clavicles. This was probably due to poor Lung function, as the "roof of the viscera." I noted, moreover, secondary infertility after two pregnancies, premenstrual syndrome, and low back pain, both on rising and when standing: these symptoms made me think of a deficiency of qi in the lower part of the body, particularly at GV-3, which governs the Large Intestine and represents the "ground of the Lung." She was in great conflict with her mother, whom she described as being "rude and bossy." It seemed to me that she did not separate from her mother's qi and moreover had copied her way of being, without being aware of it. Three sessions with CV-20, reinforced with the GV-3, significantly improved her symptoms.

The Lung also interacts with the Kidneys in a heaven/earth relationship. According to Chinese medicine, "We are recreated (Kidneys) with every breath (Lung)." This dialogue appears at the alarm points (*see* p. 143) like LU-1 and GB-25. The Lung also has a heaven/earth relationship with the Spleen. Both of them resonate with *tai yin,* the mother who is receptive and nurturing, with respiration and with food. Lung and Kidneys, and Lung and Spleen, participate in maintaining life: they are traditionally linked to "the play of clouds and rain" that symbolizes the maintenance of life, including in and through sexual relations.

THREE POWERS

Man, in between heaven and earth, links, merges with and realizes both aspects in his specificity and originality, according to his essential nature (*xing*). The vocation of man is to link, merge with, realize and manage on a daily basis the heavenly and earthly functions, each one according to their specificity, since every individual is unique.

As we saw above, these three powers will enable us to establish a relationship between zones, structures, and functions that may appear to be unrelated but are associated with the same symbol. Moreover, the attributes of the archetype in question will lead us to determine the origin of the disease and guide us toward the right diagnostic and treatment plans. This helps us to determine the points that will act on all the symptoms and on the whole person.

CLINICAL APPLICATIONS

In morphological terms, the three powers are:

- For the entire body, the head, the trunk, and the lower limbs.
- The head is divided into three parts: the top of the skull, the upper part of the face including the eyes, nose and ears, and the lower part with the mouth and chin.
- The trunk also has three parts, with the thorax, the epigastrium above the navel, and the true pelvis below the navel.
- On the limbs, the shoulders, and hips are of the order of heaven, elbows and knees of man, and wrists and ankles of earth.
- The linkage of various zones of the body with these three powers implies that each region manifests the related properties. For example, the top of the skull is "a beginning (*yuan*),[6] impetus, initiative, or influence that pervades all and causes to prosper."

(*See* p. 4 for a case history of diarrhea involving this schema.)

❖ Case History

A woman, age 55, suffered from incapacitating knee pain that had been progressing for three years. The results of all her lab tests were normal and various treatments had been ineffective. I also noted some gastric disturbances with slow digestion, heartburn, nausea, intolerance of eggs, fats, chocolate and coffee, frequent allergic rhinitis and conjunctivitis. After two ineffective acupuncture

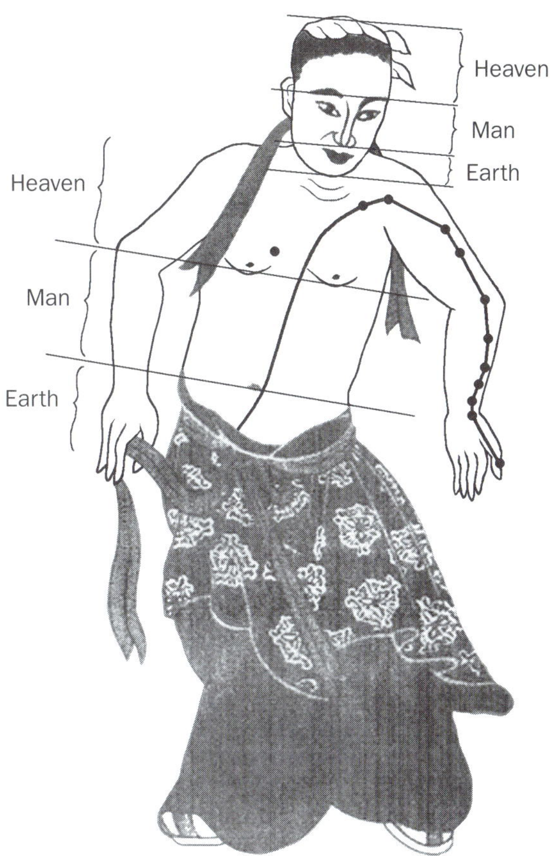

Fig. 6: Three Powers

sessions, I set aside the symptoms and observed that the three affected zones—the upper part of the face, epigastrium, and knee—all corresponded to man. I explained to her the symbolism of the three powers. She replied, "Despite my professional success and my three children, I have missed out on life, because I have not realized my femininity." Considering the extent of the digestive problems, I punctured two points that control the Gallbladder and Spleen, situated at the center of the territory: CV-11 and SP-6. Beginning with the second session, the symptoms diminished, including the knee pain, and were completely eliminated after the fourth treatment. Previously (see p. 153) I recounted a case of knee pain that was tied into the same symbolism and treated at ST-25.

Concerning the Organs

- The Lung, which is the "canopy of the yin organs," falls under the symbolism of heaven; the Kidneys, a seat and foundation, correspond to earth; the Heart and Spleen[7] at the center, to man.

- The Lung is the master of respiratory qi, which animates, circulates, covers, directs downward, diffuses and purifies.

- The Kidneys receive qi from the Lung and actualize, in the gate of vitality *(ming men)*. This is the passage from pre-heaven to post-heaven, from the invisible to the visible, from the formless to the formed, the "roots of the five organs." The Kidneys are the foundation for the spring and summer phases, for unfolding and prospering.

- The Heart and Spleen, in keeping with their human vocation, link and actualize. The Heart, on the side of unity, links, like the son of heaven, the three powers within us; as the "sovereign fire" it achieves unity in a being. The Spleen, turned toward the many, links the four limbs, and, as it controls the flesh, all structures, functions, cells and parts of the body. In its post-heaven aspect, it brings all transformations into action.

Triple Burner

Three locations, or levels, are attributed to the Triple Burner.[8] In fact, these are simply images that illustrate three functions.

- The upper burner is in the chest. It has the role of receiving the food and inhaled breath that will then be metabolized and transformed. In return, it receives the products of these transformations—the qi, blood, and fluids—which it distributes throughout the body, to warm and nourish it. As the beginning and end, it governs everything that it receives and places everything in circulation.

- The middle burner is in the epigastrium. It cooks, macerates, metabolizes, transports and extracts the essence of all that is consumed. It refines and accomplishes tasks.

- The lower burner is in the pelvis. It performs all the sorting, all the separation of the clear from the turbid in all ways, and assigns each to its proper place. It sorts, puts things in the proper place, keeps and eliminates.

The three burners manage the nutrition of a being. They correspond to heaven, man and earth.

The upper burner, linked to the Lung and Stomach, qi and blood, is related to ancestral qi *(zong qi* also known as gathering qi), which ensures that each individual, in relation to their ancestors, has a unique nature, disposition and purpose. Here, we are nourished by the Lung and Stomach, respiration and food, which produce qi and blood. Problems with the upper burner revolve around difficulties in being oneself or in having issues in relation to one's self.

❖ Case History

A 43-year-old woman was a top-level manager, single, with no children, and a practicing believer who was very oriented towards others. She suffered from eczema, allergies to cosmetics, intense cravings, circulatory problems in her extremities, waking at 3 a.m., menstrual periods that were very painful on the first day, thoracic anxiety and rare episodes of vertigo. She was shy, lacked self-confidence, and could not put herself first. Her pulses showed a deficiency in the upper burner, indicating her inability to live for herself. In fact, speaking of her own faith, she asked, "Am I free?" She found it very difficult to just be herself and understand that we have to live as both separate beings and as one with the One. Needling CV-17 brought about a significant somatic and psychological improvement.

The lower burner sorts, discerns and puts things in their proper place (e.g., it keeps or eliminates different things). It is linked with the primal source and origin *(yuan)*. Inability to connect with this primal source is the underlying cause of most problems in the lower burner. CV-7 is the alarm point of the lower burner. Located one unit below the navel, it is associated with hernial pain, pelvic pain radiating to the genitals or navel, hard and painful lower abdomen, urinary problems, genital itching or sweating, menstrual problems, infertility, post-partum problems (pain, continuous flow of dark blood), low back pain, hip and knee pain, and jumpiness and fear in persons who, in my experience, lack self-confidence. This point must not be punctured during pregnancy.

❖ Case History

Mr. G., age 46, consulted me for moments of fatigue with considerable energy fluctuations. His sleep was normal. This fatigue was accompanied by pains in the limbs, muscular trembling and a feeling of heaviness. It is worth noting that physical exercise tended to bring improvement. In addition, he reported some constipation, a burning sensation during urination, and recurring nasopharyngitis. His pulses were wiry. His tongue had a white coating.

He could not determine when these problems had begun as they were a part of a general physical and psychological malaise that had led him to begin psychotherapy three years earlier. He had a lot of energy in general, but felt scattered because of many diverse and chaotic needs.

Psychotherapy did him good, but he could not stop it for fear of relapsing.

This scattered and dispersed typology made me think of the Girdle vessel, but this cannot explain all of the signs. The Yin Linking vessel could have explained the energy fluctuations, but on a psychological level rather than on a physical one, which was not the case here.

As I continued the history, the patient told me that he had the feeling that he "was not eliminating toxins," which seemed plausible to me, since a toxic buildup could have produced the muscle pain and trembling, the nasopharyngitis (which could correspond to elimination attacks) and his low energy levels. It was interesting to see that toxin elimination through physical exercise brought improvement.

I decided to treat the alarm point of the lower burner, CV-7, and to add KI-4, the connecting point governing constipation and urinary dysfunction in the lower burner. There was a distinct improvement following the first session. By the third session, the improvement lasted a month, and then two months after the fourth session. This trend of increasingly marked and lasting improvement continued.

Of the order of man, the middle burner extracts essence in all ways, joins heaven and earth, and fulfills the natural dispositions of each person by conforming to their essence, nature and purpose. The middle burner, of the order of man, ensures the 'cooking and digestion' of foods, the extraction of essence from all forms of nourishment and the distillation of organic fluids. It has the role of fulfilling one's essential nature, including in persons. We can see that the role of the middle burner is, like that of man, to link heaven and earth in order to realize them in oneself. CV-12, at the midline epigastric area, halfway between the sternum and the navel, controls this process of the middle burner. ST-25, the second command point of the middle burner, located two inches to either side of the navel, and therefore vertically in the center of the body, links heaven and earth within us. A case history of knee pain, recounted earlier (*see* p. 153), used ST-25 in its treatment.

Regarding Qi, Blood, and Fluids

The Triple Burner produces qi, blood, and fluids. Qi corresponds to heaven, blood to man, and fluids to earth. Qi is differentiated into many types that handle all the necessary functions of life, just as heaven diversifies and is all-pervasive, "conferring upon each individual their own nature and purpose." Conversely, in keeping with its heavenly vocation, it gathers these various types of qi back into unity. The fluids, of the order of earth, imbibe, nourish and transform.

Within this scheme of things, blood, the medium of personification, embodies the symbolism of man achieving his essential nature in his specificity. In a way, qi, blood, and fluids are the post-heaven answer to the spirit, qi, and essence of the pre-heaven, indispensable to the emergence of life.

These correspondences enable us to look at certain disorders, such as headaches and migraines, according to their Chinese medicine attributions to qi, blood, or fluids.

Qi

❖ Case History

A woman, age 49, had suffered since adolescence from migraines that were of various types (wrenching, burning, and in different parts of the head), all of which were incapacitating. They were always preceded by a loss of voice (which told me to puncture one of the window-of-heaven points on the neck) and they had cleared up during her two pregnancies. She experienced conflict with her family, especially her father, and with her profession. She described herself as "illegitimate." In addition, I noted some digestive problems related to the Gallbladder, and extreme fatigue that was partially due to depression, and partially to overwork. The typical qi characteristics of these pains were consistent with this contradiction,[9] and this illegitimacy was with respect to a rule. Puncturing GV-20, at the top of the skull, which restores unity, SI-17 on the neck, which connects with the Gallbladder, and BL-48, a Gallbladder point related to the father, brought about a considerable improvement after six sessions.

Blood

❖ Case History

A 72-year-old-man said his life was "a failure, apart from his profession," and complained of pulsatile headaches alternating with ophthalmic migraines. In addition to his bloated face, his other symptoms also pointed to the blood: hypertension, hemorrhoids, and intensive congestion of the face under the influence of heat or alcohol consumption. He had had surgery for a right inguinal hernia. He was sensitive, emotional, an insomniac, and easily moved to tears. These symptoms suggested a Conception vessel deficiency and a blood disorder; it was as if he had been unable to assume (Conception vessel) the realization (blood) of an important side of his life. CV-2 and KI-23 proved highly beneficial.

Fluids

Fluid pathology can cause dehydration, edema or phlegm. This is an area in which acupuncture shows the greatest effectiveness. The reader is referred to page 59 for a case history.

The Extraordinary Vessels

The extraordinary vessels are also organized according to heaven/man/earth.

The Penetrating vessel, the central vertical vessel,[10] called the standing man, is established between heaven and earth, between the Governing and Conception vessels, which it links, integrates and completes, as it reaches for the fullness of a being.

The Girdle vessel, which is horizontal and located at the waist, girds our loins and guides us, like a compass, pointing us to our polar star, our psychic and spiritual north, the mountaintop that we aspire to reach. It links, integrates and completes the Linking and Heel vessels. The first of these, heavenly, distinguishes our yin and yang, manages our space, and therefore our selfhood and individual identities. The Heel vessels, rooted in earth, marry our yin and yang, including our femininity and masculinity, and manage our time and therefore our otherness.

CV-1, the origin of the Penetrating vessel as a central vessel, corresponds to the being established between heaven and earth. After puncturing this point I often hear patients say, "I am really living in my body again, I am beginning to exist, I feel profoundly reawakened." (*See* p. 90 for a case history involving this point.)

Water and Fire

QUALITIES ATTRIBUTED TO THESE TWO SYMBOLS

From various texts, in particular the *Book of Changes*, I have chosen the phrases that seem to best illustrate these qualities.

- Water[11] is linked to the origin of life, where all the matrices of form are found.
- Fire, heat, and light distinguish, enlighten, illuminate, discern, and separate, for example, from an enduring principle.
- Water can take all forms, from ice to vapor to rain, which it supports and maintains.
- Fire acts upon and can transform forms.
- Water, powerful and omnipresent, is the place and the source of transformations.
- Fire gives impetus to and induces transformations.
- Water, a hidden, invisible foundation, is an origin, matrix, and essence.
- Fire is an unfolding, a visible and palpable expression.

THEIR FUNCTIONS

The Water/Fire pair is an agent of transformation and change. When emerging into life under the influence of water and fire, each individual, distinguished from the indistinct, emerges from the undifferentiated, from chaos. Fire acts first: it separates, because the role of fire is to "separate from an enduring principle." Next comes water, which is origin, matrix, infinite possibility, and the primal origin of birth and life. In human beings, this involves the Kidneys and the Heart.

The Kidneys, under the symbol of water, are the matrix of all forms of creation. Moreover, a being is not created only at the time of conception, but with every new breath. Each one receives an order, a mandate (*ming*), to be created and recreated, between the Kidneys, between the second and third lumbar vertebrae, in a place known as *ming men*.

The Heart, of the order of fire, is the mirror of spirit. Spirit is primordial, original, and, by definition, expands in all directions. It is everywhere, in all places: it is at the origin of the life of the universe as well as that of every cell in our bodies. When an individual being becomes distinct, the spirit that is cosmic and universal is reflected on the mirror of their Heart; it becomes their spirit, and then expands throughout their body and radiates life. This mechanism is of the order of fire, or more precisely, comes under the symbolism of fire. It separates, so that the universal becomes the particular or personal.

There are two functions that maintain the life of this distinct individual being:

- That of their nourishment (food, respiration, affective, intellectual and sensory needs, etc.) with the Triple Burner, and the yin and yang organs, in particular by the Stomach and Gallbladder.

- Their perpetuation (with each breath) and that of the species is ensured primarily by the extraordinary organs and extraordinary vessels.

MECHANISMS THAT BEST EMBODY WATER AND FIRE IN HUMANS

In this section we will review the concepts discussed above in terms of other aspects of the body. Here they are laid out so as to put them in relation to the symbolic functions of water and fire.

Why should we attach so much importance to symbols? Primarily because Chinese medicine uses a symbolic language to describe the wonderful architecture of life and therefore of human beings. To optimally access this vision and its clinical applications, we have to utilize this symbolic language. Furthermore, in terms of understanding symptoms, this view provides a supplementary perspective and can sometimes be used to relate the mechanisms that apparently have no connection, thereby to better understand these patients and to treat them with more precision and efficiency. For example, the symbolic function of fire is to distinguish, illuminate, discern and separate; consequently, fire drives transformations. We know that the Heart discerns and illuminates when the Gallbladder decides and so they therefore drive transformations. These two mechanisms (their channels are part of a midday-midnight couple) are linked here by the symbol of fire. Simultaneous disruption of the Gallbladder and the Heart can have its origin in the loss of one of the symbolic functions of fire, as an inability to separate. When that occurs, we must treat this inability in order to treat these organs. Of course, there is no set formula on how to accomplish this; it depends of the context, the person's history, and so on.

Kidneys and Heart

In Chinese medicine, only the Kidneys are considered to be double organs; this is not so in the case of the Lung.[12] The Kidneys are called "double" because "like the original Chaos, dual in nature, they contain the two cosmic forces and, like Chaos, they are where life emerges."[13] They are in charge of the creative functions that require two parents, a father and a mother, yin and yang, heaven and earth, to unite their essence in order to conceive a being.

The Heart is the son of heaven and the mirror of spirit, as we saw above. Their relationship is essential, like that of water and fire, which temper one another.

❖ Case History

Mrs. M., age 51, was simultaneously very depressed and excited, complaining that she was afraid of everything, suffered from phobias, had constant insecurity, thoracic anxiety with agitation and tachycardia, and insomnia with difficulty falling asleep and nightmares. She was talkative, explaining that she was depressed but determined to fight her way out of it, which is what she had been doing for at least 15 years. Although she had been married for five years to a man who was profoundly gentle and affectionate, her life prior to then had been difficult, both during her childhood and during a first marriage, in which she had given birth to a child with birth defects. She said that she had felt very lonely until the last five years. Her childhood had been marred by violence, particularly from her father.

Physically, this small but sturdy-looking woman said that since adolescence, she had periodically suffered from painful, liquid diarrhea, burning pain in the bladder with frequent urination; white vaginal discharges without itching; some low back pain, connected with these episodes, that had occurred since adolescence without any apparent cause due to food, weather or psychological factors. Her menstrual periods were normal and her sex life was variable but often good over the last five years. She had the one child already noted; her pregnancy had been normal. She did not want to have more children, nor had her circumstances been in favor of more children. Without any other specific issues in her history, everything else appeared to be normal. The tip of her tongue was red. The proximal pulses were faster and stronger than the distal pulses.

We note that some symptoms were pelvic (diarrhea, bladder pain, vaginal discharges, and low back pain). On the other hand, the tachycardia, insomnia with nightmares and red tip of the tongue were evidence of an issue with Heart fire. The psychological symptoms arose from both categories. On the one hand, she suffered from fear, phobias, and insecurity, while on the other hand there was depression, agitation and anxiety and talkativeness. We know that fear can block the Kidneys' qi in the pelvis, resulting in a disconnection between the Kidneys (with pelvic symptoms) and the Heart (with thoracic symptoms). There was an excess of Heart fire: it was not being tempered by the water of the Kidneys.

That the proximal pulses (pelvis) were stronger than the distal pulses (thorax) suggested that there was a pelvic blockage of the Kidney qi. Point GV-5, located below the spinous process of L1, causes the qi to rise from the Kidneys.

In this case, the best point for tempering, liberating and unblocking the Heart fire is CV-15. I punctured this on her third visit, after starting with two treatments to release the Kidney qi. The first two sessions were two weeks apart. There were distinct signs of improvement in the Kidneys. With the third treatment, which included CV-15, the cardiac symptoms began to improve as well.

Maintenance of Life with Nutrition

The Triple Burner is the leading mechanism in charge of nourishing a being. It is a function that, as it says in the *Classic of Difficulties,* No. 25, "has the name but no form." The 17th-century text, *Thread Through Medicine,* states that the ministerial fire is at the behest of the gate of vitality, which to us means that it is something like the "minister of the gate of vitality," mediating between the gate of vitality and the body, it is simultaneously fire ("burner") and also "pathways of water" so it can be seen as a cauldron in which water boils under the influence of fire and generates vapor, or qi. It controls the mechanisms that ensure our nutrition. The alarm point of the Triple Burner is CV-5, on the midline, at two units below the navel. We will return to it shortly. Its associated point is BL-22, located laterally two units from GV-5, the pivot point, the mediator that causes the qi to rise from the Kidneys. At the same height, at a distance of four units, is the point BL-51, which controls lactation, as well as the nourishing mediation between mother and child. Note the "mediating" relationship of these three points.

Gallbladder and Stomach Participate in the Same Symbolism

In the middle regions, the Stomach is on the side of water, while the Gallbladder is on the side of fire. The Stomach receives, cooks and digests food, and is the locus and source of transformations, so it is of the order of water. It is the sea of water and grains and provides for the entire body, thus making the *yang ming,* according to Chapter 44 of *Basic Questions,* "the sea of all the yin organs and yang organs." Thus, the qi of the five organs is always blended with the qi of the Stomach and cannot act alone. It is the sea of qi, blood, and all the yin organs. Together with the Spleen, it is in charge of the granaries. With its affinity for the Kidneys and water, it is the source of qi for the Kidneys. It is in opposition to Heart fire: an excess of Heart fire can cause a Stomach ulcer.

❖ Case History

Mr. L., age 23, told me that for about five years he had been suffering episodes of intense fatigue for no apparent reason. These lasted several weeks or several months. The episodes occurred gradually and he then felt drained and worn out, which drove him to conserve his strength to the best of his ability. He tried not to speak too much or make too many gestures, and he kept his activity to a minimum. Yet however little energy he spent, his condition worsened very quickly, both on a psychological level (when he had worries or had to concentrate) and on a physical level (when he practiced physical exercise, sport or had sexual intercourse). He felt better in bed and when resting. This fatigue was obviously linked to an essence deficiency.

It is a deficiency because the condition is aggravated by the least effort and improved by rest. A fatigue of an excess type is aggravated by rest and improved by physical exercise; a fatigue of a stagnation type occurs in the morning and gradually lessens during the day and disappears in the evening.

It is a deficiency of essence because of his difficulties with concentration and the aggravation of the fatigue following intercourse.

Other symptoms also occurred during these episodes:

- dull headaches with a sensation of fullness in the head, especially at work
- an aversion to noise of any kind and to bright lights
- pronounced difficulties in concentrating without particular memory issues
- slight depressive episodes with a need for company, sadness and gloomy thoughts
- an aggravation of all these symptoms by alcohol.

All of this suggested that another factor was involved, namely, an excess of yang above, especially in the head (headache of the excess type, aversion to noise, light and heat).

Moreover, he reported:

- digestive problems: constipation (he also had a few episodes of diarrhea due to emotional stress, e.g., before he took an exam), slow digestion with post-prandial fatigue, a fairly frequent burning sensation and cramps in the stomach, difficulties in digesting starchy foods
- a slight loss of hearing and sexual problems.

When I saw him, Mr. L. was a first-year university law student because he had failed the competitive exams that would have allowed him to go to the more prestigious schools. He was naturally anxious and worried, tried to hide his timidity, acknowledged he was meticulous, precise and methodical (he came to my practice with a well-written list of his symptoms).

His childhood was a happy one, and so was his adolescence. After minor troubles at school initially, he got high grades until he was in tenth grade. At that time, he changed high schools and realized that he was just an average student, which he could not face.

I thought a Stomach disturbance was the origin of his digestive problems, with difficulty digesting starchy food and stomachaches, which are typical *yang ming* signs, and can lead to essence deficiency: "the Stomach is the sea of water and grains" (*Basic Questions*, Chapter 33).

He also showed Kidney signs: hearing problems, depressive episodes, recent sexual difficulties. The Kidney disorder was then secondary to the Stomach deficiency. The relationship between the Stomach and the Kidneys is well known. Both pertain to water and both are the root of the five yin organs, as the Kidneys are the root of production of the five organs and "the five organs all receive qi from the Stomach" (*Systematic Classic of Acupuncture and Moxibustion*, Chapter 1).

I needled two points on the external branch of the leg *tai yang*, BL-50 (Stomach) and BL-52 (Kidneys). The function of most of the points on that branch is to store up the essence and spirit of the corresponding organs. An improvement was noticed after the third session and the symptoms had disappeared after the sixth treatment.

The Gallbladder in the middle regions is of the order of fire. It has the role of taking the initiative, starting the process of transformation (including but not limited to digestion). It ensures that these occur in the right time and place, like the emperor who initiates the beginning of the year in the east in the spring, bringing together the corresponding time and space. It is the only 'pure' yang organ that has no contact with food, and is among the extraordinary organs, which serve to perpetuate existence. The Gallbladder and Heart, both of the order of fire, are strongly related in terms of physiology, pathology, and their midday-midnight pairing. (*See* p. 37 for a case about headaches and digestive problems.)

We note that initiative and decision are related to the fire of impulse, which initiates a process that separates one from a previous state.

Maintenance of Life: the Perpetuation of Life by the Six Extraordinary Organs

The six extraordinary organs in charge of perpetuating human beings and the species include "the brain and marrow, bones and vessels, Gallbladder and the gestational envelopes." In each of these pairs, one organ is placed under the symbol of water (marrow, bones and gestational envelopes) and the other is placed under that of fire (brain, vessels, and Gallbladder).

The pair of Gallbladder/gestational envelopes illustrate this relationship. The Gallbladder decides, in the sense of "cutting" through indecision. It separates things and sets them in motion. It is responsible for all beginnings, including the beginning of life at the time of conception, in that first moment of gestation where a being becomes separated, in the midst of the indistinct, from an enduring principle. As we have seen, the mechanism that distinguishes a being from the midst of chaos, and that begins a life, is of the order of fire. The Gallbladder, which separates and initiates, is related to this initial moment, so I place it under the symbol of fire. A disruption of this particular function of the Gallbladder results in functional infertility, an inability to gestate. BL-48 corresponds to this function.

The gestational envelopes, which are the place of all transformations, are of the order of water. They are controlled by the point CV-5, and are not limited to the uterus; they comprise all types of gestation carried out by anyone, which all involve the same mechanisms, in different ways. For clinical purposes, it is connected with infertility, sexual assault, abortion, etc. We have already seen this point as the alarm point of the Triple Burner. It governs the nutrition and perpetuation of the being. We can see that it is a foundation stone, as its name suggests: *shi men*, or "stone door."

(*See* p. 68 for a case history using CV-5 in this way.)

EXITS AND ENTRANCES, GOINGS AND COMINGS

Exits and Entrances

The word 出 *chu*, to exit, be born, or to engender, is etymologically a young plant that emerges from the earth and begins to spread out.[14] The word 入 *ru*, to enter, go into, or to disappear, is "that which penetrates from the exterior to the interior."

This pair is connected with life and death. In fact, there is a traditional Chinese expression that refers to "exiting into life, entering into death." *Exiting into life* means to emerge into a visible form, to have form, an appearance, a name, after becoming distinct amidst the chaos. *To enter into death* is to no longer have a form, a name; it is to return to being without form, to being without name, to the indistinct.

The entrances and exits are governed by a mechanism called the corporeal soul, linked to the Lung, respiration, and to the embodiment of qi. The corporeal soul is the autumnal function that causes qi to be embodied in a tangible form as it exits into life, and to disperse as it enters death, when it returns to being without form. The corporeal soul is connected with the Lung, to the breath in the space between heaven and earth that permits the condensation, transformation and circulation of qi. The points that correspond to it—BL-13 and GV-12—according to Chamfrault and Soulié de Morant, include the symptomatology of "a desire to die or to kill." When a part of a being's qi that is allotted for their embodiment cannot accomplish this, it turns against itself with its purpose of life or death. This explains the desire to die or to kill, accompanied by psychological or pulmonary symptoms.

Which are the functions or points related to the corporeal soul? The Lung, its channel and points, its paired arm *yang ming* channel and its points; ST-25, the alarm point of the Large Intestine, and, according to the *Great Compendium of Acupuncture and Moxibustion,* the abode of the corporeal and ethereal souls; and, according to Soulié de Morant, ST-37, which treats the corporeal soul while ST-39 treats the ethereal soul.

Below is a case illustrating the relationship between the arm *yang ming*, the corporeal soul and pregnancy.

❖ Case History

Mrs. B., age 49, was a literature teacher. To outward appearances she was calm but there was some sort of repressed violence in her eyes. She complained of insomnia and fatigue. She was stocky, muscular, and spoke with a weak voice. She often suffered from hoarseness and throat problems and was prone to frequent pharyngitis and laryngitis.

Depending on the day, she either had problems falling asleep or woke up at three in the morning. Her sleep was light and she would wake at the slightest noise. She repeatedly dreamed that she was flying in the air.

This dream showed that one type of energy was not descending; perhaps it was Lung or Heart qi, or the energy of one of the three yang. The empty proximal pulses and the full pulses at KI-3 confirmed this. Had there been a deficiency below, both of these pulses would have been empty, regardless of the etiology.

Mrs. B felt that her fatigue was not normal and could not be explained by her insomnia, much hard work (she was preparing for the highest competitive exam for teachers in France), her psychoanalysis, which was very demanding, or by the problems she had with her 12-year-old daughter. This fatigue, mainly physical, was more intense in the morning and was aggravated by her (usually heavy) periods and accompanied by a sensitivity to cold and by hypotension with some dizziness. She rarely had significant sweating during the day or night.

A yang or qi deficiency seemed plausible. If it were blood deficiency, she would have had a pale complexion, nocturnal sweating and scanty periods.

What was the significance that the fatigue was worse in the morning? Roughly, either a disturbance of the "morning audience" of the Lung, a disturbance of the Gallbladder, which governs all beginnings, or a disturbance of the initial movement of the yin (CV-4) or of the yang (GB-25).

She was both painfully distended and yet had no urge to pass stools; she had no urinary symptoms. Her periods, every 35 to 40 days, were heavy, painful and tiring. On the other hand, she digested well all sorts of food and drink. She also noted a recent tendinitis of the left thumb, located along both the *tai yin* and *yang ming* channels, a frequent pain on the medial side of the left leg, seemingly on the foot *shao yin*, and rarely, lower back pain.

Psychologically, although she wanted to live, socially and even spiritually, she did not know where she stood. Her everyday life was a burden to her. She was not correctly related to her own body, which she did not know well, and it was difficult for her to be tuned in to her sensations. Spontaneously, she said that she was overly sensitive to injustice. Often feeling insecure and not properly protected by her father, she had sometimes been "flirting with death." Her anxiety attacks, either felt in the throat or the solar plexus, had been decreasing since she had started her psychoanalysis.

An unwanted child, the pregnancy of her mother had been difficult and the first months of her life as a baby had not been easy. Her mother had told her of a serious accident during the seventh month of her pregnancy that gave her quite a shock. This general picture pointed to a disrupted communication with the corporeal soul because of the combination of her failed relationship with her body and her sensations, her permanent flirting with death, and above all of her difficulties in "exiting into life."

The Lung or its channel was not involved for there were no signs of organ or channel disorders, and the thumb pain overlapped the arm *yang ming* and arm *tai yang*. Many things spoke in favor of the arm *yang ming* channel, including the intestinal disorders and the foot *shao yin* impairment, its paired channel in a midday-midnight relationship. For me, the arm *yang ming* is linked to what precedes birth, that is, pregnancy. In fact, this patient, an unwanted child, described the difficult pregnancy of her mother, with difficult moments during the seventh month, and said that she had "difficulties in exiting into life." This convinced me to treat this channel. I chose the well point, LI-1, which holds, like a germ, the whole evolution of the arm *yang ming*. The improvement was obvious right after the first session, with the patient having two dreams about resurrection! It was confirmed after the three following sessions, respectively one, three, and six months later. On several occasions, she used the word "resurrection."

CLEAR/CLOUDY OR PURE/IMPURE (JING/ZHUO)

This is a pair about sorting, distinguishing and separating. In this context there is no inherent superiority to the clear or pure (*jing* 淨) nor inherent inferiority to the turbid or cloudy (*zhuo* 濁) as they are two sides of the same coin. The importance lies in their interrelationship.

This pair assigns things to their proper places. As the Daoist classic *Liezi* states, "The clear, light qi rises and forms heaven; the turbid, heavy qi descends and forms earth; the middle qi forms man."[15] Inevitably, we are constituted of the clear and the turbid, which in some contexts can be considered pure and impure. The important point is to keep each in its proper place, the pure above and within, the impure below and without. Pathology does not reside in the existence of clear and turbid, but in the fact that they are not in their proper place, for example, that the turbid is above or that the clear is on the outside. This pair governs the exchanges between distinct elements. In a human being, the pure qi is absorbed, or retained; the turbid qi is channeled to the next sorting point or toward the outside. The clear qi rises to the thorax, where the Lung and Heart reside, and to the brain. The turbid qi descends to the Stomach, Intestines and Bladder, to the lower orifices.

The mechanisms categorized under the symbolism of clear and turbid sort, distinguish, place and exchange. These structures are the lower burner (responsible for sorting), the Gallbladder (the only pure yang organ), and the Small Intestine (in charge of separating liquids and solids in food, "water and grain," and, in nutritional terms, the clear from the turbid).

The diaphragm is also emblematic of this pair. It separates and unites the abdomen and thorax, and therefore also everything that is of the order of instinct and feelings. In addition, it permits that which is pure and heavenly to rise to the Lung, Heart and brain, and prevents that which is impure and earthly from rising. The diaphragm separates in order to reunite, filters in order to blend, and keeps the pure and the impure in their proper places: it has the function of maintaining wholeness, that is, the harmonious relationship between all the structures of a being. For an example, see the case discussed in the section on the diaphragm above (*see* p. 161).

CHAPTER NINE

DIAGNOSIS AND TREATMENT

Causes of Disease

The seven emotions and perverse qi are seen as the causes of disease in Chinese medicine. To me these are related to the combination of heredity (the container), a history of trauma and suffering (which fill the vase), and external aggressions (which make it manifest).

MY EXPERIENCE

Practicing acupuncture has taught me to observe that we have two types of memory, psychic and somatic, that record all of our experiences—pleasure, pain, trauma, anxiety, suffering, etc.—in a constant dialogue beginning at the time of conception. It is not psychosomatic in the sense that our physical symptoms are caused by our psyche. The body itself is a memory and our symptoms are its language. The body is constantly conversing with the psyche. Acupuncture has two things to offer here: an original perspective for interpreting this body language and the means to treat the parts of the body where these memories have been stored. Scars will remain, of course, because one cannot undo the past, but they will be less painful. Furthermore, this pain will become "unstuck" from the places to which it has adhered so that it becomes accessible to the psyche. The ideal treatment is one that addresses both types of memory, for example, a combination of psychoanalysis and acupuncture. Such a combination makes it possible to transform this unproductive dialogue into a productive one and may lead to a lasting cure in some chronic cases.[1]

Here is an example of this body memory.

❖ Case History

A 52-year-old man came to see me for intense pain in his right hip, localized in the groin and in the greater trochanter, that was incapacitating and unrelenting since its appearance 17 months before. He was quite surprised at this because he had never been sick. All of the tests had been negative and all treatments had been ineffective. He had not experienced any trauma, either physical or emotional, in the preceding months. Considering the results of the tests, I decided to immediately look at it from an acupuncture point of view. I did not find anything that could explain the pain. I was perplexed, and at the end of the visit, a phrase came to mind: "The hip is the place where adolescent energies are concentrated." I quoted this to him. "You've found it!" he cried. "When I was 14, my parents, who had seemed to get along up to that point, when through a very intense conflict, including physical violence. They split up. Neither one of them wanted to keep me. They gave me to a single aunt, who really loved me, but who was a bigot and could not give me any guidance through my emerging sexuality. This aunt died three weeks before the pains appeared."

His body had remembered his adolescent suffering in the corresponding place; he spoke when an event reminded him of this difficult time. Apart from understanding what had happened, puncturing the point that corresponds to adolescence, GB-29, cleared up the pain in 48 hours. Here we can see the extraordinary continuity of acupuncture: one point provided an effective response to this suffering.

This case history seems to illustrate what acupuncture and, more generally, Chinese medicine can contribute to the West in the 21st century. Our bodies remember our entire lives, from the moment of conception. This expresses itself in different ways, including symptoms. Acupuncture provides an original way of reading this language of the body. In addition, because of the points, it gives us a way to dialogue with these places of suffering. When doing so, "The symptom is no longer just an obstruction to be released, or a wound to be healed, but a memory to be recollected and, above all, an invitation to turn towards the future and realize your potential."[2]

IMPORTANT ETIOLOGIES

Except in cases of serious deformity, heredity merely defines weaknesses, a potential for disease that may or may not end up occurring.

Aggression, Stress and Psychological Suffering

These are what Chinese medicine refers to as the seven emotions: elation, anger, sadness, pensiveness, melancholy, fear, fright. Any psychological attack or emotion that is excessive or repeated is liable to create an obstruction or diversion of the qi (that is to say, of a function or information) in certain parts of the body, which are different for each individual according to heredity (weaknesses), the type of suffering, and the period in which it occurs. This obstruction or stagnation begins at an organ or channel but its manifestation can become complicated depending on the various pairings of the channels (e.g., interior/exterior, midday/midnight) or relationships among the organs, or sufferings or other aggressions suffered subsequently. At first it can lead to functional disturbances; if the imbalances remain untreated, it can progress to organic lesions.

How can we protect ourselves? First, by causing our qi to circulate harmoniously, regulating our functions and stimulating our defenses (*wei qi*) with such treatments as acupuncture, *taiji*, or *qigong*. It is also important, in my experience, to understand where, how and when we are fragile.

❖ Case History

An important captain of industry, who was being treated for overwork, seemed impervious to anxiety, even in the midst of major conflict. One day he asked me for an emergency visit. "I am ashamed. I am very worried about a silly little thing. I cannot seem to overcome this anxiety that ties my stomach in knots and keeps me awake, all because of a registered letter sent by a neighbor woman, threatening to have two of my trees cut down because they are hanging over her lawn. It's ridiculous!" I asked him if this reminded him of a painful event. "Yes," he replied, "It's strange! When I was young we were very poor. My father, an alcoholic, did not work most of the time. The bailiff would often show up to seize what little property we owned; he would regularly threaten to seize the tree from our courtyard, a precious place where I always took refuge to dream of better days; this utterly terrified me." We all feel strong until the moment some event touches one of these weak spots within, no matter how minor it may be: then it can be an opportunity to become strong through better self-knowledge.

Other External, Bacterial or Viral Attacks

Traditional Chinese medicine combines these under the description of pathogenic climatic energies such as wind, heat, cold, dryness and dampness. But it is, above all, a matter of how humans adapt to their natural milieu and its variations and stressors. Clearly, wind and heat and so forth may be excessive and thereby harmful. But in most cases they are not inherently pathological. They only become so when humans do not know how to defend or adapt themselves against such excesses or insufficiencies. Apart from cataclysmic events, they need to be able to adapt to all climatic variations. In Chapter 1 of *Basic Questions* the sages of ancient times are said to have emphasized timely avoidance of the pernicious effects of exhaustion and "robber" winds and, through calmness and concentration, to maintain one's natural respiration in a docile state and to contain one's spirit within. This is the way to be immune to disease. These ancient sages are not people who were living thousands of years ago: they are within each one of us, in the depths of our very being.

Here we are basically being told of our responsibility in all events, and of our necessary capacity for adaptation and anticipation. There is no use in accusing the wind or viruses, bacteria, other agents, or fate. Of course, there are attacks that are so intense and sudden that they overwhelm our defenses and anticipation, but these are rare.

Take note: sometimes, especially in the spring, a season when the body cleans itself, it is necessary to distinguish between a viral attack and the elimination of toxins in the pulmonary, intestinal and urinary systems. The symptoms are often similar. Those suggesting elimination are excretions (sweat, urine, and stool) that are especially foul-smelling and a relatively low fever around 38°C. It is important to recognize this situation because, in cases of elimination, the wrong action would be to prescribe antibiotics (which would bring more toxins into the body); instead, one should favor elimination of the toxins through herbal therapy and acupuncture. LR-10 is often a useful point.

Lifestyle

"The people of high antiquity, those who knew the *Dao,* modeled themselves after yin and yang, conformed to the calculations. Their eating and drinking were moderate, they rose and rested with regularity, and did not wantonly overwork. Therefore they were able to keep their form and spirit together and exhaust the years [given to them] by heaven so that they did not pass on until they had spent one hundred years." (*Basic Questions,* Chapter 1)

Lifestyle affects the "nutritive and protective" qi and therefore our immunity. Indeed, the quality and integrity of these energies depend on it. Reckless, prolonged overwork, for example, results in the exhaustion of the nutritive and protective qi and, as a result, aside from fatigue, it diminishes one's defenses against external stressors. In the same manner, extreme or repeated anxiety attacks weaken our system of defense; thus the importance of acquiring good psychological balance, peacefulness and the ability to keep a distance from what happens.

Conclusions

It is necessary, on a diagnostic level, to take into account all of these different factors such as heredity, memories of painful moments, humiliations, etc. On a therapeutic level, we must understand that it is indispensable to provide support to each patient and help them to protect and maintain themselves both physically and mentally, unless their somatic and mental resources have been overwhelmed. This goes against the prevailing trend of doctors who tend not to trust the defensive capacities of the patient and therefore systematically prescribe antibiotics or psychoactive drugs.

Clinical Examination

EMPTINESS AND THE MEDICAL CONSULTATION

Like yin and yang, emptiness or the void is a notion and reality that has profoundly influenced me.[3] As emphasized by François Cheng, "Emptiness, in correlation with other notions such as vital breaths [qi] and yin-yang, is without doubt the most original and the most constant affirmation of a dynamic and holistic vision of life that ever came out of China."[4]

Emptiness is fundamental to Chinese tradition. It is an essential condition for life and its guarantee. According to Chapter 4 of the *Daodejing*, "The Way is empty." Its importance is reflected in its frequent evocation, through words such as 虛 *xu* (emptiness/deficiency), 無 *wu* (nothingness), and 空 *kong* (emptiness, void). These are concepts that appear not only in ancient texts such as the *Daodejing*, *Zhuangzi*, and *Huainanzi*, but also in those by contemporary writers such as François Cheng of the French Academy. Moreover, their importance is confirmed by modern physics. As Klein writes, "The Void is not empty, it contains energy. ... The Void thus appears as the basic substance of matter, which contains the potentiality of existence and from which it emerges without ever cutting the umbilical cord."[5]

What is emptiness? What is it not? It is neither deprivation, nor absence, nor nothing, nor nothingness: it is the condition, the guarantee of the fullness; it contains all of its potential. The guarantee of freedom of movement and the transformation of qi, emptiness is silence, an availability that allows all things possible, and in particular, it arises spontaneously, naturally, at a given time and place.

Let's take the tempo in music as an example. Two musical notes must be distinct for each to exist fully. The interval between them should not be too short, should not merge them, or they will not be fully heard. However, it should also not be too long, or the relationship between them would disappear. The same is true of human relationships of any kind, romantic, friendly, therapeutic, or other.

Personally, my experience is that emptiness, represented here by the intermediary generation in the family, explains that it is "the grandfather who transmits to the grandson," as a well-known Chinese saying goes. The same words are not meant and understood in the same way by a grandfather and a grandson. There is no empty space between a father and son because they are too close and too united for their energies and their words to circulate freely, for the saying and the listening to be accurate. Achieving emptiness, momentarily of course since it cannot be a permanent state, calls for reticence, refraining from the assertion of one's own will (the Chinese principle of "nonactive action" *wu wei* 無為), in order to allow that which spontaneously seeks to arise. This means effacing one's own self, self-will, ambition, and desires for the sole purpose of avoiding any interference with the emergence of what is natural, so that the word, gesture, or point that needs to arise can do so freely. This is important—even crucial—in any medical consultation, and especially so in acupuncture. It is a foundation of the *art* of medicine.

Emptiness: the very Heart of the Consultation

As a human being and a physician, I realize that, in the world we live in, we have to do things, make decisions, and take action. However, I understand the Chinese tradition as telling us to stop for a moment, just for that moment; to set aside your desires, ambitions, wants, worries, and decisions; to try to perceive that something that is spontaneously and naturally, at this very moment, in this place, trying to arise, and that you might not have thought about yourself; and to stop trying to prevent it from occurring; to give yourself a short time, just a few minutes. All you need to do is let go and, just for the moment, stop willing anything other than to allow the right thing to occur, here and now.

To me, this invitation is one of the most important lessons offered by this tradition: let's stop preventing the right things with our own will, and learn how to allow things to happen by taking the time to do so. It reminds me of the advice given me by Professor Aubry at the end of my first year of medical studies in 1954: "I want to tell you a secret; you may realize it yourself in 20 or 30 years' time. Meanwhile, remind yourself every single day (as I have). When you have given up the desire to be effective and the overarching will to cure, and content yourself with offering humble support, often without understanding, then you will become a true physician and start to become truly effective." I was reminded of this by a patient about 15 years ago. In parallel to the psychoanalytic work that she was pursuing, I was providing monthly treatments. Her symptoms barely changed. I felt irritated by my own ineffectiveness and I asked her if she really wanted to continue her treatment. She answered, "Doctor, would you please be so kind as to allow me to keep my symptoms and understand that you are still doing me a world of good, regardless?" I thank her to this day: she reminded me that not all things can or should be cured. Our role is to provide support.

First of all, how do you *allow* this emptiness to be present in a consultation? By allowing genuine silence to occur, at the beginning or at any time during the visit. "Genuine" implies that this silence must permit complete availability; peaceful, with your weight comfortably centered in the pelvis, and breathing easily, so that both people are prepared to listen or allow any thoughts to be expressed: a word, a gesture, a look, an attitude, anything, including, for the acupuncturist, the one or two points that need to be punctured at that particular time. Our reasoning always approves and rationalizes these insights immediately, even if it did not produce them. Obviously, this cannot be expected to occur at every visit. We cannot always be in this available frame of mind; far from it, and besides which, the silence is the product of two persons, the practitioner and the patient. We cannot do everything.

This emptiness, this silence, is what *ensures* the right type of relationship between the practitioner and patient, just as it ensures the free flow and transformation of qi in life. It even ensures the accuracy of the diagnosis and treatment: the right posture, the right word, and the right point, the right therapeutic action (puncture, surgery, prescription) all depend on it because these different elements cannot be separated. They comprise an inseparable whole.

Emptiness is also the necessary condition for accurate technique in acupuncture. Once I have decided on the point, I have to locate it precisely, by massaging the depression in which it is located to determine the corresponding special skin texture, the opening, its direction and depth, and, in a manner of speaking, to ask for permission to puncture it. Then, in an attentive, concentrated and relaxed posture, well-anchored in my pelvis, free from any thoughts or emotions, spontaneously and naturally, I allow my hand to painlessly introduce the needle, which will reach the bottom of the well on its own. Just like the butcher in Chapter 3 of the *Zhuangzi* who wrote that he who knows how to thrust the thin cutting edge of the knife into the interstices handles it with great ease because he puts it into empty spaces. The acupuncturist must do the same as he deals with points that are empty of specific anatomical structures but full of qi, of energies. This emptiness has an impact on the *effectiveness* of any treatment, not just acupuncture.

PRACTITIONER'S INTENT AND ATTITUDE

Patients arrive in my office. If they have not already consulted other doctors, I begin with a modern biomedical diagnosis, using diagnostic tests and specialist consultations as needed. This is rarely the case, as I mostly see patients who have been suffering for many years; they have had all the necessary tests and present either with a diagnosis or knowing that biomedicine has no diagnosis for them.

Inspection

As the patient arrives I observe their posture, gait, gestures, face, voice, and appearance. For example, if their spine is hyperextended, I think of a possible deficiency of the Governing vessel. If they have a thoracic kyphosis, I think of a chest that does not open and perhaps GV-10. I give them time to settle in and get acquainted with the surroundings: this is a moment of emptiness that permits a flow and exchange of qi, thoughts, words and feelings between us. Next, I ask the patient to undress; I observe their morphology and the color and tone of their skin; I look at their conjunctiva, and their tongue, including its color and any coating.

History

I question the patient, asking them to describe their symptoms in detail; a biomedical diagnosis (such as biliary dyskinesia) is not enough to tell me which point to needle. However, descriptions like "heartburn, with slow digestion, nausea, and intolerance of coffee and chocolate" are more useful to me. I examine the entire body, leaving psychological and behavioral symptoms for last, as at that point it will be easier for me to see how they fit in and it is important to first understand the body's own language. I try to relate these somatic symptoms to the mechanisms of Chinese medicine: yin organs, burner, extraordinary organs, channels, movements of qi, etc. This is how I orient my questions and my information gathering. One thing that I do that many practitioners do not is to ask patients about their dreams; they may evoke a movement of qi that is not occurring, an organ that is not functioning properly, etc. For example, if the patient often dreams that they are flying away, I would deduce that there is qi that is not descending, such as the qi from the Lung, Heart, or one of the three yang warps.

We first have to understand, for each patient, which mechanisms are disturbed, their relationships and their connections. As seen before, it is only afterwards that we can relate them to the specific history, traumas, life of this human being. From there we can understand which points will be most appropriate for the concerned body areas and mechanisms. Indeed, acupuncture is a system for interpreting symptoms as the language of the body and the means of access to the places where suffering is anchored.

Palpation and Pulses

I palpate the body, search for painful areas, and note the temperature of various zones in passing: for example, a cold zone suggests there is a qi deficiency in the area. I also ask the patient to remove their watch simply because I will need to take their pulse and a watch usually compresses the wrist.[6] Obviously, this investigation is more complex than the assessment of the pulse in conventional Western medicine, but we must always take into account the individual anatomical variations and anomalies.

First of all, I examine the main peripheral pulses of the carotid (ST-9), posterior tibialis (KI-3), dorsalis pedis (ST-42) and radial arteries (LU-9) at the wrist. This gives me information about the qi, its superficial and deep circulation, exchanges between above and below, and the status of their reserves. I then palpate the carotid pulse at ST-9 (reflecting primarily the state of the superficial, external, and yang organs) and LU-9 (reflecting primarily the state of the deep, internal, and yin organs). The comparison between the pulses at ST-9 and ST-42 tells us whether there is equilibrium between the upper and lower body. The pulse at LU-9 tells us about the state of the circulating qi, especially the nutritive and protective qi, while that at KI-3 tells us about the reserves of qi, especially of the Kidneys. I also compare the pulse at KI-3 with the Kidney pulses at the wrist. If the Kidney pulses at the wrist and the pulse at KI-3 are both weak, it signifies a Kidney deficiency. If the radial Kidney pulse is weak, but that at KI-3 is strong, it means that the qi is not descending.

The mechanics are as follows: I place my middle finger on the pulse position level with the styloid process, the index and ring fingers above and below, the wrist being slightly in extension. The area around the styloid process is the middle position; between the styloid process and the hand is the distal position; and the position located toward the elbow is the proximal position. These radial pulses are located on the *tai yin*, Lung and Spleen, related to breathing and food, qi and blood being therefore assimilated and flowing.

First, I investigate the overall pulse, its strength, speed and rhythm, its superficial or deep characteristics, and other different parameters (excessive, insufficient or normal, considering the patient's gender and age, as well as the context). This is how I evaluate a patient's qi:

- strong or weak, full or empty *(shi/xu):* to know the quantity of qi
- floating or sunken *(fu/shen):* to know whether the qi is superficial or hidden deep inside; the superficial qi can be either from an external pathological qi or normal qi reflecting the very nature of the person
- rapid or slow *(shuo/chi):* to know if there is heat or cold in body qi or in the external-ly-contracted qi
- long or short *(chang/duan),* the pulse either overspills its normal place (long) or does not fully occupy its place (short): to know if there is a normal fullness or an emptiness
- wiry or slack (normal pulse) *(xian/huan):* the wiry pulse, tense like a string, gives information on the Liver and the Gallbladder; the term *huan* usually means a normal pulse that is not too tight, but sometimes in context it means overly slack
- leathery *(ge)* is tense like the skin of a drum and signals an interior tension, due to constrained qi that cannot express itself
- slippery *(hua),* "like a string of beads slipping under the fingers," signals the presence of phlegm.

These notions must be corroborated with the clinical examination and with the individual's behavior. For example, I often find that a deep pulse corresponds to a reserved, introverted attitude; superficial pulses correspond to an extroverted personality, if there is no invasion of external pathological qi.

Next, I check whether the pulse is correct for the season, based on the scheme in *Basic Questions,* Chapter 18: wiry *(xian)* in the spring, overflowing *(sheng)* and hook-like *(gou)* in the summer, floating *(fu)* or featherlike *(mao)* in the autumn, sunken *(chen)* or stone-like *(shi)* in the winter. An anomaly means that there is a dysfunction in the corresponding phase.

Li Shi-Zhen's *Pulse Studies of the Lakeside Master* is for me a primary source in terms of pulse diagnosis. I analyze the right and left sides according to the scheme laid out in Chapter 2 of this book for an overall assessment of the yin (right) and yang (left) qi of the body, always originating in the Kidneys, the root of production of the five organs. A yin deficiency with fatigue, insomnia, night sweats, signs of heat and weaker pulses on the right side needs to be tonified through the Kidney yin, for example, with

BL-52 and KI-2. A yang deficiency with fatigue, daytime sweating, signs of cold and weaker left pulses calls for tonifying the Kidney yang with GV-4 and KI-3.

Next, I perform a bilateral examination of the distal (*cun*), middle (*guan*) and proximal (*chi*) positions. In this case, I may find the same anomaly again, for example, the same weakness, in both distal positions, in both middle positions, or in both proximal positions, left and right. This lets me investigate three things:

- First, the *three burners*. A deficiency in both distal positions implies a deficiency in the upper burner: This should be confirmed with clinical examination, which would reveal physical and mental fatigue, insomnia, anxiety, sense of oppression, feeling of suffocation, and palpitations. I can encounter short pulses that do not fill up the proximal and distal positions, which most often signals a constraint in the middle burner with digestive disorders (CV-11 or 12) or anxiety (e.g., CV-14, 15 or 16).

- It can signal a deficiency in the *upper, middle or lower parts* of the body or the trunk (thorax, epigastrium, and pelvis). A deficiency in the pelvis or the lower part of the body is manifested by empty proximal pulses.

- Next, the *up-and-down movements* of qi in the body and particularly in the trunk. A deficiency in one of the two distal pulses implies that qi is not rising to the thorax, because, for example, LR-14 is not functioning: one of its tasks is to make qi rise from the abdomen to the thorax. Empty proximal pulses with normal KI-3 pulses tell me that different types of qi cannot descend to the pelvis, either because their movement is constrained or because the pelvis does not receive them properly. The general context will permit diagnosis.

Here I refer to a case history mentioned earlier.

❖ Case History

Mrs. G., age 56, was a midwife who consulted for "a lack of drive and enthusiasm." "I'm sinking," she added. She complained of a sensation of epigastric heaviness and oppression radiating to the back, between the shoulder blades. Her back and her shoulders felt heavy. Her chest felt closed. These symptoms coincided with the time of menopause. She had few other symptoms. Her sleep was all right. Her proximal pulses, as well as the KI-3 pulses, were deep.

How could I treat this "sinking" impression? On her first visit, needling CV-5 seemed the best thing to do. After I had needled CV-5, she felt tired for three days and dreamed of "a black baby." I thought this may link back to the Kidneys and gestation. She was more lively. Maybe she was "sinking" a bit less. The KI-3 pulses were then back to normal. This evolution of the pulses showed that qi was not descending, probably because it was constrained in the chest, which GV-10 can treat.

Finally, I examine each of the three sections individually, both superficially and deep, on the right and left sides. This makes a total of twelve positions that correspond to the yin organs:

- distal position: right = Lung and Large Intestine; left = Heart and Small Intestine
- middle position: right = Spleen and Stomach; left = Liver and Gallbladder
- proximal position: right = gate of vitality or Triple Burner yin; left = Kidney and Bladder or Heart Master yang

For each of these, I observe whether the pulse is relatively superficial or deep in its own position, excessive or deficient, and a number of other specific findings. The pulse is deep on the right proximal position, the Triple Burner or the gate of vitality is weak; the clinical examination will permit a differential diagnosis. When the pulse is "tight as a drum" (*ge*) in the left middle position, then the Liver or the Gallbladder are affected by deficiency and cold. When the pulse is "like a string of beads slipping under the fingers" (*hua*) in the right distal position, there is either bronchitis or pregnancy; the differential diagnosis is easy enough.

Diagnostic and Therapeutic Conclusions

The next step is a diagnostic summary of all this information, pinpointing the disrupted mechanisms (from a Chinese medical point of view), their complications, their relationship to the personality and history of the patient, and then arriving at an understanding of which two or three points to puncture on this patient at this particular time.

Practicalities

The basic facts are that acupuncture points are treated by puncturing (with a needle), warming (with an artemisia moxa stick or cone) or by massaging (especially for small children).

NEEDLING BASICS

Before puncturing, I massage to familiarize myself with the point, sense the surface opening and the underlying direction. I always use fine single-use stainless steel needles, choosing the specific one based on the depth of the point, using slightly thicker and longer needles for deeper points. With the needle in hand, as I said above, I clear my mind and allow the needling motion to occur spontaneously at the same time as the pause that occurs at the end of exhalation.

Needling must be painless. The point is a well. The acupuncture needle penetrates through the orifice of the well and goes down to the bottom, without deviating or going further down. The practitioner, like the calligrapher or the jade cutter, instinctively knows what will happen after the needle has been inserted and he knows where to stop, without meeting any obstacle and without touching any sinews, veins, nerves, and so on. The emptiness of the acupuncturist communicates with the emptiness of the point. The patient experiences a painless numb or swollen sensation called *de qi,* which starts at the needled point and can radiate along the channel.

TONIFICATION AND DRAINING

I only use tonification or draining techniques in acute cases. Otherwise, I trust the regulation and restoration capacities of the body, and limit myself to inserting the needle in the best possible way, as described above. To tonify, I insert the needle following the direction of the channel and turn it slightly clockwise. To drain, I insert the needle contrary to the direction of the channel and turn it slightly counterclockwise.

Most often, I use what is called a harmonizing method. I very seldom rotate the needle, especially when there is significant deficiency or cold.

DURATION OF NEEDLING

This varies according to the aim pursued, the nature of the disorder and the season; needles are kept in place longer when tonifying than when draining. If the disorder is not recent, and is linked to deficiency or cold, I leave the needles in for 20 to 30 minutes. If the disorder is recent, and is linked to excess and heat, I leave the needles in for 10 to 15 minutes. The duration is longer in winter, when the qi is deeper, than in summer, when the qi is more superficial. It is also longer when the body's qi needs to get rid of a perverse qi.

MOXIBUSTION AND OTHER FORMS OF STIMULATION

Moxibustion

The purpose of moxibustion is to provide heat in case of yang or heat deficiency. It is also indicated in case of cold excess, either in the exterior or interior. In these cases, I use moxa sticks.

To tonify, I do not hold the end of the stick close to the point. In this way, it causes a medium rather than an intense heat, and thus can stimulate a fairly large area. I ask the patient to be aware of the heat sensation and I stop as soon as it has reached the necessary place and depth. For instance, when I moxa CV-6, I wait until the heat sensation reaches the entire pelvis and even the lower limbs.

To drain, in case of an invasion by pathogenic cold, I hold the stick closer to the skin and vigorously heat the area (without burning it) for a very short time, then repeat 10 or 30 times according to the duration of the disorder or invasion.

Massage

I limit myself to massage of the points and not the more complex and refined traditional Chinese massage, known as *tui na.* I mainly massage a point when I treat children younger than seven years of age, or to prepare the point for needling, in order to get to know it better. I massage clockwise. I do not press too hard, but lightly, as I just want to stimulate the qi. In fact, I breathe in to the point from my pelvis (CV-6). As the massage continues, I can focus a more precise sense of the center of the point. At the beginning, I have the feeling that it is an empty basin that gradually fills up as the massage proceeds. I stop when I feel that it is full.

Electrical Stimulation

I never use this technique. In the 1970s I did use it strictly as an analgesic technique. I did not find it very efficacious for treating pain, quite to the contrary, so in my experience it was not useful.

REACTIONS TO TREATMENT

- What does it mean? What can happen?

After a session, especially after the first session, some symptoms may be aggravated, starting 1-3 days later. Flare-ups that occur later are probably not a reaction to the treatment, although this cannot be completely excluded. A reaction to the treatment lasts from 1-4 days, not longer. If it does last longer, it should be taken not as a reaction but as an aggravation of the condition, which compels us to use a different treatment.

I cannot explain these reactions, but they often constitute a positive sign; they show that the patient is receptive to acupuncture and that the points chosen were the right ones. The earlier they appear, the better the prognosis. They can even start when the patient is still on the table. A pain that worsens ten minutes after the needle is inserted will soon be cured.

- Are they necessary, do they just happen sometimes, or can you predict when they will occur?

They are unpredictable and unnecessary. Some patients get better very quickly without any reaction.

- Do patients need to be warned about them? If so, how?

I always warn the patients that they may have a reaction. I tell them it is not necessary, and that not having one does not mean the session was ineffective. I ask them to call me if it is too intense or if it worries them.

PRACTICE DETAILS

Treatment Frequency

- The second session always takes place 3-5 weeks after the first one, when the body still has a memory of the information triggered by the needles.

- The interval between the following sessions varies according to the nature of the disorder and its evolution. The second one often takes place 4-6 weeks later, as do the following sessions if there is no evolution of the symptoms.

The principle at work is to have only a few treatments and to sufficiently space them out to see their effects. I always ask the patient to phone me if they do not notice any change after two weeks.

- When the patient is much better, the interval between two sessions is eight weeks to six months.

Session Duration and Follow-up

As seen before, I leave the needles in place for 10-30 minutes, according to the case. The first session, including the history, the needling and the answers to the questionnaire at the end of the treatment, lasts about one hour.

If nothing has changed after a few sessions, contrary to my expectations, I sometimes ask the patient to consult one of my colleagues, who will have a new perspective on the case. After a few sessions, it is often difficult to change the vision we have of a patient.

PREVENTIVE TREATMENT

I recommend a preventive treatment in two cases. First for seasonal diseases, for example, hay fever. I ask the patient to come about one month before the anticipated beginning of the pathology. Second, in chronic conditions, when all is well, I prescribe a session every 6-12 months, around the time of the spring and autumn equinoxes (March 21 and September 21) because at those times the different types of qi are more mobile and accessible.

CHAPTER TEN

SUMMARY: IGNORE THE SYMPTOMS AND TREAT THE PERSON

THE MOST EFFECTIVE APPROACH is to always treat the person rather than the symptoms. It is important to have as complete a vision as possible. This is evident necessarily when a symptom has been present for a long time or has already been treated. But it is also true in certain acute cases where one might be tempted to think that a predetermined protocol would bring the quickest results. When faced with any symptom, and particularly if it is an enduring one, the thing to do is to successively apply the following principles:

- Search for any possible regional causes of local problems.
- Situate the local and regional problem within an overall imbalance that maintains and serves as the basis of the problem.
- Ignore the symptom and attempt to understand the person, then translate this perception into points.

Possible Regional Causes

Searching for possible regional causes of local problems is related to an old principle in Western medicine: when faced with any type of pain, especially if it persists, search above, below, before, behind, within or without, that is, the opposite. For example, in the case of pain in the back of the neck, look at the front of the neck, for a window-of-heaven point; for a case of an arthrosis of the thumb, investigate the elbow; for a knee, investigate the hip; for a sacroiliac joint, investigate the groin; for a shoulder, the nape of the neck; for the upper back, the chest.

Here's an example from an actual case.

❖ Case History

I had been treating Mr. L., age 42, for a long time. He is a philosophy teacher and consulted me for episodes of depression, insomnia, headaches, paravertebral pains and bronchial frailty.

In 2000 he came to see me for an acute sprain of the right ankle sustained by falling from the ladder in his library six days before. The pain was very intense on the leg *shao yang*, around the external lateral ligament and on the medial malleolus; the ankle was swollen; there was a small bruise on the forefoot. The x-ray showed everything was normal. He had been treated with a splint, which he wore during the daytime. What did the bruise imply? A sprain may involve a channel sinew or a primary channel, with bruising in the latter case. So there was no reason to treat the channel sinew by the distal well point. I decided to treat the proximal river point, GB-38, which is indicated for impairment of primary channels, because its role is to promote the irrigation of tissues that are dependent on the corresponding channel. I paired this with the unblocking point, GB-36.

I saw him again four days later. The pain was just as intense. It had even increased on the inside of the ankle, and continued to the knee. Because the pain was extending internally, and in order to bring into play the connecting-source system that links the channels in external-internal pairs, I decided to puncture GB-37, which controls the longitudinal connecting point of leg *shao yang* and goes to the ankle and foot via LR-3. Five days later, the pain was even worse on the inside of the ankle; it was even radiating to the back of the calf!

Were there any other points to try in the ankle area? No, since the pain was localized on the leg *shao yang* and leg *jue yin* channels. It was better to let go of that approach and try another. I said to myself that if treating the painful area did not work, I needed to look above or below. There was nothing on the forefoot. I investigated the knee and the hip, even though these joints showed nothing. On the knee, I could not find any particularly painful points. The inner side of the hip also showed nothing. However, LR-11 was hyperalgesic and triggered pains on the inside of the knee that connected to the pain radiating from the ankle. Puncturing LR-11 considerably improved the pain in the ankle and leg within 24 hours. When he was getting out of bed, he even heard a cracking sound, as if everything were shifting back in place. A second treatment of LR-11 reinforced with LR-6 cleared up the symptoms completely. LR-6 is the cleft point of leg *jue yin*.

The traumatic tendonitis in the groin was preventing the ankle from healing. It had gone undetected, as is often the case, because it was not spontaneously painful.

❖ Case History

This squat, introverted man, age 42, was referred to me by his chiropractor for a back pain between T3 and T6 that had started four months previously. It was located on the midline, constant, worse on waking, and was unaffected by either physical exercise or by the weather. It appeared after a particularly painful breakup which led him to experience loneliness similar to that which he had experienced as a child.

As this specific area had already been treated by a competent chiropractor, I had to look elsewhere, above, below or on the front. The areas above and below the cervical and lumbar spine had already been treated. The anterior of the body, that is, the inside of the chest, had to be considered. The history revealed slight feelings of constriction of the thorax. Moreover his girlfriend had sometimes noticed that he appeared to occasionally stop breathing while asleep.

His medical history included a thyroidectomy subsequent to a cancer. He was an emotional, sensitive and quite introverted man. His tongue was normal. The Heart pulses were deep.

Which is the mechanism that concerns both the thorax and the Heart? On consideration of the constricted feeling and the fact that it was worse on waking, I thought of a stagnation which could also explain the difficulties he had expressing his emotions (including his tears or grief) and perhaps also the sleep apnea syndrome.

HT-1, which sets the chest yin into motion, was the point to be chosen. I often needle it in certain cases of angina or asthma, of subdeltoid bursitis, of frozen shoulders (frequently in association with SI-11). The backache disappeared after the second treatment. It came back a few months later, when he had been vexed. Needling this point made the pain disappear within 12 hours.

IMPORTANCE OF CONTEXT

A local or regional disturbance is not enough to make a problem chronic. For that to occur, there must be a general problem that is maintaining the disturbance, creating a vicious cycle, as seen in the following case history. A local problem will only persist if a more general one prevents it from healing. For example, if I have a Stomach weakness and therefore a weakness in the Stomach channel, a trauma to the area crossed by this channel will take much longer to heal; treating the Stomach will then be necessary.

❖ Case History

Mrs. L., age 56, came to see me in March 1995 for epicondylitis that had begun in November 1994 after a case of food poisoning from eating oysters. It could not be blamed on any sports activity or any other particular effort. The epicondylitis was bilateral, unaffected by the weather, barely influenced by movements of the forearm or wrist, but always aggravated by a heavy dinner. Rheumatological treatments and physiotherapy had no effect. Her digestive history included constipation with no urge to defecate, and rare instances of nausea without food intolerances.

The woman was a political science teacher who had little self-confidence. She was always tied up in knots and tense, and reported that she often had a lot of tension in her neck and shoulders. She was so tense that she was often surprised to see herself tightly gripping her steering wheel. She even wondered if this might be the cause of the elbow pains.

Her history included an appendectomy, two normal pregnancies and a few cases of pharyngitis, and nothing more. The woman was cheerful yet keyed up: the muscle tension was visible during the examination, her tongue trembled and had a slight yellow coating, and the Liver pulses were tense (*xian*). The proximal pulses were weaker.

The atypical nature of this bilateral epicondylitis, the conditions of its occurrence and the aggravation after a full meal, made me decide to ignore the symptom and focus on the general problem. The general tension and muscle contractions connected with the Liver and affecting its functions of draining and detoxifying seemed clear enough.

- In this woman, who had a high degree of professional recognition, the tension was secondary to her lack of self-confidence. The weaker proximal pulses corresponded to this deficiency, which is often related to a deficiency in the lower burner, particularly its function of sorting out and eliminating the impure. I needed to puncture a point that would tonify the pelvic qi, lower burner, and her self-confidence.
- The poor drainage and detoxification of the Liver led to an accumulation of impurities, heat and toxins. These became localized in the muscles (which are associated with the Liver) because of their constant state of tension and contraction.
- In addition to this general state of tension, there was also another layer of tension in the neck and shoulders, due to her need to constantly maintain control, especially in her emotions. We know how such contraction of the neck and shoulders can lead to pains in the upper limbs, such as shoulder pain, elbow pain, etc.
- The intense gripping of her steering wheel was the final straw for her; it concentrated all of this tension in her elbows.

Thus I decided to begin by treating:

- The pelvic deficiency connected to her lack of self-confidence, at the lower

burner that governs the sorting of pure and impure and protects the Kidneys and Liver, by CV-7 *(yin jiao* or "yin communication").
• Then, by working on the Liver's draining function at the cleft point, LR-6.
• And finally, by relieving the contraction of the neck and shoulders with a point located on *yang ming* (the channel that traverses the lateral epicondyle), ST-12.

The improvement in the constipation, the overall tension, the contraction of the trapezius muscles, and the epicondylitis was spectacular. We repeated the treatment two weeks later. By the third visit, one month later, everything was even better: there were only a few pains in her elbows after heavy meals. We advised her to have maintenance treatments each year at the equinoxes and to see an herbalist for detox teas to take at the same time.

❖ Case History

Mr. N., an analyst and writer of 68, stocky, obviously full of energy, both exuberant and reserved, consulted me in December 2002 for long-term pains aggravated by a fall on the ice ten years before. The pains were all located on the right side of the body and affected the neck, shoulder, trunk, groin and lower limb. The influence of the weather on these pains was clear. He was also acutely sensitive to the atmosphere conveyed by people or groups of people. These influences suggested TB-5, a connecting point of the arm *shao yang* and an opening point of the Yang Linking vessel.

He had no other physical symptoms. However, he said that he was often depressed and had less enthusiasm and drive since he was compelled to flee from his country in 1979. The grief linked to this exile was still very sharp. He did not complain of anxiety and slept well. He had been married but had no children.

His tongue looked normal. His pulses manifested his great energy; they were deeper on the left distal position, the pulses of the Heart. Which Heart point should be chosen? I rejected using the arm *shao yin* points, especially HT-4, HT-5, HT-6 and HT-7, because there was no anxiety, no insomnia and no signs specific to this channel. For similar reasons I discarded CV-14, CV-15 and CV-16. Because his depression was transient, I also set BL-44 aside.

I was left with GV-4 and CV-19. I chose CV-19, which I think "reconciles" because of the important inner progress of this man. After two treatments two weeks apart, the pains clearly improved, the depression less so. He once said, "I feel compressed by anger and grief," which made me, a month later, replace CV-19 by CV-18, as this point includes the idea of compression of time, space and psyche (compression of the eight organs). The result was spectacular. He quickly recovered his drive again, began working with enthusiasm and even started tracing his genealogy. After the fifth session, he felt well: "My body is less of a barometer," he said.

Mr. N. came back four months later: "Grief and tears are buried here," he said (pointing to his chest), "and each night I cry silently." Which is the point in relation to TB-5 that includes this idea of "crying silently"? GB-41, a confluent point of the Girdle vessel with which it is paired, provided much relief.

The patient came again in August 2004 for an important and stubborn urticaria that had appeared five weeks before after eating fish. For consistency, I chose GB-31, which is a point on the *shao yang* linked to the Gallbladder and very much indicated for pruritus. It proved efficient on the second day, after having caused a sort of pain in the left thigh along the leg *shao yang*.

He came again in October 2005 with this question: "How can I reintroduce the left part of my body, excluded when I was 16 when my father was sent to exile?" I chose a point on the Yang Linking vessel, on the hip, which is related to adolescence, GB-29 on the right. According to the patient it caused "an energetic and psychological cataclysm on the table with profuse sweating," after which improvement was quite apparent.

He came back in June 2006 with a particularly severe left leg pain. The localization was a classic one, on the *yang ming*, on the anterior side of the thigh. What was less usual was the alternation of hyperalgic phases and complete remissions with no known precipitating factor. The pain started after a very violent quarrel. The MRI scan revealed a significant disc hernia at L3-L4 on the left. Because of the location of the pain, I needled ST-31 on the left because this point benefits the hip after a person is back on his feet thanks to the use of ST-30. I linked this problem to the recent quarrel. I got no result whatsoever. Remembering the October 2005 treatment and the Yang Linking vessel, I then needled the next point on the left on that same channel, SI-10 on the shoulder. This is based on a perception of a three-fold evolution of the being with three corresponding areas of the body: childhood and the ankle (BL-61), adolescence and the hip (GB-29), adulthood and the shoulder (SI-10). SI-10, on the shoulder, just above the trunk, involves another phase in the evolution of the being, a maturity, a distance, an invitation to transcend history to access, in the head, a wider vision of life, to a meta-history. BL-61 and GB-29 are points of the Yang Linking vessel; SI-10 is shared by the Yang Linking vessel and the Yang Heel vessel.

Forty-eight hours later the pain had disappeared and he was only left with a left paravertebral discomfort and a cardboard-like sensation on the thigh. This pain reappeared, although less intense, at the end of September 2006. Needling the same point had an immediate positive effect and the pain only came back in late December.

It's worth emphasizing how the progress of both the patient and the practitioner was consistent with the different treatments.

TRY TO UNDERSTAND THE PERSON

❖ Case History

Mrs. M., age 73, came to see me in January 1996 for a case of urticaria that appeared in 1992, shortly after the death of her only son, who had been killed in an accident at the age of 37. The urticaria had been more or less constant for the last four years, neither improved nor aggravated by the seasons, weather, food, temperature or psychological factors. It prevented her from sleeping, which led her to use sleeping pills. The mechanisms of urticaria are usually described as a release of wind-heat in the skin (wind-heat from the Liver, Heart, or blood) or the internal non-closure of *yang*.

There was little else to report. She had an appendectomy at the age of 22. Her periods, one pregnancy and menopause had all been normal. There had been some circulatory problems in the extremities, with cold hands and feet, a slight case of Raynaud's syndrome, and occasional numbness in the hands at night. There was also repressed anxiety in the solar plexus, with agitation, that had increased significantly since the death of her son but had always been present, especially when waking in the morning. The accidental death of her son had been the only difficult event in a "conventionally" happy life.

Her tongue was normal. Her pulses were on the whole tense and had an imbalance in the distal positions, with a weak Heart pulse and a deep, tense Lung pulse.

I diagnosed a Heart obstruction, with release of wind-heat, and chose CV-15 and HM-4. CV-15 was chosen to release the Heart fire repressed within, while HM-4 acts on both the nervous agitation and the circulatory problems in the extremities. Two treatments of these points produced a worsening of the urticaria, lasting for two weeks after the second treatment.

I then tried ST-15, which returns the *yang* to the inside and is indicated for certain cases of urticaria. Its name, *wu yi* or "roof screen," contains the word 翳 *yi,* which means a screen that stands in front of a house and protects it. This patient showed no signs of insecurity, nor any other *yang ming* signs. Once again, two sessions had no effect.

In my thinking, I now set aside the usual mechanisms. I was faced with a case of urticaria, a cutaneous manifestation that had appeared after the accidental death of the patient's son, accompanied by anxiety with internally constrained qi. Could this not be a case of obstructed Lung qi due to the perceived injustice of the accident, the mourning, grief and unacceptability of this death of a 37-year-old son who was also an only child? The Lung pulse was deep and tense. KI-22, whose indications include sensitivity to injustice, and which governs the diffusion of Lung qi to the outside, was clearly indicated. After the first treatment, the urticaria disappeared for ten days; after the second treatment, it disappeared for three weeks. Two months after the third session, the patient declared herself cured. Her anxiety had receded. The circulatory problems had not changed. The pulses were normal. We advised her to come back at the fall equinox, which she did even though the urticaria had not returned.

So it turned out that the Lung was the cause, although we first thought it was the Heart. Was the morning anxiety a warning sign?

Conclusion

As seen in this book, Chinese tradition describes a beautiful and unusual architecture of the living world and in particular the relationships of human beings to it. This tradition describes a natural order that encompasses all manifestations of life: cosmic, human, animal, plant and mineral. All forms of life are governed by the same laws that are reflected in their structures and their functions and relationships. According to Etienne Klein, "Physical laws are timeless, they have remained constant since the beginning of the universe."[1] Chinese tradition expresses this natural order through symbolic language: heaven/human/earth, water/fire, hard/soft, and resonances between numbers, among others. As often occurs with traditions, symbols, myths and rites serve as intermediaries between the symbolic "celestial" laws and their symbolic "terrestrial" manifestations, between the infinity of structures and living beings in the universe. Since the beginning of Chinese civilization, relationships between the descriptions of earth and the human being, and between the functions of the human body and the government of the Chinese empire, have been established.

This vision is on a celestial level, according to Chinese medicine, and not on a terrestrial, anatomical, or historical level. Therefore there is no need to describe terrestrial manifestations, such as the precise anatomy of the viscera, because this medicine utilizes symbolic language to reflect the laws governing the function of the universe at all levels, including the empire, the human body, and the viscera, even the smallest levels of microscopic life. This vision is not necessarily superior to others, since these two traditional views of Chinese and Western medicine, yin and yang, the physical and the metaphysical, the meta-historical and the historical, the terrestrial and celestial levels, are complementary to each other.

The genius of the Chinese medical tradition is that it illustrates the continuity of the relationship reaching from a symbol to a specific diagnostic and therapeutic action, to the insertion of a needle in a precise point of the body, to relieve or heal, depending on the case.

How is this symbolic approach to be utilized pragmatically in the everyday practice of medicine ? At least in four ways.

- First, this symbolic vision has important clinical and therapeutic implications and applications which enable us to link apparently unrelated mechanisms and symptoms, in terms of both physiology and pathology. A better understanding of the language of our patients' bodies allows us to see beyond their symptoms, to welcome them totally and to give them our support, thereby permitting us to treat our patients in a more effective and more profound way.

- This highly symbolic vision of the universe, expressed through acupuncture, also helps us understand and explore the dual aspects, psychological and somatic, of the human memory. These memories record all of the experiences and their associated emotions maintaining a constant interaction, which we have lived since conception—pleasure, pain, trauma, anxiety, suffering, etc. It is not "psychosomatic," meaning that the physical symptoms are not induced through emotional causes. The body has intrinsic memory; our symptoms are their language. The body interacts constantly with the psyche. Acupuncture offers us two things: an original way to read the body language and a way to gain access to areas where the suffering of the body was locked in. Also, it can help to stimulate the circulation and release of qi, thereby freeing the symptoms. The scars remain of course, because you cannot erase what has been, but they become less painful. Moreover, these areas of pain are "unleashed" and become accessible to the psyche. The ideal treatment should address itself to both memories, for example, through the combination of psychoanalytical work and acupuncture, since this offers a chance to transform this dialogue and make it less painful, which can lead to a permanent cure in some chronic cases.

- Furthermore, in both the West and in East Asia, the study of all the aspects and mechanisms and points of Chinese medicine is far from complete. To make progress in this area, it is necessary to explore the traditional Chinese symbols that are associated with the points more deeply. Our understanding of the acupuncture points and their applications will be enhanced by these efforts. Thereafter, the research in conjunction with a Western biomedical approach can be expanded. But first, a thorough understanding of what Chinese medicine has to offer is necessary; otherwise, we remain only on the surface.

- Last but not least, one more aspect of Chinese medicine must be emphasized: it is based on a philosophy of life, the conviction of the inter-connectedness and therefore solidarity with all manifestations of life. Solidarity need not be sought, since it simply is an inevitable and natural fact. It is not emotional, charitable or in the realm of love, but a basic physical law and a cosmic reality. Even our slightest gestures, feelings or thoughts have an impact on the furthest reaches of the universe and will rebound to us. All living beings embody the same archetypes and are subject to the same laws, since all living structures reflect the same fundamental architecture, in various forms.

The archetypal structure of microcosms corresponds to that of the macrocosm. It is simply a fact, whether we like it or not, that we are all interdependent not only with other human beings, with the entire human race, but with all living things and with the entire universe.

POINT FUNCTIONS

Introduction

THE FOLLOWING ARE MY personal observations on the utility of a select number of acupuncture points. I have limited my comments to those points that I myself use regularly and with which I have significant experience. Similarly, as these are my personal observations, this is not a systematic review of the point functions, and the amount of detail will vary greatly from point to point. The points are ordered in this index according to the order of movement of qi in the primary channels.

Lung Channel

■ LU-1

Called the "Middle Palace" *zhong fu*. Related to the center, particularly CV-12, the alarm point of the middle burner, which is the origin of the Lung channel.

Emblematic point of the autumn harvest. In autumn the fruit has fallen from the tree and will never be on the tree again. We see here definitive separations, such as death. This point treats mourning and grief.

Helps with two movements toward the interior: toward the middle burner and into the chest,

My profound appreciation to Louise Aghassian, who was kind enough to perform the arduous task of translating this appendix.

— qi rises up, counterflow: chronic impairment of the nose or throat, vomiting, especially when it occurs during coughing fits

— qi is not harvested and so the qi, blood and body fluids do not move inward but accumulate in the periphery with such problems as edema affecting the face or the four limbs: anorexia, and shoulder and back pains

Problems of the Lung,

— including the anatomical lungs and bronchi

— cold in the diaphragm, insomnia with waking at around 3 a.m.

Insufficiency of the "morning audience" of the Lung

■ LU-2

Called "Cloud Door" *yun men*. At the top of the thorax, it governs the exit of qi from the Lung upward toward the clouds, through the upper part of the body (nape of the neck and head) and limbs, with peripheral heat signs.

Deals with a sensation of fullness in the chest, as the qi does not go out and accumulates inside the chest with frequent sighing.

Most often, this blockage is due to repressed anger, a violent experience, or an intense repressed emotion.

Here too, the symptoms include waking at 3 a.m.

■ LU-3

A window-of-heaven point on the arm *tai yin*. It serves to facilitate the descent of the respiratory Lung qi.

If this descent does not work, the Lung qi accumulates upward with allergic rhinitis, asthma, epistaxis, congestion in the upper part of the body. These problems occur more during the spring when qi rises like the sap of trees.

While both this point and KI-27 facilitate the descent of Lung qi in the treatment of problems such as allergic rhinitis, KI-27 is more for seasonal allergies, while LU-3 treats problems that occur all year.

■ LU-7

Connecting point

Has a pulmonary effect.

Indications: heat in the heel of the hand or the palms; yawning, coughing, dyspnea, frequent urination; sadness, grief

Large Intestine Channel

◼ LI-1

This is the well (*jing*) point and, as such, it acts on all functions of the channel. I will sometimes puncture a well point to facilitate the effect of another point on the same channel.

Also, as it is a well point, it treats the channel sinew.

Works on the orifices of the face.

◼ LI-4

Used for acute viral infections.

Coupled with LU-7 to work on the Lungs, with SP-6 to harmonize the qi and blood, with ST-36 to regulate all of the *yang ming*, and with LI-3 to eliminate toxins and treat allergies in general.

◼ LI-6

The collateral point of the Large Intestine. As such, if it does not function properly, the yang does not go into the yin but stays outside. People with this problem are sensitive, active, easily excited, and reactive.

Painful gums, grinding of teeth, cavities and toothaches; deafness

Painful obstruction of the diaphragm, sensation of cold in the teeth and gums

Mental problems, excessive talking

◼ LI-9

Used in neurology. An interesting symptom is "cold feeling inside the bones and marrow." (Chamfrault)

◼ LI-10

Named *shou san li* or "Three *li* on the Hand" and thus corresponds to ST-36 *zu san li* or "Three *li* on the Leg."

LI-10 governs the upper part of the body, especially in the context of direct attack by external pathogenic wind affecting head, upper limbs, throat, voice, teeth, and neck.

◼ LI-15

On the arm *yang ming* channel, it governs the entry of yang qi of the upper limb into the trunk of the body on the shoulder. Used when a painful shoulder is due to an excess of yang, marked by the pain being aggravated by rest, heat, and pressure.

This point is effective in some cases of pruritus and rashes. We think of this point if there are other *yang ming* signs.

■ LI-17

LI-17 is a window-of-heaven point and contains the character for heaven (*tian*) in its name: *tian ding*. It is used for "sudden muteness."

LI-17 is also effective in shoulder pain, particularly that which is alternately anterior, lateral, and posterior.

■ LI-18

According to Nguyen Van Nghi, the *Great Compendium of Acupuncture and Moxibustion* states that it brings the protective qi out from the trunk to the periphery.

If the implication of the arm *yang ming* seems likely in a case of sudden horseness, this is the main point to use.

■ LI-19

I often use this for nasal problems, especially for anosmia if LI-20 is not effective enough.

Stomach Channel

■ ST-1

As the meeting point of the leg *yang ming* with the Yang Qiao and Conception vessels, I use it if all these vessels are affected.

For spasms or facial paralysis and some types of conjunctivitis.

■ ST-3

The meeting point with the Yang Qiao vessel.

Very important point for facial neuralgias (barrier point).

■ ST-4

Its name is *di cang* or "Earth Warehouse."

The meeting point with the Yang Qiao vessel; connects to GV-26 and CV-24.

Important point for facial spasms and paralysis. Should be heated by moxa for yin paralysis (when the eye cannot be closed).

▪ ST-7

Called *xia guan* or "Below Gate," under the zygomatic arch, it corresponds to GB-3 which is called *shang guan* or "Above Gate," which is above this bone.

It is a barrier point that allows the yang to descend from the skull to the face, particularly to the temporomandibular joint (TMJ) and the ipsilateral mandible.

I use it for problems in the TMJ and dental pains, especially for the molar and premolar teeth.

For its preventive action, I needle this point before teeth are pulled or implanted, as it hastens healing and decreases the side effects of these procedures.

▪ ST-8

Headaches and migraines that are deep and feel as if the head was about to blow up, while also spreading to the eyes

Wind in the eyes with conjunctivitis

▪ ST-9

Facilitates the connection between the body and the head. A dysfunction of this point therefore leads to "excess in the chest, dyspnea" and symptoms of throat and neck: difficulty speaking, nausea, throat pain and/or swelling, goiter.

▪ ST-11

Barrier point which facilitates the qi descending into the trunk from the neck. This is a type of "interiorization," therefore the symptoms it treats include:

Swelling of the throat with difficulty swallowing, food going down the wrong way

Hiccups (may only require massaging this point, and not puncturing it)

Stiff neck, goiter

Difficulty in being aware of one's emotions and feelings

▪ ST-12

The crossing place for all yang meridians and the *yin qiao.*

A link between the head and thorax, and even the trunk, because the deep part of leg *yang ming* and leg *shao yang* channels go to ST-30 above the pubis.

Think of using it for some upper limb pains, or neck pains along the pathway of the *yang ming*, and for some types of insomnia, dyspnea, or intercostal neuralgias.

Also for the person who cannot let go of emotions, people, attachments, etc.

■ **ST-13**

The name of this point is *qi hu* or "Qi Door" in which *hu* is specifically the inner door of a house.

The Stomach points from ST-13 through ST-16 all relate to the idea of insecurity due to issues of faulty closing off from the outside, which manifests as problems relating to protection and insecurity. Remember that closing in or shutting in from the exterior to the interior is one of the functions of the *yang ming*.

Its signs are pulmonary (cough, dyspnea), diaphragmatic (hiccups), and loss of taste.

■ **ST-14**

I will specifically choose this point for four problems:

— all sequelae of trauma, whether physical or psychological and whether the effects are somatic or affective. If the point is only tender on one side, which is usually the case, I only use that side.

— allergies that are aggravated by heat

— a patient who cannot tolerate being touched or even looked at

— protective obesity: these people wrap themselves in fat as a protection against an environment perceived as aggressive or dangerous, but also to protect themselves from intimate contact with others.

■ **ST-15**

The name of this point is *wu yi* or "Roof Screen," with the second character also having the meaning of concealment. It is for people who are insecure and tend to feel themselves under attack.

For cases of urticaria that are aggravated by moist heat, which can be via the skin (e.g., after a hot shower) or via damp-heat food and drink (e.g., alcohol).

I also needle this point for allergies of a dampness pattern, which are intensified by exposure to water, bathing, and sweat.

■ **ST-16**

This point is in the same atmosphere of insecurity as the other points in this group, with moderate pulmonary signs and diarrhea.

■ **ST-20**

The name of this point, *cheng man,* means "Receiving Fullness." So I will needle this point when the Stomach "cannot contain" and does not accept food, as if it were already too full. Drooling is a good sign of this disharmony, as it reflects a Stomach qi that does not descend.

■ ST-21

I needle this point for gastritis, when the Stomach does not digest food and also does not empty, therefore there is no undigested food in the stools.

■ ST-23

To me this point is related to the Small Intestine and, through that connection, coupled with the Heart, makes it a type of "Heart earth."

I consider this point particularly connected with the Heart spirit.

It is used for diarrhea or intestinal troubles connected with stress and anxiety.

■ ST-24

Another point that I consider related to the Small Intestine and coupled with the Heart. Like ST-23, it is a "Heart earth," but connected with Heart fire. ST-24 treats Heart fire that affects the Small Intestine.

Used for diarrhea, intestinal pains heightened by cold (deficiency of fire), abdominal external cold, cold drinks or cold food, especially raw vegetables.

■ ST-25

The name of this point is *tian shu* or "Pivot of Heaven." It is located two units on either side of the navel, and therefore vertically in the center of the body. It links heaven and earth within us. It is, at the same time:

- reunion in the body of heaven (above the navel) with that of earth (under the navel)
- home to both ethereal and corporeal souls (as noted in Chapter 31 of the *Great Compendium of Acupuncture and Moxibustion*)
- alarm point of the Large Intestine
- according to the *Classic of Difficulties,* No. 31, it is the second alarm point of the middle burner (along with CV-12). The functions of the middle burner are to join (ST-25) and to refine, to accomplish (CV-12).
- corresponding to autumn, it receives; it harvests from the earth the influences that have descended from heaven.
- symptoms are related to fullness above and emptiness below and include those involving the digestive tract, menstruation, and insomnia (often marked by dreams of flying).

■ ST-27

The location of this point is at either side of CV-5, which can be seen as the foundation stone of the abdomen. As such, it reduces the intensity and frequency of attacks of diarrhea.

It also treats heat in the thorax that can present with insomnia as well as intestinal, urinary and genital problems.

■ ST-28

The name of the point is *shui dao* or "Water Way" and it is located at the level of CV-4, the emergent point of the Penetrating vessel.

Its symptoms tell us of a yin excess in the pelvis with regional issues manifesting as premenstrual back pain or pelvic fullness and bloating.

■ ST-29

This point is located at the level of CV-3, where the qi returns to be stored in the pelvis.

It treats an excess of yin in the genitals with *yang ming* signs such as impotence, menstrual irregularities, internal cold in the uterus, cold and perineal pain, prostatitis, orchitis, pain of the penis, hernias due to the *yang ming* not closing the yang in the pelvis.

■ ST-30

The name *qi chong* or "Qi Surging" contains the same *chong* as the Penetrating (*chong*) vessel. I use it in three ways:

— with ST-36 for problems of the "sea of drink and food" for fullness when excessive, or inability to eat although hungry, when deficient

— as a Penetrating (*chong*) vessel point (often matched with SP-4)

— in relation to the deep branches of the leg *yang ming* (as reflected in ST-12) and the leg *shao yang* (GB-21)

■ ST-31

The name of this point is *bi guan* or "Hip Barrier." It controls the entry of yang qi from the leg into the pelvis. It is used for thigh and hip pains due to a yang excess.

A great point for knee pain.

This point is often involved in somebody who has the impression of being unable to move ahead even one more step in his life or who has the sensation of one's legs being cut out from under them.

■ **ST-35**

For pain in the knee joints.

Also used for more pains in the peripheral ligaments along the *yang ming*.

■ **ST-37**

In the *Great Compendium of Acupuncture and Moxibustion*, it relates to the corporeal soul.

A special connecting point with the arm *yang ming* Large Intestine channel. In Chapters 4 and 19 of the *Divine Pivot*, it is used to treat Large Intestine diseases due to an external pernicious influence.

When punctured along with ST-36 and ST-39, it releases *yang ming* heat.

■ **ST-38**

Treats poly-articular attacks *(bi)* aggravated by dampness.

■ **ST-40**

As a connecting *(luo)* point between the leg *yang ming* and *tai yin*, it treats phlegm regardless of where it manifests: it may be punctured or, preferably, tonified with moxa.

When its functions are disrupted, the yang stays blocked upward and outward (resulting in the symptoms below). This also leads to a poor knowledge of the interior, of the intimate.

Symptoms include mental disturbances, epilepsy, madness, hysterics, overexcitement, hallucinations, actions such as dancing on tables or throwing off one's clothes.

Spleen Channel

■ **SP-3**

The source point that receives qi from ST-40. These two points can be needled together when signs of both *yang ming* and *tai yin* are present.

■ **SP-4**

As the collateral point of the leg *tai yin* (*tai* = opens), which helps the *tai yin* open toward the outside or *yang ming*. When dysfunctional, the person is introverted and has a tendency to not express feelings and emotions.

Acute intestinal pains, vomiting, diarrhea

Abdominal swelling, large stools

Sighing and complaining, melancholy, schizophrenia

— the opening point of the Penetrating vessel

■ **SP-6**

The name is *san yin jiao* or "Three Yin Intersection" that reflects where all the leg yin channels cross. It causes the qi of these channels to ascend.

It has an effect on blood in the pelvis, particularly as it relates to uterine and prostate problems.

It also affects the Gallbladder.

Gives a feeling of the whole body being heavy; this is a frequent sign accompanying dysfunction of the leg *tai yin* Spleen.

■ **SP-7**

This is the third connecting point on the leg *tai yin*, in addition to SP-4 and SP-21.

It is important to facilitate the smooth opening and receiving functions of the leg *tai yin* (e.g., it is helpful in treating dyspareunia).

It is useful also for Spleen or leg *tai yin* dysfunction with dampness and has a valuable diuretic effect.

■ **SP-8**

As the unblocking cleft point, it works on treating energetic or psychological blockage of this yin organ or meridian.

I use it in emergency situations if urination is difficult.

■ **SP-10**

The name of this point is *xue hai* or "Sea of Blood," and it is the only point that has the word "blood" in its primary name.

It purifies the blood, specifically the pelvic blood.

Used if the blood is "toxic" or "impure" with rashes, including eczema, menstrual blood, nausea, etc.

■ **SP-12**

A secondary name of this point is *shang ci gong* or "Upper Palace of Kindness," where the word *ci* has the connotation of the kindness that is shown by a mother, that is, a type of motherly love.

Tai yin is "mother" and therefore can be involved when she is "missing" (e.g., with lactation difficulties) and with *tai yin* signs and a yin excess in the pelvis.

■ SP-14

Located at the level of CV-6 and as such is related to issues of the lower fire. Because it is at this level, SP-14 is for abdominal symptoms exacerbated by external or alimentary cold.

We must think of this point when there are abdominal, digestive troubles, heightened by cold either in the environment or in the food and drink.

■ SP-15

At the level of the umbilicus, near K-16 and ST-25.

For gastric and intestinal troubles that are associated with a variety of issues related to the four limbs and with *tai yin* symptoms.

■ SP-17

Directs the pure Spleen qi upward.

Its pathological signs include accumulations under the diaphragm: growling and rumblings with a splashing sound at the level of the diaphragm.

■ SP-21

The great connecting point of the Spleen.

When this point in involved in cases of excess internal cold, the entire body is painful (source: *Systematic Classic of Acupuncture and Moxibustion).*

In case of deficiency, the joints are loose (source: *Gathering of the Blossoms of Acupuncture).*

Heart Channel

■ HT-1

Treats yin stagnation in the chest and sets the chest yin in motion.

Indications: anxiety, sadness, absence of joy, precordial pains, angina, thirst

Although traditionally not mentioned for asthma, I have often found this point useful when patients experience a feeling of constriction in the chest during an asthma attack, as it opens up the chest and Heart.

Useful locally for difficulty in raising the arm, as well as for a sensation of cold in the upper arm and elbow.

HT-4

The name of this point, *ling dao*, means the "Way of the Spirit" or of the divine.

It is used for depression, sadness, fear, excitability, muteness or aphonia; it is particularly effective if there is a cold feeling in the bones.

This point, HT-5, and HT-6 can all be used for groaning, precordial pains, pain of the elbow, and speech disorders.

HT-5

This is the connecting point of the Heart channel, treating an inability to speak due to being overwhelmed by emotion and fullness in the area of the diaphragm.

This point connects us to the meaning of our lives, our reason for living.

In addition to treating emotional lability, tight sensation in the Heart, lack of self-confidence, agoraphobia, and inexpressive face, this is a very useful point for treating stage fright.

HT-6

This is the cleft point on the channel and treats obstructions along the channel and of the Heart.

It treats fright and different types of fear along with neurasthenia with significant night sweats.

HT-7

The name of this point, *shen men*, means the "Gate of the Spirit."

It is the main point of the Sovereign Heart and opens a profound connection with the spirit. The primary indications are major disturbances of sleep and memory.

Small Intestine Channel

SI-3

As the confluent point of the Governing vessel, it calms psychological troubles or seizure disorders due to Governing vessel dysfunction.

SI-7

It is both the connecting point and, according to Chamfrault, an alarm *(mu)* point for the Stomach.

Indications: loose joints, difficulty moving elbows; skin issues: styes, excrescences on the neck and face, warts; psychopathy, madness, apprehension, overexcited speech

■ SI-10

As this is on the shoulder, just above the trunk, it relates to the phase in one's evolution that is maturity with detachment: an ability to transcend history in order to access, in the head, a wider vision of life.

A meeting point of both the Yang Girdle and Yang Heel vessels.

Can be used for acute or chronic pains of the shoulders or the hips.

■ SI-11

Often indicated for periarthritis of the shoulder with an inability to raise the arm.

Must be combined with HT-1 if there are signs of stagnation.

■ SI-12

A wind point, its name is *bing feng* or "Grasping Wind."

Often indicated for scapular pain due to the effects of external or internal pathogenic wind. The internal pathogenic wind must be expelled via the leg *jue yin* (coupled with the arm *tai yang* according to the midday-midnight rule).

■ SI-16

The name of this point, *tian chuang*, means "Heavenly Window." As an arm *tai yang* heaven point, it connects the trunk to the head, the heaven in the human being.

It is related to problems affecting the face and head by wind and cold and has an impact on eye and ear function.

Often indicated for stiffness of the neck or cervicobrachial neuralgias along the *tai yang* trajectory.

At the same time, we generally observe throat pain, as with all window-of-heaven points.

■ SI-17

Governs the ascent of yin from the body to the head.

The name of this point, *tian rong*, means "Heavenly Appearance." As an arm *tai yang* heaven point, it connects the trunk to the head, the heaven in the human being.

Connected with the Gallbladder (as noted in Chapter 5 of the *Divine Pivot* on the roots and nodes) and the Liver (by its divergent channel).

Governs the ascent of yin from the body to the head.

Indicated for headaches due to yin deficiency with occipital radiation or initial pain in the occiput.

■ SI-18

Related to problems of the nose and mouth.

Indicated for some facial neuralgias or toothache of the upper maxillary.

Bladder Channel

■ BL-1

The node of the *tai yang*, it links leg *tai yang*, arm *tai yang*, leg *yang ming*, and the Yin and Yang Heel vessels.

It is related to the eyes and vision.

BL-1 is the terminus of the Yin Heel vessel, by which the qi of the Yang Heel vessel goes to GB-20.

BL-1 is the entrance of qi into the brain.

■ BL-2

Indicated for nasal problems.

For *tai yang* headaches due to wind.

For overexcited behavior of a *tai yang* nature. Note that TB-23 also corresponds to overexcited behavior. Overexcited *tai yang* is very reactive and the emotion is skin-deep, while *shao yang* overexcitement leans more toward being impulsive and angry.

■ BL-3

Clears the yang of the eyes and nose.

Used for nasal congestion, headaches, some epilepsy attacks.

■ BL-5

Often useful for *tai yang* headaches or migraines due to an excess of yang.

Pain is marked by a breaking or tearing sensation due to an excess of yang.

Has a differential diagnosis with BL-6 (radiation toward the lower maxillaries), BL-7 (heaviness in the head), and BL-8 (insanity).

Sometimes associated with dim vision and/or a stiff back.

■ BL-6

Tai yang barrier point from the skull to the face, thus it is marked by headaches with radiation toward the mandible.

■ BL-7

The name of this point, *tian tong,* means "Heavenly Connection."

Headaches due to an excess of yang with heaviness of the head.

Stiff neck with a tearing sensation in the nape of the neck *(tai yang* characteristic).

Problems here often are accompanied by problems along the leg *tai yang* as well as with the nose and eye.

■ BL-8

Releases endocranial yang with vertigo and insanity *(dian kuang).*

Symptoms include panic, a need to run, and abdominal distention accompanied by dyspnea.

■ BL-10

The name of this point, *tian zhu,* means "Heavenly Pillar." It is a window-of-heaven point.

BL-10 favors the descent of yang from the cranium downward. If this window of heaven does not function properly, it results in a cranial excess of yang with a deficiency below, for example, headache due to the excess of yang going through the nape of the neck toward the back and limbs. The indications in *Grand Compendium of Acupuncture and Moxibustion* include vertigo with weakness in the legs, extreme pain at the top of the skull, and weak legs that cannot support the body.

This point stores the memory of the difficulty of finding and actualizing our own expression of universal laws.

■ BL-11

An alternate name of this point (as well as GV-14) is *bai lao,* "Hundred Labors," which refers to this point's use in treating people who are very tired because they are overburdened physically or psychologically. Also it is a point of the sea of blood of the channels *(Divine Pivot,* Chapter 33), which makes it useful for patients who feel very heavy for no particular reason.

The meeting point *(hui)* of the bones, as an extraordinary organ. I often use it for patients with polyarticular pains.

Indicated for vertebral pain and knee pain in those who are overburdened, either physically or psychologically.

■ BL-12

The name of this point, *feng men,* means "Wind Gate."

Indications include attack by exterior or interior pathogenic wind affecting the leg *tai yang,* especially the nape of the neck and lower limbs, as well as the lungs, eyes, nose or skin.

■ BL-13

Back associated point of the Lung. Note that all of these points are more focused on acute conditions.

Main symptoms: lung or skin problems, back issues (such as scoliosis), and, based on its connection to the corporeal soul, either suicidal or homicidal tendencies.

■ BL-14

Back associated point of the Heart Master

Indications: chest pain, heart diseases, circulatory troubles in the extremities, hiccups

■ BL-15

Back associated point of the Heart

Indications: acute or subacute Heart problems accompanied by psychological disorders, poor memory, and muscular contractures

Another interesting indication is delayed speech development in children.

■ BL-16

Back associated point of the Governing vessel; it has the alternate name of *gao gai,* "High Canopy."

It opens the chest and I use it to make the Heart qi descend when blocked in the diaphragm or thorax.

■ BL-17

Back associated point of the diaphragm

Meeting point of blood and governs the blood

Linked to the *jueyin* organs, Heart Master and Liver

Indications: blood deficiency, stasis, and blood heat with pruritis, nettle-rash, eczema, hemorrhages

One useful sign when this point may be indicated is a heavy and painful body with a desire to lie down.

■ BL-18

Back associated point of the Liver

Indications: psychological problems, insomnia (somnambulism, night terrors), eye disorders, gastric problems, muscular disorders (cramps, contractures), and menstrual disorders

■ BL-19

Back associated point of the Gallbladder, considered here as an ordinary yang organ

For gallbladder troubles, eye disorders, a bitter taste in the mouth, jaundice, abdominal cramps

■ BL-20

Back associated point of the Spleen

Many digestive signs including lassitude, edema, and remaining thin despite eating a lot of food

Hemorrhages (as the Spleen is responsible for keeping the blood inside the vessels)

■ BL-21

Back associated point of the Stomach

For digestive disorders, emaciation, muscle contractures

■ BL-22

Back associated point of the Triple Burner

Abdominal distention, anorexia, emaciation with other signs of Triple Burner dysfunction

■ BL-23

Back associated point of the Kidneys, to be tonified for Kidney deficiency or treated with moxibustion for deficiency cold in the Kidneys

For a variety of Kidney problems manifesting as urinary, digestive, menstrual, or sexual disorders, especially lumbar problems, edema, and spermatorrhea

▪ BL-25

Back associated point of the Large Intestine

Intestinal and urinary problems, cystitis due to intestinal disorders. These patients are often thin even if they eat a lot.

▪ BL-29

A barrier point that controls the exit of yang from the trunk to the pelvis and lower limbs

A blockage of this point is always aggravated by coughing and often manifests as pain radiating along leg *tai yang* to the lower limb.

▪ BL-39

Lower uniting point of the Triple Burner and a connecting point of the leg *tai yang*

Useful in certain cases of prostatitis, cystitis, or diarrhea with burning during urination and/or defecation, if the pulse in both proximal positions is deficient.

▪ BL-40

Lower uniting point of the Bladder, used for urinary incontinence

Governs the skin, and especially the blood in the skin: cutaneous diseases, loss of hair, loss or thinning of eyebrows

Effective in sciatica affecting the *tai yang* as well as pain in the lumbar region that goes up to the nape of the neck. Bleed if possible.

▪ BL-42

The name of this point, *po hu*, means "Door of the Corporeal Soul."

As the corporeal soul "matches the essence in its entrances and exits" (*Divine Pivot*, Chapter 8), this point aids the Lung essence in severe exhaustion of the Lung qi and is used for pulmonary issues, difficulties in fully embracing life, and a desire to kill.

▪ BL-43

Back associated point of both the noble fats (*gao*) and nutritive heat (*huang*)

BL-43 suggests great physical and mental exhaustion, loss of memory, and is also indicated for cases of separation or the loss of loved ones.

▪ BL-44

The name of this point is *shen tang* or "Hall of the Spirit." As a connection with the

Heart spirit, it contributes as a modest but useful adjunct to the treatment of major mental disorders such as manic-depression.

It governs the essence of the Heart and should be used for nervous exhaustion with depression, insomnia, poor memory, and an empty Heart pulse.

▪ BL-46

The name of this point is *ge guan* or "Diaphragm Barrier."

As a diaphragm point, it treats esophageal dysphagia and hiccups, particularly if there are other *tai yang* signs.

Indicated for intercostal neuralgias.

▪ BL-47

The name of this point, *hun men,* means "Gate of the Ethereal Soul."

It controls the Liver's relationship with its spirit, the ethereal soul that ensures all of the "comings and goings": day and night, muscular and energetic, visual and imaginary, etc. It is like tree sap that flows readily and freely from the furthest ends of the roots to the tips of the branches. In this way it is the command point for all Liver functions.

Hepatic troubles, insomnia, somnambulism, talking and screaming while asleep, contractures, muscular cramps

Preventive for early tics and jerks, such as in some choreiform disorders

▪ BL-48

Governs the Gallbladder as an extraordinary organ. This point is related to the father.

The mechanism that distinguishes a being from the midst of chaos, that begins a life, is of the order of fire. The Gallbladder, which separates and initiates, is related to this initial moment, so it is placed under the symbol of fire. BL-48 corresponds to this function and thus treats functional infertility.

▪ BL-49

The name of this point, *yi she,* means "Abode of Intention." This point controls the Spleen's relationship with its spirit, the intention *(yi)*.

Moreover, it restores the essence of the Spleen when exhausted. This type of fatigue is both intellectual and physical (not psychological or sexual) and is accompanied by digestive problems.

■ **BL-50**

The name of this point, *wei cang,* means "Stomach Storehouse." It and BL-48 are the only points related to the yang organs on the lateral branch of the leg *tai yang* channel.

Indicated in gastric disorders, with no appetite for life, edema, and lower back pain.

■ **BL-51**

The name of this point, *huang men,* means "Gate of Nutritive Heat."

It is indicated for lactation disorders, mastitis or other breast diseases.

■ **BL-52**

The name of this point is *zhi shi,* "Chamber of Resolve," and it stores the Kidney essence and spirit, that is, the resolve (*zhi,* sometimes translated as will or ambition) connected with the survival instinct. It is the quality of our resolve that enables us to survive in physically or psychologically difficult conditions. Without it, we are physically, intellectually, and sexually fatigued and, above all, lacking in drive and the will to live.

In Kidney exhaustion due to deficiency of essence (from a chronic disease, overworking, etc.) we can observe intestinal, urinary, renal, and/or genital problems along with edema and low back pain.

■ **BL-53**

The name of this point is *bao huang,* "Envelope of the Nutritive Heat."

Its symptomatology is mainly pelvic, with significant genital implications. This point is related to the pelvic envelope, the qi/blood balance in the pelvis and, as a result, the uterus. Its pathology is connected to a blockage of qi and of blood in the pelvis, and this blockage is closely linked to the genitals, prostate, menstruation, pregnancy, etc.

■ **BL-58**

The name of this point is *fei yang* or "Flying Yang." It connects the relatively superficial leg *tai yang* with the deeper leg *shao yin.*

The symptoms of this connecting point are:

— stuffy nose, runny nose, nosebleeds, pains on the top of the head and in the back

— depression, hysteria, madness

In my experience, patients with a dysfunction affecting this point often dream that they are flying away and are quite edgy and quick-tempered.

■ **BL-60**

The name of this point is *kun lun.* The Kunlun are legendary mountains in Chinese tradition. It is indicated for a verticalization of the being and pains or muscular cramps due to a lack of verticality.

In obstetrics, this point treats difficult labor and aids in delivery of the placenta.

■ **BL-61**

The gate of early childhood, linked to GB-29 and SI-10.

I needle it in children who want to remain baby-like as well as for growing pains.

■ **BL-62**

Governs the Yang Heel vessel and thus helps one to exteriorize. In this way it expels heat from the skin (furuncles, acne, etc.) and also calms some everyday joint pains.

■ **BL-63**

This is the cleft point used to unblock the leg *tai yang.*

As the starting point of the *yang wei* vessel, it can reinforce the effects of TB-5 on the functions of this vessel.

■ **BL-67**

The name of this point is *zhi yin,* "Utmost Yin." It governs all head and face disorders.

Treats pains due to anything disrupting the leg *tai yang* channel sinew, including shoulder pains.

With a heated needle, helps to turn a malpositioned fetus if used between 32nd and 36th weeks of pregnancy.

Kidney Channel

■ **KI-1**

The name of this point is *yong quan,* "Gushing Spring." This well point sets the yin in motion.

Important in severe deficiency of leg *shao yin* and therefore of all the yin of the body. Symptoms can occur that may be related to any of the five yin organs and often include some forms of exhaustion (physical, psychoemotional, intellectual, and/or sexual), along with dizziness, sore throat, vertex headaches, and intense frights. Also used for loss of consciousness.

■ **KI-2**

I use it to simultaneously reinforce the leg *shao yin* and Yin Heel vessel.

■ **KI-3**

If the proximal pulses and the KI-3 pulses are both weak, this would imply a weakness in the lower half of the body (e.g., of the CV-5 or Yin Heel type), or a general deficiency of yin and yang in the Kidneys.

If KI-3 pulses are full, this suggests that some type of qi cannot descend.

■ **KI-4**

This is the connecting point of leg *shao yin* and treats reduced urination accompanied by anxiety, and mid-thoracic back pain that radiates to CV-17. These people often have a sense of inferiority and of failure, lack of authority, lack of joy, timidity, nervousness, apprehension, and a desire to seek solitude and "close the door to shut out the world." Their Kidney qi is in most ways normal, but is not deployed, that is, it does not rise throughout the body, both physically and psychologically.

In my experience this point also governs the lower burner and treats low back pain, constipation, and urinary disorders.

■ **KI-5**

This is the cleft point on this channel and is very effective in regulating menstruation, particularly to help young women with amenorrhea or irregular menstruation. It can also regulate the Penetrating and Conception vessels.

■ **KI-6**

The name of this point is *zhao hai* or "Shining Sea" and it is the starting point of the Yin Heel vessel.

Indications: night-time erratic pains in the joints, insomnia, constipation, dysuria, premenstrual syndrome, melancholy (being without light).

■ **KI-8**

A cleft point of the Yin Heel vessel that is related to issues of confidence and betrayal. This is found in its name *jiao xin,* "Exchange of Trust."

■ **KI-9**

The starting point and cleft point of the Yin Girdle vessel. This makes it very useful at the beginning of a pregnancy.

▪ KI-11

Governs the Kidneys in their role as the root of production of the five organs. This explains the signs of deficiency in the Kidneys, with a lack of sperm, amenorrhea, etc. There will also be symptoms of exhaustion of the four other yin organs.

While KI-1 has a similar focus, there are more leg *shao yin* symptoms, while KI-11 has more symptoms of the other yin organs.

▪ KI-12

This is the leg *shao yin* Kidney point at the level of CV-3. That point governs the withdrawal of qi into the depths and this point deals with the same movement.

It acts on the genitals and on sexuality. It is used for lack of virility, impotence, and genital diseases in both men and women.

▪ KI-13

The name of this point is *qi xue* or "Qi Hole." As the meeting point with the Conception and Penetrating vessels, it protects and favors pregnancy and controls the ebb and flow of the Kidney qi.

At the same level as CV-4, these points share the alternative names *zi hu* or "Child's Door" and *bao men* or "Envelope Gate." This shows how closely related are the functions of these two points.

▪ KI-14

Alarm point of the Triple Burner, it governs the gestational envelopes.

Regulates the pathways of water (source: Guillaume, 1995) while controlling the storage function of the Kidneys and marrow.

I needle it to reinforce the amassing of essence by the Kidneys and to strengthen the marrow.

▪ KI-15

This point is in charge of draining the Kidneys.

I needle it to supply the lack of purification by the Kidneys, producing an accumulation of intestinal, urinary, and genital impurities. Commonly the Kidney pulse is slippery and empty and there are heat symptoms such as dry yet foul-smelling stools, cystitis, or vaginitis.

■ KI-16

As a *huang* point near the navel, it is related to pregnancy.

I needle it in cases of fetal growth deficiency and repeated miscarriages due to poor nutrition of the embryo.

I also use it in cases of people who did not receive sufficient affection as children and who present with cold symptoms affecting the digestive and urinary systems.

■ KI-17

The name of this point is *shang qu,* which I take to mean "Trade Bend." I understand this point as handling the transport functions of the Spleen. When this is deficient, there is an accumulation of Stomach qi in the abdomen leading to such problems as hernia from excess, hiccups, stomachache, abdominal accumulation, and uterine congestion.

■ KI-18

In my experience this point drains the Spleen in order to cleanse it and eliminate toxins.

Symptoms include digestive and urinary accumulation of damp-heat with some connection to the Spleen.

■ KI-20

Drains and decongests the Liver for symptoms of digestive and urinary accumulation of damp-heat with some connection to the Liver.

It is particularly effective for vomiting due to a Liver disorder, including morning sickness.

■ KI-21

This point resolves Liver qi constraint and loosens areas of contractions.

It controls the Liver function of evening out and regulating the qi of the body and the functions of the yang organs (also an important point for vomiting and motion sickness), moodiness (particularly bad moods, aggravated by anger), and poor memory.

■ KI-22

This point governs the diffusion of Lung qi to the outside.

It is linked to fairness and judgment or justice and therefore, pathologically, to injustice. It is particularly effective in cases of someone suffering from injustice with pulmonary and gastric signs.

■ KI-23

This point is named *shen feng,* meaning "Spirit Seal," and is often useful in purifying the
Heart blood.

The damp-heat in this area has cardiac, circulatory and cutaneous symptoms marked by
facial congestion aggravated by heat (sun, alcohol, etc.).

■ KI-25

The name of this point is *shen cang* or "Storehouse of the Spirit." The word storehouse
refers to winter and the storage functions of the organs.

Its symptoms manifest as a counterflow of both the Lung and Stomach qi.

Soulié de Morant added two important signs: "lingers on the unpleasant side, doesn't
like life."

■ KI-26

This point clarifies the qi and fluids of the Lung and serves as the purification point of
that organ.

As a purification point, it treats damp-heat which has symptoms that relate to the Lung.

■ KI-27

This point directs both the Lung qi and the liquids that converge in the thorax downward to treat fullness in the upper part of the body with such problems as allergic
rhinitis, asthma with mucus, dyspnea with high, short, superficial breathing, and
severe insomnia.

It is also one of the most effective points for pain on the anterior shoulder and the upper
limbs, along the pathway of the arm *tai yin* channel sinew.

Heart Master (Pericardium) Channel

■ HM-1

As LU-3 serves to facilitate qi exchanges with the head, so HM-1 serves the same role
with the blood.

Symptoms include congestive headache, diaphragmatic spasms, and difficulty in moving
the limbs.

■ HM-2

The name of this point is *tian quan* or "Heavenly Spring." As a heaven point, it facilitates
the entry of yin at the shoulder. Symptoms include pain in the arm and upper back.

■ **HM-3**

This point is necessary to treat those with a propensity to fright and Heart Master symptoms.

With HM-2, HM-3, HM-4, and HM-6 there is counterflow of the Lung, Stomach, and Heart qi with cough, dyspnea, palpitations, nausea, and belching.

■ **HM-4**

As the cleft point, it serves to relieve obstruction after somatic or psychoemotional trauma.

For fear and anxiety, cardiac disorders and diaphragm spasms.

■ **HM-5**

Related to the central mechanisms: spirit, Heart, middle burner.

It helps to center people and is useful for "off-center" patients who have problems such as mania, agitation, laughing dementia, and who appear to be "possessed."

■ **HM-6**

The name of this point is *nei guan* or "Inner Pass." It is the connecting point of the arm *jue yin* and the confluent point of the Yin Linking vessel.

It controls the upper burner and facilitates the relationship between the upper and middle burners. As such, it frees the diaphragm and is used for heartburn and pains in the solar plexus.

It is also used for stiff neck and for such psychoemotional problems as mental fatigue, forgetting words, indecision, anxiety due to yin deficiency, diminished motivation with anxiety, laziness.

■ **HM-7**

One of its secondary names is *xin zhu* or "Heart Master," which is a secondary name of both the arm *jue yin* channel and the Heart organ itself.

Indicated for insomnia and psychoemotional disorders marked by frequent and extravagant laughter. Usually the palms are also hot.

■ **HM-9**

This is the well point and so governs the arm *jue yin* channel sinew. Treats chest wall pain and pain of the root of the tongue. The arm *tai yin* channel sinew can also treat chest wall pain, but without tongue involvement, and this chest wall pain can reach as high as KI-27. Often I try one, and if it is ineffective, I use the other.

It serves as a general "sweep" of the channel. If it is clear to me that a certain channel should be treated but I cannot decide which specific point to puncture, I will treat the well point, as it acts on the entire channel. Often after that, symptoms specific to a particular point will manifest.

Triple Burner Channel

■ TB-5

The name of this point is *wai guan* or "Outer Pass." It is the connecting point of the arm *shao yang* and a confluent point of the Yang Linking vessel.

As a connecting point of arm *shao yang,* it is used to treat issues relating to problems in communication between this channel and the arm *jue yin* Heart Master channel with patients who are being overly excited or are exhibiting tremors.

It is a point that concerns relations with the outside world and protects the body from the influence of exterior climatic pathogenic qi.

As the confluent point of the Yang Linking vessel it is indicated for barometric pains, that is, changes in the patient's pains that allow them to forecast the weather.

Also for spasms in the elbow or a weak elbow.

■ TB-7

The name of this point is *hui zong,* "Meeting of Ancestors." It is the cleft point of the arm *shao yang* channel.

Indications: painful skin, upper extremity pain, cramps, epilepsy, deafness

■ TB-13

The name of this point is *nao hui,* "Upper Arm Meeting."

The barrier point of the upper limb: for arm pain along the path of the *shao yang* and for neck swellings.

■ TB-14

For shoulder pain and inability to raise the arm due to a stagnation which is improved by movement and heat.

■ TB-15

On the Yang Linking vessel and a barrier point for flow going toward the face.

Indicated for stiffness of the neck, shoulder pain, and arm pain.

■ **TB-16**

The name of this point is *tian you,* or "Window of Heaven," and it connects the trunk to the head, which is the heavenly part of the human body.

Indications: recently impaired vision or hearing; cervicobrachial pains along the *shao yang* pathway; night terrors, somnambulism, and strange dreams, such as dreaming of falling into an empty space

■ **TB-17**

The name of this point is *yi feng,* "Wind Screen."

For facial problems due to exterior or interior pathogenic wind such as facial paralysis, trismus, and ear disorders.

■ **TB-20**

This point is related to the neck and face, not the ear.

Useful for disorders due to wind affecting the face, and for swellings of the neck.

■ **TB-21**

The name of this point is *er men,* "Ear Door," and thus it primarily focuses on the ear.

For tinnitus (particularly if it is high-pitched, like the call of a cicada) and deafness.

■ **TB-23**

This point relates to the eye and is used for eye pains.

Often used for *shao yang* headaches, migraines, and frontomaxillary sinusitis.

It is often used for people who are restless.

Gallbladder Channel

■ **GB-1**

Important for eye disorders, particularly of the conjunctiva and cornea, or for visual disorders due to wind-heat.

Useful for supraorbital neuralgia.

■ **GB-2**

Very useful for ear blockages and headaches.

Often there is awakening at 3 a.m., restlessness and sadness.

◼ GB-3

The name of this point is *shang guan,* "Upper Barrier." It governs the ipsilateral temporomaxillary joint along with ST-7, *xia guan* or "Lower Barrier."

A *tai yang* pain in the temples can come from either a *tai yang* disorder or a blockage of this point.

◼ GB-5

The name of this point is *xuan lu,* "Suspended Skull."

Corresponds more to pain that radiates to the outer canthus of the eyes, nose and teeth, due to its connections with the arm and leg *yang ming* channels (noted in Chapter 22 of *Divine Pivot*).

Indicated for an accumulation of impurities (such as toxins or damp-heat) manifesting as heat in the brain with headache or migraine, stuffy nose, red eyes, nervousness accompanied by a sensation that the body is hot, neurasthenia, etc.

Difficult to differentiate its indications from those of GB-6.

◼ GB-6

The name of this point is *xuan li,* "Suspended Tuft of Hair."

The indications are very close to those for GB-5, but tend to be less about an accumulation of impurities and more about heat in the middle burner.

◼ GB-8

Important point for oral-related problems, especially the treatment of tobacco addiction (used with GB-1).

Dissipates inebriation when used with GV-25.

Useful for rheumatism due to alcoholism.

◼ GB-13

The name of this point is *ben shen,* "Root of the Spirit." It connects with the Yang Linking vessel.

Can be used in psychiatric disorders and epilepsy.

◼ GB-14

For significant ocular symptomatology due to an excess of yang.

The barrier point indicated for frontal headaches due to an excess of yang or for *tai yang* facial neuralgia.

■ **GB-15**

The name of this point is *tou lin qi,* "Head Next to Tears." It is related to GB-41, the name of which is *zu lin qi,* or "Foot Next to Tears."

Treats *shao yang* headaches due to a stagnation of yang with stuffy nose and pain of the eyes.

■ **GB-20**

The name of this point is *feng chi,* "Wind Pool." It is indicated for exogenous or endogenous wind attacks into the head or to the back of the neck.

Indicated for both superficial and deep headaches and/or stiff neck.

Puts into motion excess *shao yang* in the upper part of the body.

■ **GB-21**

The name of this point is *jian jing,* "Shoulder Well."

It is used locally for problems of the neck and back.

As is directs the *shao yang* qi downward toward the pelvis, it is also used for pelvic problems. Examples include expediting delivery with difficult labor or for stopping uterine bleeding due to qi deficiency.

■ **GB-22**

Meeting point of the three upper limb channel sinews and entering point of the three upper limb yin divergent channels into the thorax.

Thus it alleviates axillary problems such as swelling, adenopathies, or an inability to raise the arm, and also puts into motion yang that has stagnated in the thorax.

Moxibustion is forbidden.

■ **GB-23**

An alarm point of the Gallbladder, which is linked to spring, it releases constrained qi in the body.

This point has a relationship with the *tai yang* while GB-24 is linked to the *tai yin.* This means that there may be additional *tai yang* symptoms with a blockage of GB-23 or additional *tai yin* symptoms with a blockage of GB-24.

A blockage at this point leads to fullness in the chest, sighing, acid regurgitation, inability to stay still in bed, a desire to run around, and difficulty with interpersonal relationships.

▪ GB-24

The second alarm point of the Gallbladder is linked to spring with symptoms somewhat similar to GB-23, but with a yin blockage: in fact, it is connected with the *tai yin*.

Gallbladder disorders are more obvious here, with symptoms such as constipation, hiccups and indecisiveness.

Externalizing *(tai yin)*, it is a good point to treat kidney stone colic.

▪ GB-25

An alarm point of the Kidneys, it relates to the winter-like activation or setting into motion of the yang qi of the body at midnight.

Associated with winter, it activates the Kidney qi by putting it into motion. If this qi is not in motion in the pelvis, we have low back pain that makes it difficult to stand for long periods, muscle spasms in the lumbar region and hips as well as in the shoulders and upper back, diarrhea, flatulence, dysuria, and even nephritis.

▪ GB-26

The name of this point, *dai mai* or "Girdle Vessel," shows that it is a main point on this vessel.

If the vessel does not function, we observe pelvic disorders with cramping or spasticity, especially gynecological disorders. The patient is scattered and tries to do a hundred things at once, neither systematically nor orderly.

▪ GB-29

A meeting point of both the Yang Linking and Yang Heel vessels, this point affects issues related to the passage through adolescence and its difficulties.

Symptoms emerge when a special event (such as an old friend's death) serves as a reminder of this difficult period.

A wide range of symptoms can appear: lower back pain, hip pain, or disorders of the pelvis, including pelvic pains, cystitis, or orchitis.

▪ GB-31

This is a wind point, the name of which, *feng shi,* means "Wind Market." As a wind point it is very useful for pruritus.

It has a good effect on stagnation in a knee marked by joint issues with effusions.

■ GB-33

The name of this point is *xi yang guan,* "Knee Yang Barrier," and an alternate name is *han fu,* "Mansion of Cold."

It is a barrier point of the knee: for pain along the *shao yang* with an inability to flex and extend the knee due to yang deficiency or cold.

Combined with LR-7, it is used for radiation toward the medial aspect of the knee.

■ GB-34

The united point of the leg *shao yang* channel.

Very effective for Gallbladder issues related to digestive problems or inflammation.

■ GB-35

The cleft point for the Yang Linking vessel.

Can be needled to reinforce the effects of TB-5.

■ GB-36

Cleft point of the leg *shao yang* channel that is especially indicated in cases of acute physical or psychological blockages.

■ GB-37

The name of this point is *guang ming,* "Bright Light." It is the connecting point.

Indications include:

— cold hands and feet

— powerless, flaccid legs such that one cannot rise unassisted from a seated position

— epilepsy, palpitations, intense emotional reactivity, as the yang is blocked up externally and does not go into the leg *jue yin*

— inability to stand up for long periods of time; the point is also useful for eversion ankle strains and sprains, combined with GB-44 or GB-38 if there is a hematoma

— very effective for eye disorders and to improve the vision

■ GB-39

This is the group connecting point for the three leg yang channels, according to the *Great Compendium.* It causes their qi to descend.

Its symptoms are related to stagnant qi that affects not only the respiratory and digestive functions, but also rheumatism due to dampness with swelling.

It is also the meeting point for the marrow and is very useful for moderating the side effects of chemotherapy.

■ GB-41

The name of this point is *zu lin qi,* "Foot Next to Tears." It is related to GB-15, named *tou lin qi,* "Head Next to Tears." It can reinforce the latter for *shao yang* headaches.

It is the stream (wood) point of *shao yang* and is yang that causes the yin to circulate in cases of yin stagnation, particularly when the *jue yin* is affected.

Confluent point of the Girdle vessel.

■ GB-44

The well point and therefore the governing point of the leg *shao yang* channel sinew.

The name of this point is *zu qiao yin,* "Foot Orifice of Yin." Thus it is related to GB-11, *tou qiao yin,* "Head Orifice of Yin."

As is true of all the well points, this serves as a general "sweep" of the channel, meaning that it acts on the entire channel and helps to clarify which particular point should be selected for the precise treatment.

Liver Channel

■ LR-2

Dispersion point of the wood phase. I use it when there is a desynchronization between a person and the macrocosm with an excessive wood motion that needs to be dispersed.

■ LR-3

Stream and source point of the leg *jue yin;* often used in combination with GB-37, the connecting point of the leg *shao yang.*

Combined with LR-10 to purify the blood for such problems as pruritus, eczema, foul-smelling menstrual bleeding with cramps, and some types of infertility.

Indicated for allergies, nettle-rash, eczema, etc., especially when coupled with LI-4. This combination is known as the "four gates."

■ LR-4

The river point of the leg *jue yin.*

Mostly used for urogenital problems (both male and female) and also for low back and ankle issues.

■ **LR-5**

Connecting point of leg *jue yin,* it is used for:

— extreme and painful erections and a sudden onset of genital itching

— an introverted or internalized person with a lack of joy, melancholy, frequent sighing, and/or worry

— low back pain with tightened muscles, like the string of a bow

■ **LR-6**

The primary name of this point is *zhong du,* "Central Capital." An alternate name is *tai yin,* "Great Yin." This demonstrates the importance and profound nature of the *jue yin.*

This is the cleft point, which is especially indicated in cases of acute physical or psychological blockages.

■ **LR-7**

When the pains are located on the inside of the knee, it is often advisable to puncture LR-7, the name of which is *xi guan,* "Knee Barrier."

■ **LR-9**

The name of this point is *yin bao,* "Yin Envelope." It governs the pelvis with such symptoms as dysuria, irregular menstruation, and low back pain that extends to the lower abdomen.

I have found it is effective for some pain due to endometriosis.

■ **LR-10**

This is a major point for detoxification, especially in the springtime.

The psoas muscles, which many osteopaths label the "garbage cans of the body," are also related to LR-10.

■ **LR-11**

This is the barrier point on the leg *jue yin* that activates the entry of yin qi at the hip.

While not noted, to my knowledge, in the Chinese literature, I have found this point remarkably effective for certain types of sacroiliac pain and sciatica. Numbness of the ipsilateral big toe is a sign that this point will be useful.

■ LR-13

The name of this point is *zhang men,* "Completion Gate." It is the alarm point of the Spleen, the meeting point of the yin organs (*Classic of Difficulties,* No. 45) and a point on the Girdle vessel. It is basically on the same transverse line as KI-16, ST-25, and SP-15.

From our point of view, LR-13 governs the Spleen, the terrestrial side of the center, which is space where life occurs (much like the terrestrial globe). It is in constant dialogue with the celestial side of the center, the sovereign Heart, which is the source of life.

Its indications include lack of qi, weakness, emaciation, sallow complexion, and ice-cold extremities.

■ LR-14

The name of this point is *qi men,* "Cycle Gate." It is the alarm point of the Liver.

It corresponds to the spring and therefore to the end of night, and the end of any yin phenomenon. For example, in women, it governs the end of the menstrual period, the end of pregnancy (postpartum difficulties, expulsion problems). It is effective at the time of menopause, the end of the procreative phase of life, to treat problems such as hot flashes. It governs the end of the qi movements that rise from below, from the depths of the yin zones to the upper areas of the thorax, the qi rising from the abdomen to the chest.

It is therefore indicated when something that must end does not end, or ends badly, whether it is a case of bronchitis, a menstrual period, a pregnancy, a procreative period, a separation, etc., as if the night (yin) could not end to allow the day to appear.

Conception Vessel

■ CV-1

The name of this point is *hui yin,* "Meeting of Yin." It is also the origin of the axial aspect of the Penetrating vessel.

After puncturing this point it is not uncommon to hear patients say something like, "I am really living in my body again, I am beginning to exist, I feel profoundly reawakened."

■ CV-2

This is a "master point" of the Conception vessel as it acts on the entire vessel, the primary function of which is to support and take responsibility.

Indications: lower back pain, male or female infertility, inguinal hernia, hydrocele, varicocele, leukorrhoea, as well as extreme cold due to deficiency

It governs the skin as the limitation of our body, as opposed to the limitation related to our name, which is ruled by the Governing vessel.

It is a reunion point of sinew channels of the legs, and I add this point whenever I have to treat them as it prevents the diffusion of any related pathogenic qi.

◼ CV-3

Alarm point of the Bladder.

It corresponds to the retreat of qi to the depths, to storage, and to the seed that germinates underground.

Indications: gynecological masses (cysts, fibromyomas, etc.), problems with the birth of the placenta; urinary tract problems for either sex, infertility, depression; impotence

◼ CV-4

This point corresponds to the summer, to setting yin in motion. It is a meeting point with the Penetrating vessel and also the alarm point of the Small Intestine.

This point has several summer functions. It sets pelvic yin qi into motion and treats general stagnation of yin.

As the alarm point of the Small Intestine, it has the function of fructification (a function that corresponds to summer) and of digestion of the products absorbed through eating food, which explains the symptoms of digestive and urinary problems connected with this yang organ. Thus the point combines two summer seasonal actions.

The name of the point is *guan yuan,* "Barrier of the Primal." It is associated with the primal qi, yang and fire of the Kidneys, putting the yang of the Kidneys into motion. It is the first point on the Penetrating vessel. When it malfunctions, there is exhaustion with deficiency, with a deep sense of inner cold, premature aging, and genital and sexual problems, with deep and short pulses, as well as tooth marks on the sides of the tongue. It is a point that tonifies the entire body.

It must be stressed that CV-4 is the convergence of three functions: it sets the yin of the body and the fire of Kidneys into motion; it governs the Penetrating vessel; and it serves as the alarm point of the Small Intestine.

◼ CV-5

The name of this point is *shi men,* "Stone Door," as in a foundation stone. It is indicated for breakdowns, when, under certain life circumstances, a person has the feeling that everything is crumbling. In this case, the pulses in both of the proximal positions are deep and broken down too. The breakdown can contribute to knee or foot pain, since the feet and knees are also the footing and foundations of the person.

It governs the gestational envelopes (*bao*). These are involved in cases of infertility, miscarriages, and in certain sexual dysfunctions, including the after effects of assaults. In such cases, acupuncture can reduce the psychological scarring.

It is also the alarm point of the Triple Burner and therefore corresponds to all that maintains life, nutrition and perpetuation.

We must think of this point when treating acute isolated abdominal pains which have no organic grounds.

■ CV-6

The name of this point is *qi hai,* "Sea of Qi," as it is related to the fire in the midst of water that generates qi.

It is indicated for physical and psychological exhaustion, as well as for a deficiency of essence that is marked by an empty pulse in the proximal positions.

■ CV-7

This is the alarm point of the lower burner that sorts out the impure from the pure and puts each in its proper place.

Its indications include pelvic, intestinal, urinary disorders, low back pain, lack of self-confidence, and an empty pulse in the proximal positions.

A differential diagnosis has to be done for the pelvic points of the Conception vessel, which all share empty pulses in the proximal position.

■ CV-9

The name of this point is *shui fen,* "Water Separation."

It is said that this point corresponds to the separation of food into fluids (going to the Bladder) and solids (going to the bowels) and, in the case of Small Intestine, the separation of pure and impure fluids.

Its indications include abdominal disorders with diarrhea; ascites and edema; stiffness and paravertebral contractions, especially in the lumbar area.

I must say that I am not sure that this point has any particular effect on edema, whether needled or treated with moxa; or any effect that it does have is short-lived.

■ CV-11

The Stomach, Gallbladder and Spleen are in the middle, which is governed by CV-11. I needle this point when I want to act on systemic issues, such as fatigue and general achiness, as well as digestive issues of these three organs simultaneously.

■ CV-12

The name of this point is *zhong wan,* "Middle Cavity." It is the alarm point of the Stomach and the middle burner.

It controls the accomplishment function of the middle burner. It is also indicated in essence deficiencies in the middle burner caused by overwork or exhaustion with intense fatigue, nausea, digestive problems, especially epigastric problems, and a short pulse that is hard to feel in the proximal and distal positions.

This is also the meeting *(hui)* point of the yang organs, the origin of the arm *tai yin* channel, and the root of *tai yin.*

When this point is involved, in addition to any other symptomatology, epigastric pains and digestive disorders are normally present.

For these indications it can be needled by itself, but more commonly it is used in combination with another point: ST-36 for Stomach issues, SP-4 for middle burner problems, and either LU-7 or SP-1 for *tai yin* dysfunctions.

■ CV-13

The name of this point is *shang wan,* "Upper Cavity," and it aids in movements from the middle burner toward the upper burner.

A digestion point, it governs problems due to phlegm.

■ CV-14

As the alarm point of the sovereign Heart, it is connected with Heart fire in a state of deficiency.

Pathologically, it corresponds to an eclipse of the sun, causing symptoms of deficiency, lack of energy, melancholy, anxiety, sadness, and a deep sense of cold.

■ CV-15

This point is connected with the Heart fire in a state of excess, because it cannot *externalize*; this point releases Heart fire that was repressed internally. This is why it is said that it governs the expressions of the Heart.

Indications include: psychological, mental, and cardiac issues, as well as dysfunction of the diaphragm (hiccups). This is a major point in the treatment of epilepsy.

■ CV-16

This point is connected with the Heart fire in a state of excess, because it cannot *return* to its home, the Heart, remaining blocked externally.

This inability of the Heart fire to return results in an intense sense of excitement, insomnia, tachycardia, and a patient who simply is not centered.

■ CV-17

This point controls the upper burner. Its indications are:

— in cases of excess: a feeling of fullness in the thorax, oppression, dyspnea that improves with exertion, anxiety, and full and strong pulses in both distal positions

— in cases of deficiency: intense physical and psychological fatigue, depression, insomnia, dyspnea with exertion, weak voice, palpitations, anorexia, and small, thin pulses in both distal positions

This point also controls externalization and distribution throughout the body of the ancestral qi *(zong qi)*, which is located in the chest. It is the upper sea of qi (related to BL-17, the upper sea of blood), and is used for intense somatic and psychological fatigue.

■ CV-18

This point serves as the *jue yin* node that permits flexible, easy flow of qi in all areas and directions, including from one's ancestors to descendants.

It describes a compression of the energy in the chest, with chest pain, functional cardiac disorders, as well as dyspnea.

■ CV-19

The name of this point is *zi gong,* "Purple Palace," which relates to the imperial palace, the center of the empire, and so is connected to a reconciliation of a person to their real self.

■ CV-20

The name of this point, *hua gai,* "Magnificent Canopy," is the canopy that covers the emperor's chariot. It refers to a covering like a roof where two sides join together. Thus it governs the heavenly function of the Lung, the "canopy of the organs," and helps to direct the Lung qi downward.

This point is used when separations that should have occurred did not take place, for example, in an adult cutting all ties with the energy of the mother when the normal mother-child separation had not previously taken place.

According to Chamfrault, this point is the starting point of Conception vessel qi.

■ CV-22

The name of this point is *tian tu,* "Heavenly Chimney."

It governs the relationship between the thorax and heaven. It is effective in aphonia, in certain cases of asthma, or in spasms of the diaphragm. The face is often ruddy and very hot.

■ CV-23

This point is the node of the *shao yin* and can be indicated in case of a severe break in this vessel, with acute signs along the arm and leg *shao yin.*

It is a meeting point of the Conception and Yin Linking vessels. It gathers the qi of the Kidneys, Spleen and Heart and can be needled to act on these three vessels or organs.

Governing Vessel

■ GV-1

Starting point of the Governing vessel, often indicated for scoliosis.

When the Governing vessel is deficient, the patient becomes stooped with a heavy head and there are also intestinal and urinary disorders, often including impotence.

This point augments both somatic and nervous strength, so that the person not only becomes physically stronger but also feels more powerful in general.

■ GV-3

This point controls the Large Intestine in its role as the "earth" of the Lung.

It corresponds to the Large Intestine, the Kidneys and the gestational envelopes of the pelvis, and receives the qi sent down by the Lung from CV-20.

The name of this point is *yao yang guan,* "Lumbar Yang Barrier," and it enables the yang qi to descend to the pelvis, sacrum and lower limbs.

■ GV-4

The name of this point is *ming men,* "Gate of Vitality [Life]."

Applying moxibustion here treats fire from deficiency of the Kidneys with sensations of the body burning, a sense of feverishness with no rise in body temperature, prolapse of the rectum, urinary incontinence, leucorrhea, impotence, and an empty right proximal pulse.

- ■ GV-5

The name of this point is *xuan shu,* "Suspension Pivot." This relates to the Kidney qi being suspended here, as it is at this pivot that it ascends.

GV-5 brings up the Kidney qi. When it is blocked, there is an obstruction of Kidney qi in the pelvis, preventing it from rising to the other organs. This leads to a sense of blockage in the pelvis.

Like other Governing vessel points on the lower back, this point treats symptoms involving the lower back and the intestinal and genitourinary systems, in particular leiomyomas, which it can reduce in size.

An interesting aspect of this point is that it is associated with dreams that include snakes.

- ■ GV-6

We have seen that GV-5 brings up the qi from the Kidneys, the roots of production of the five organs, from the level of the prenatal origin, towards the other viscera. This process begins with the Spleen, whose back associated point is at the level of the post-natal qi at GV-6.

Indications are the same pelvic fullness that occurs due to a blockage of GV-5 along with signs of Spleen deficiency.

- ■ GV-7

The name of this point, *zhong shu,* or "Central Pivot," is related to the Gallbladder, which is noted as the *zhong zheng* organ in Chapter 8 of *Basic Questions*. On one level these terms mean "just and moderate," but literally they mean "central" *(zhong)* and "upright" *(zheng)*. I believe that the Gallbladder has the function of keeping a person upright and centered, and needling this point helps it accomplish this task.

- ■ GV-8

Located at the level of BL-18, the back associated point of the Liver, this point treats the stirring of Liver wind.

Indications: contractions, cramps, convulsions, mania, hysteria

■ GV-10

The name of this point, *ling tai,* or "Spirit Platform," is another name for the Heart. Martial arts practitioners concentrate on this point to feel the presence of an opponent, even those behind them.

Its function is to open the chest. When it is working correctly, the person is stable and peaceful, so they can breathe freely and have a sense of openness in the chest.

■ GV-11

The name of this point is *shen dao,* "Spirit Path." It is a point that relates to the Heart as the ruler.

Indications include psychological and cardiac symptoms as well as those of the Governing vessel in general, such as scoliosis, depression, and confusion.

■ GV-12 -

At the same level as the back associated point of the Lung, this point is related to the corporeal soul and the Lung, with the exit into life, and manifests with pulmonary and related psychological signs: severe psychological symptoms including both homicidal and suicidal desires, madness, hallucinations, and delirious speech.

■ GV-15

The name of this point is *ya men,* "Gate of Muteness." This reflects its indications for speech disorders, including those that occur after a stroke.

It is also for excessive yang of the Governing vessel manifesting with opisthotonos, headaches, or merely stiffness of the spine.

■ GV-16

This point is located under the occipital protuberance, from which vessels enter and exit the brain. It mobilizes all of the brain qi.

The protective qi is concentrated at this point to protect the brain from external wind. It is also a meeting point of the Governing and Yang Linking vessels.

The name of this point is *feng fu,* "Wind Mansion." It is a wind point and treats both exterior and interior wind.

Indications include headaches, vertigo, torticollis, and stiffness of the neck with pain radiating from this point to the two shoulders, convulsions, madness, or stroke.

■ **GV-18**

Treats endocranial phlegm with such symptoms as ophthalmic migraines accompanied by difficulty in getting the tongue to work.

■ **GV-20**

The name of this point is *bai hui,* "Hundred Meetings." As it is located at the vertex, it is where all the yang qi of the body meets with the leg *jue yin.*

It treats an excess of yang in the upper part of the body and causes the yin to ascend. It is a major point for insomnia.

In the *Great Compendium,* this point is associated with heaven, while CV-17 is associated with humans and KI-1 with earth.

It also governs the sea of marrow, with GV-17.

■ **GV-22**

It controls the circulation of blood in the head and therefore treats bursting headaches due to blood deficiency, aggravated by alcohol, heat, and menses, but improved by pressure on the eyes and local application of cold.

■ **GV-23**

The main name for this point is *shang xing,* "Upper Star." A common secondary name is *gui tang,* "Ghost Hall."

It treats congestive headaches due an excess of blood, with nasal obstruction, as well as eye pain that is aggravated by direct pressure over the eyes.

■ **GV-24**

The name of this point is *shen ting,* "Courtyard of the Spirit." It seems to unify and calm the person.

A frontal spirit point, it is particularly effective in cases of depression arising from the Heart, as it stimulates the person's psychological and mental strength.

■ **GV-25**

This point restores consciousness and awakens one from drunkenness.

■ **GV-26**

Its name is *shui gou,* "Water Ditch," which refers to the philtrum. Another standard name, *ren zhong,* refers to the same location, and literally means "Middle of Man."

This is a resuscitation point: it brings the soul back into the body, re-establishes the relationship between yin and yang when their separation has induced a loss of consciousness, and also calms the mind. It is indicated for epileptic seizures; it calms down delusions, madness with agitation, mania, fright or hysteria.

This point unites body and soul, yin and yang, and the Governing and Conception vessels.

Miscellaneous Points

■ M-HN-3 *(yin tang)*

Clears the upper facial region, for example, in allergies affecting the nose and eyes, as well as facial neuralgias.

It also is useful in calming the spirit.

■ M-HN-7 *(yu yao)*

This point is very effective for eliminating heat from the eyes with such symptoms as pain, redness, swelling, keratitis, conjunctivitis, and dimming of the vision.

CHANNEL ILLUSTRATIONS

Part 1: Fourteen Primary Channels

Key to Part 1 Figures:

DOT-DASH-DOT BLACK = external pathway of channel

GREY = internal pathway of channel

RED = connecting pathways

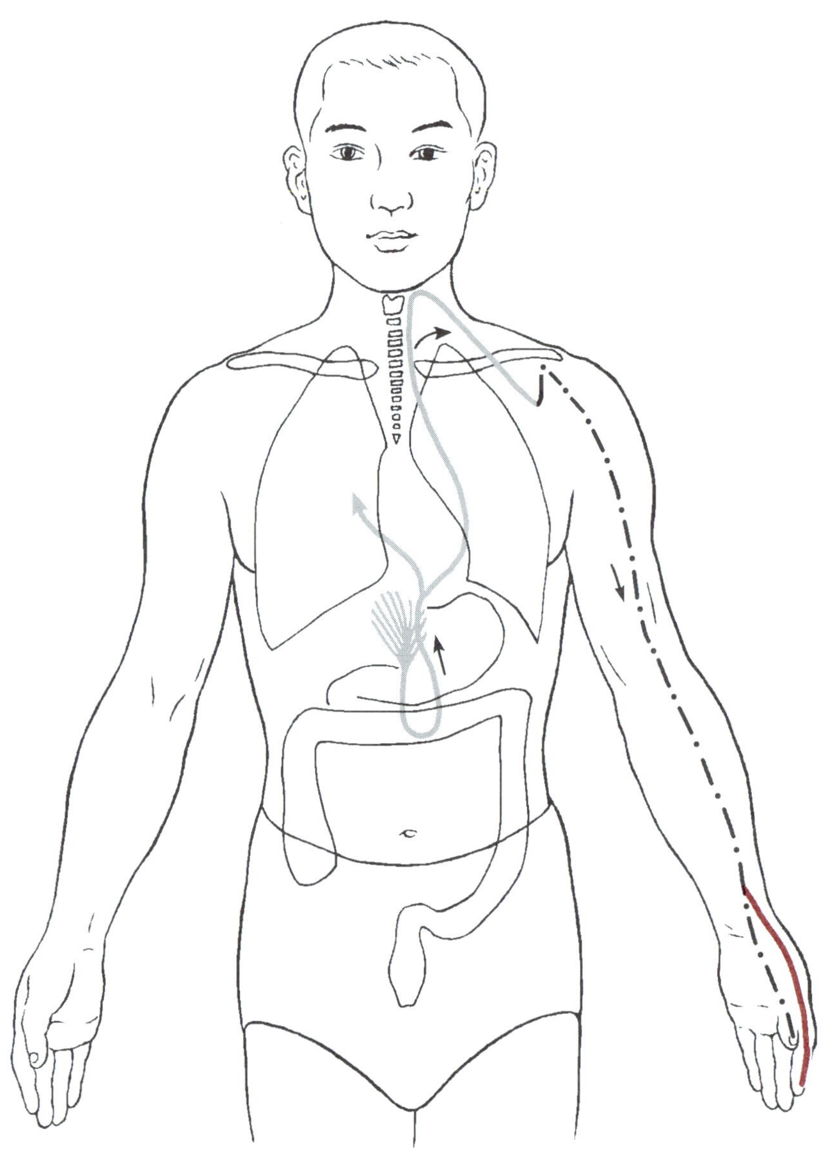

Arm *Tai Yin* Lung Channel

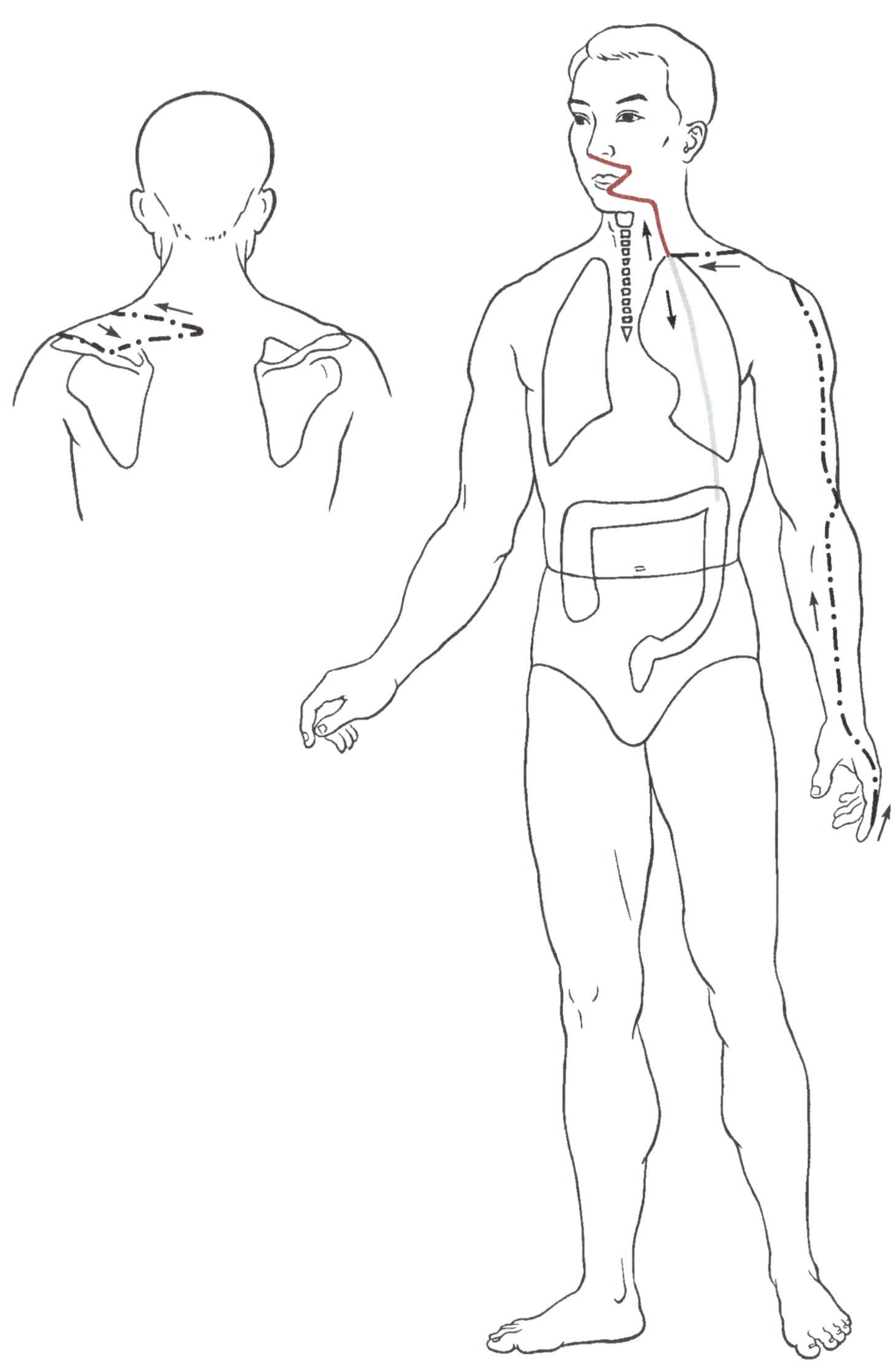

Arm *Yang Ming* Large Intestine Channel

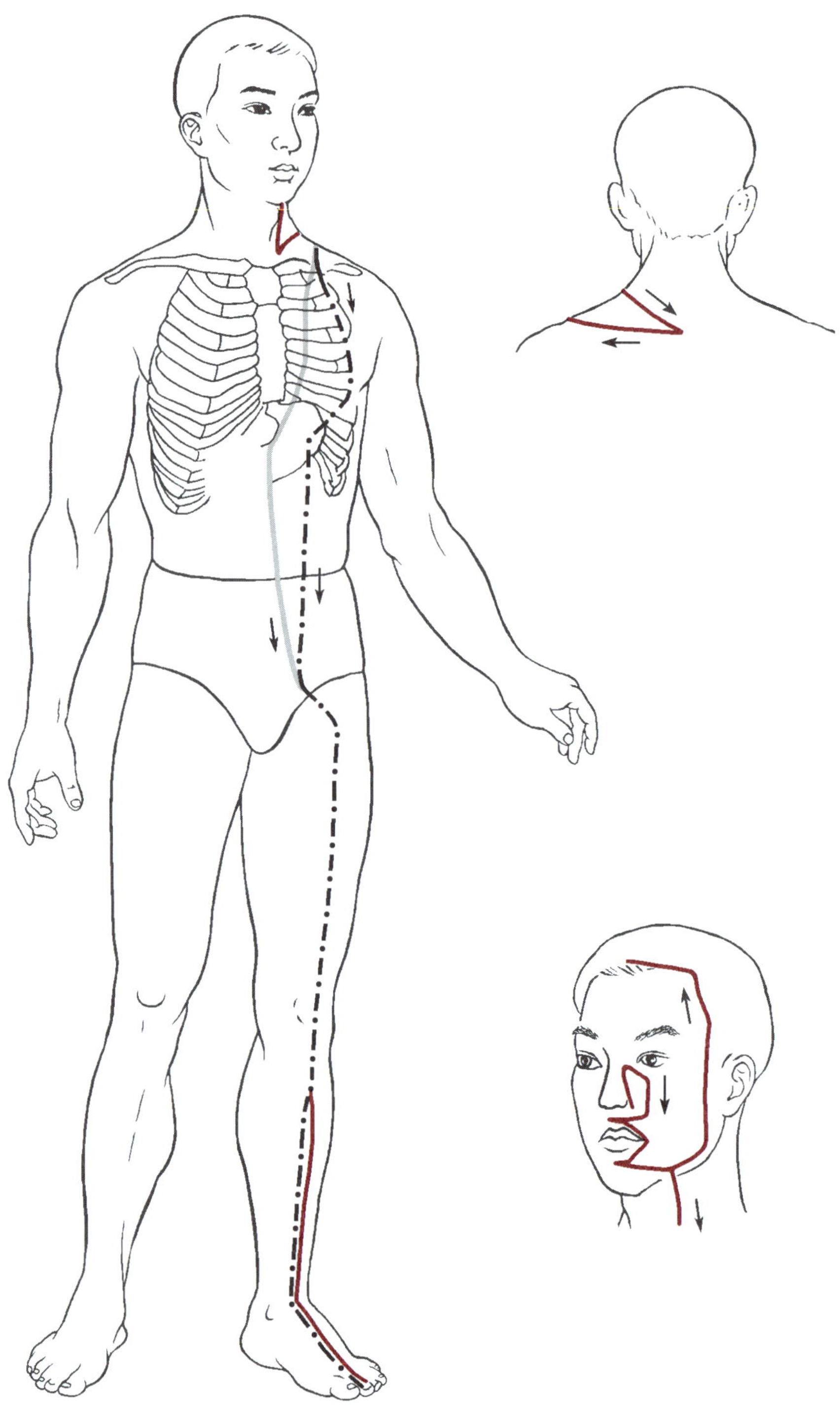

Leg *Yang Ming* Stomach Channel

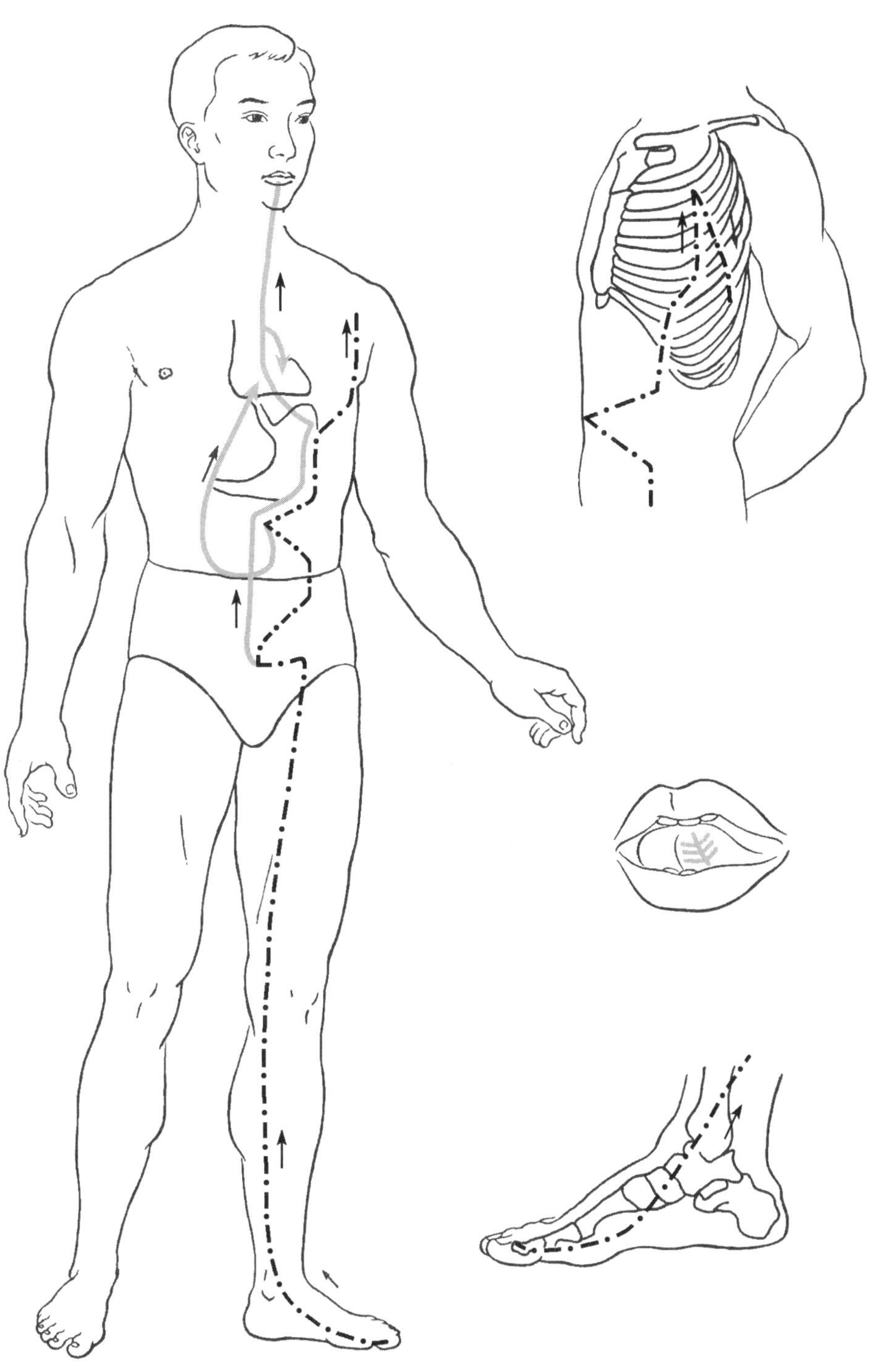

Leg *Tai Yin* Spleen Channel

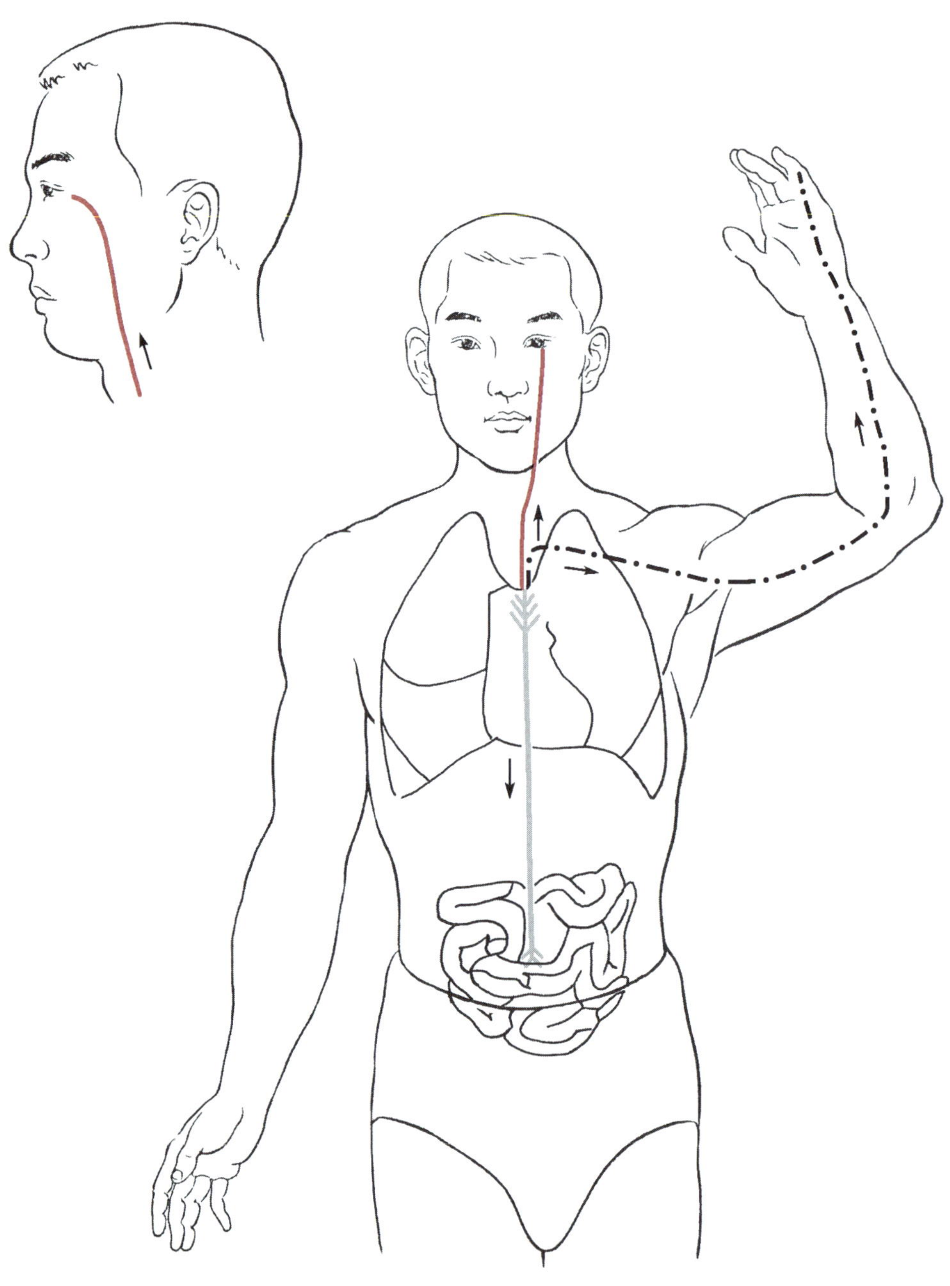

Arm *Shao Yin* Heart Channel

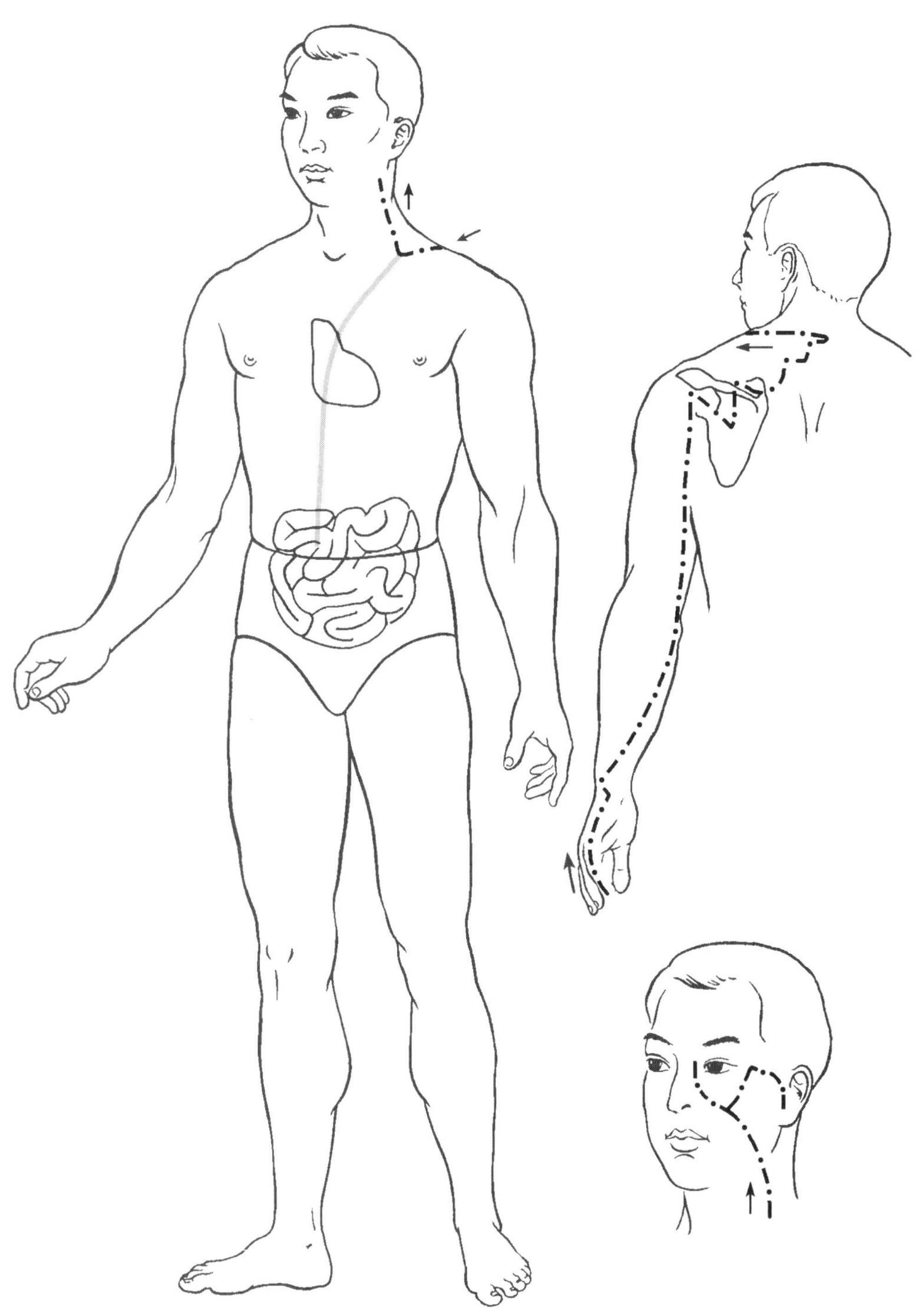

Arm *Tai Yang* Small Intestine Channel

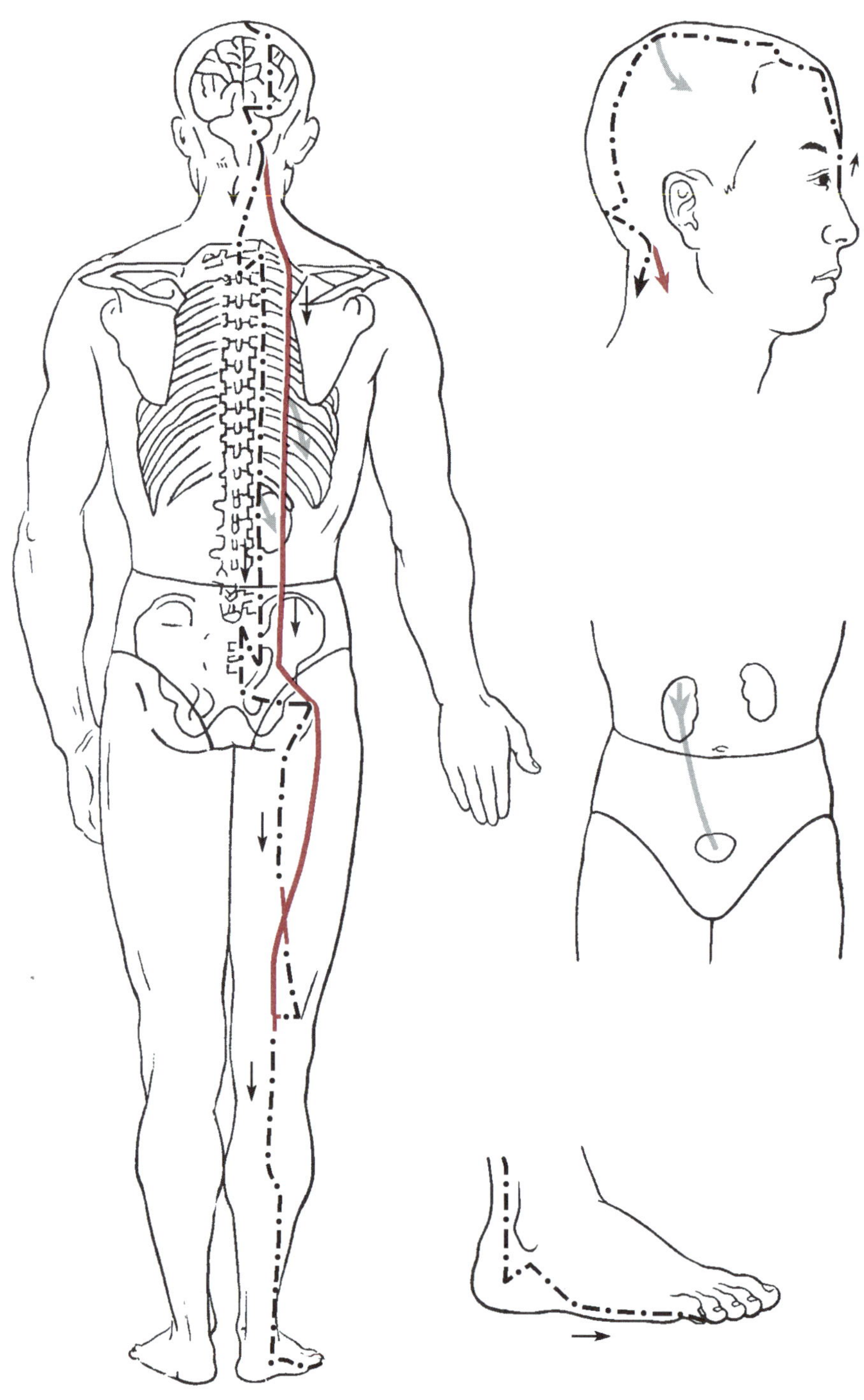

Leg *Tai Yang* Bladder Channel

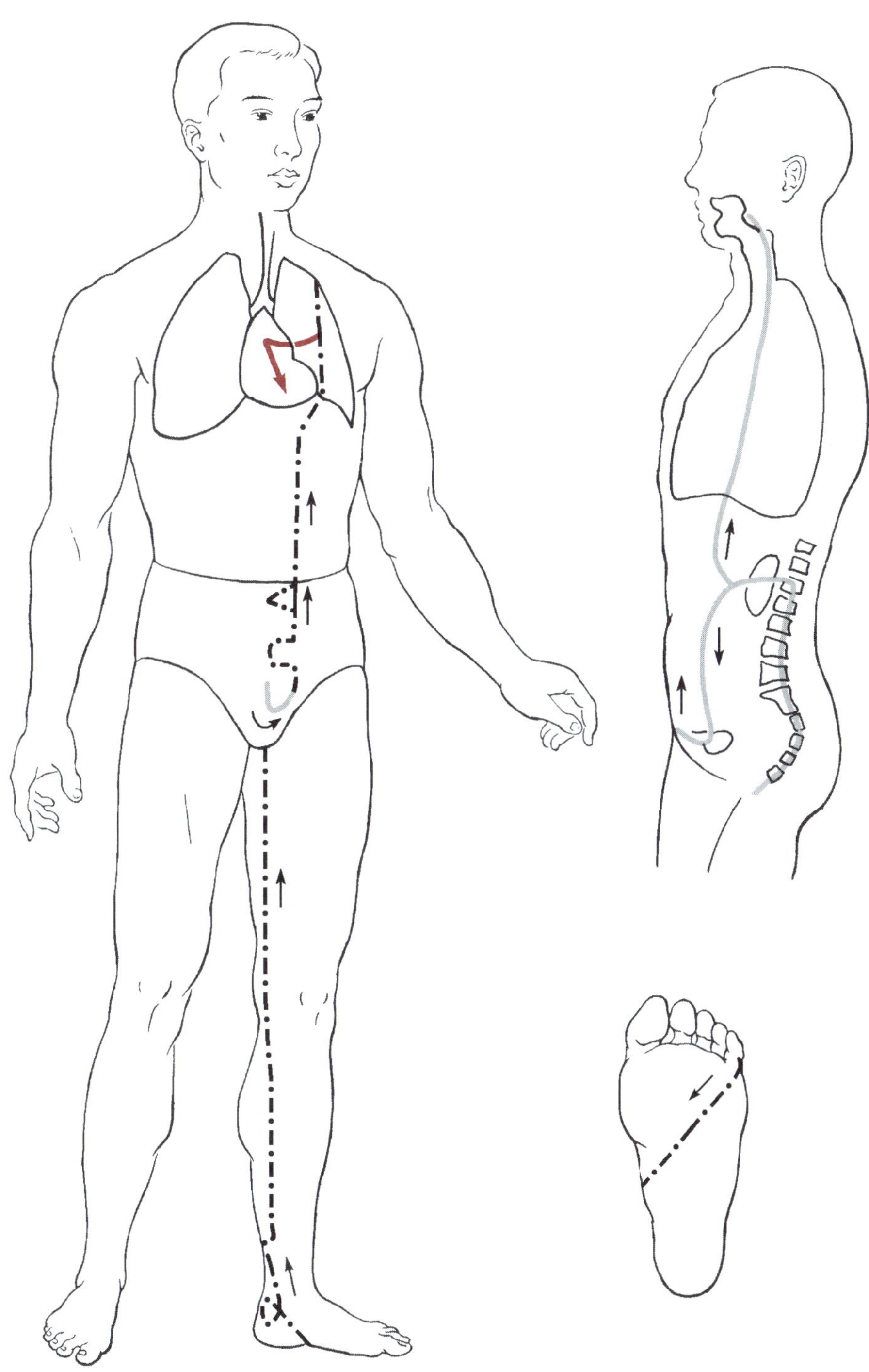

Leg *Shao Yin* Kidney Channel

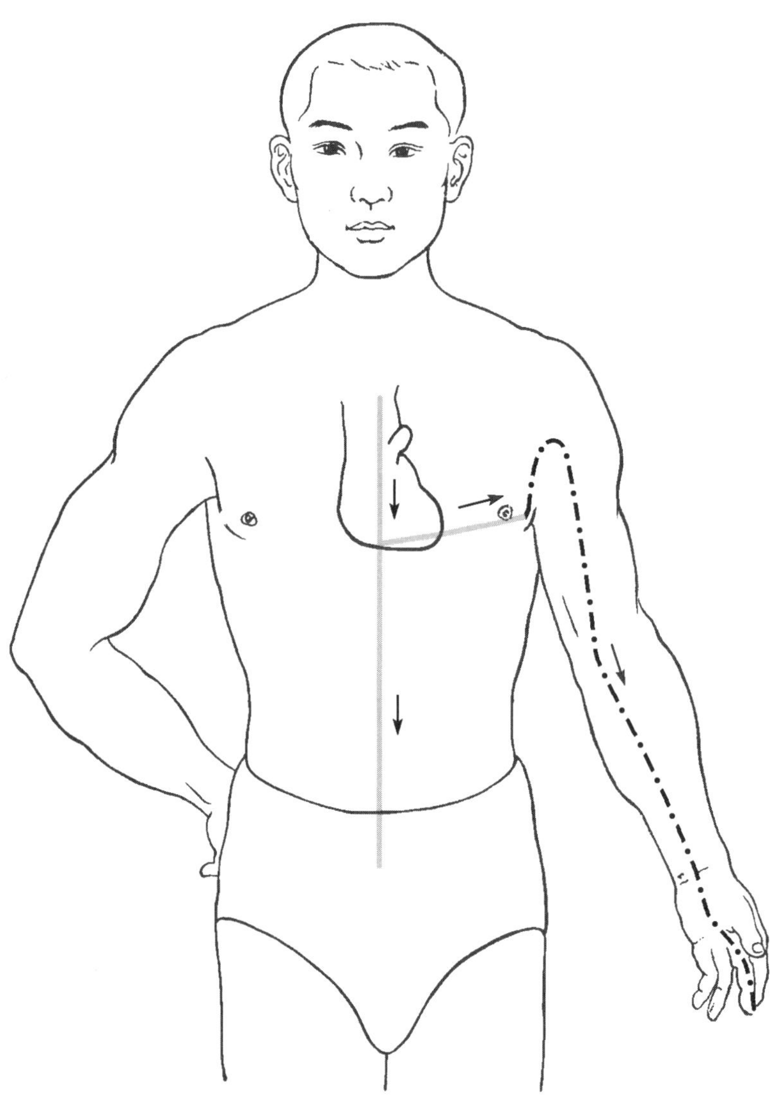

Arm *Jue Yin* Heart Master (Pericardium) Channel

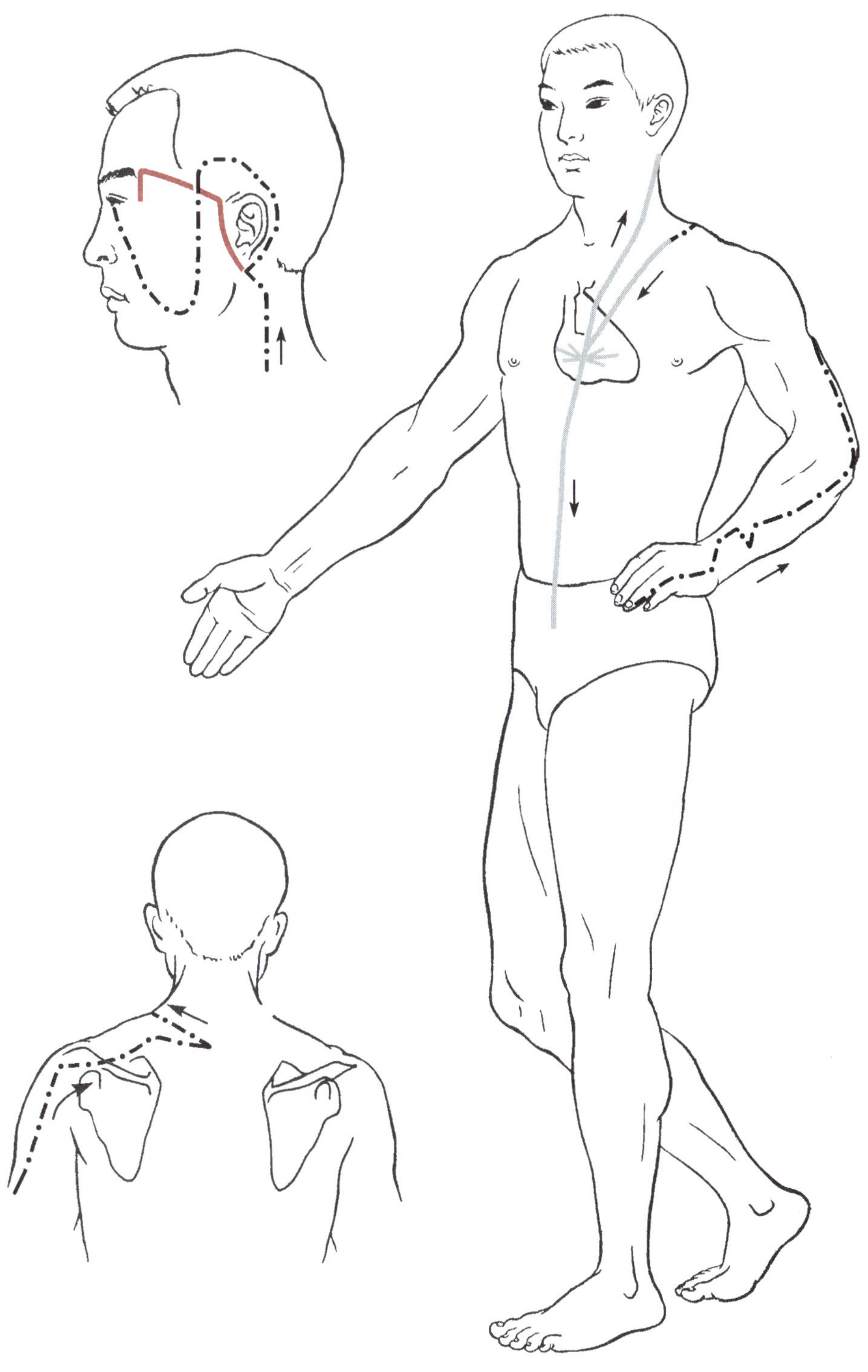

Arm *Shao Yang* Triple Burner Channel

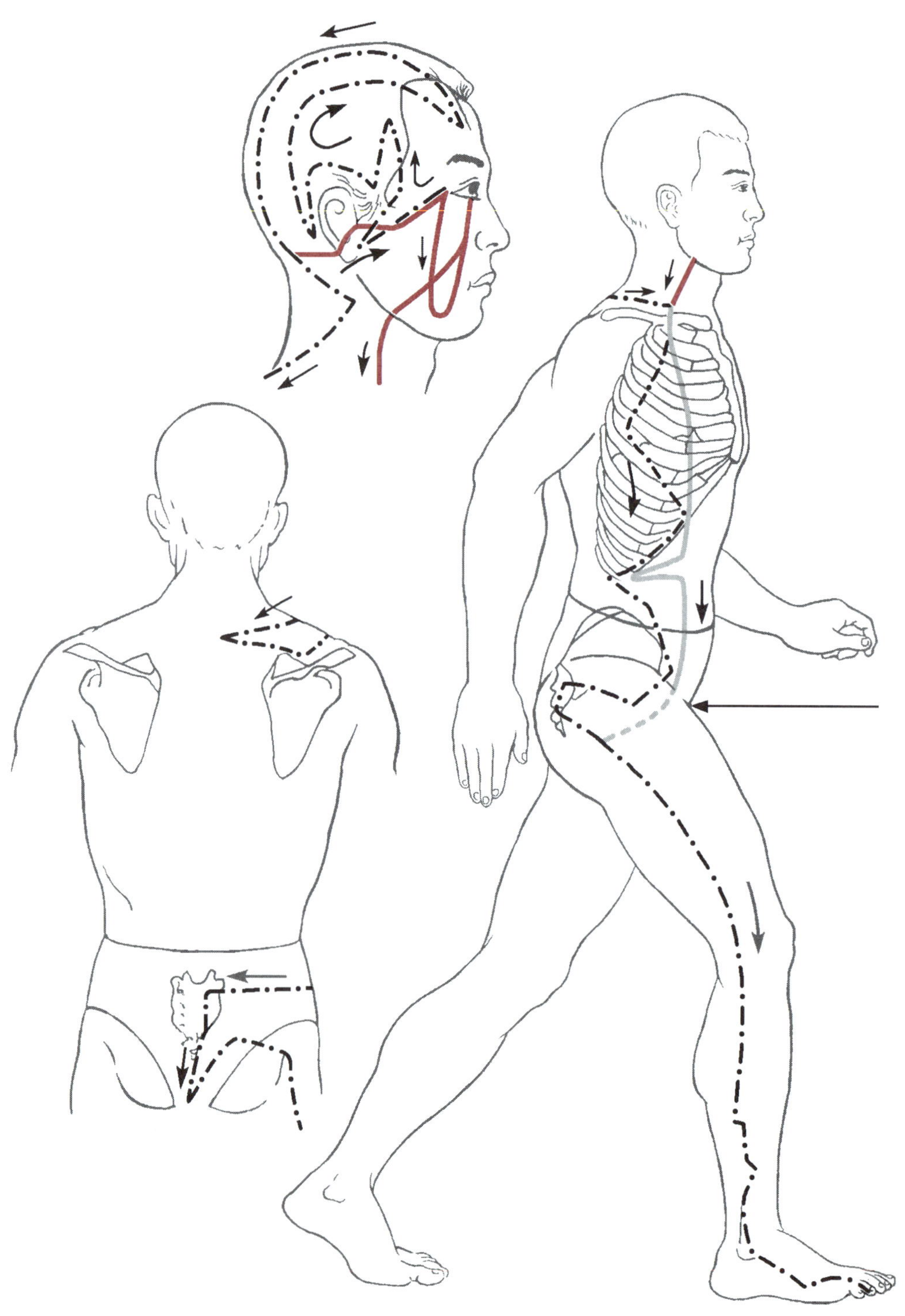

Leg *Shao Yang* Gallbladder Channel

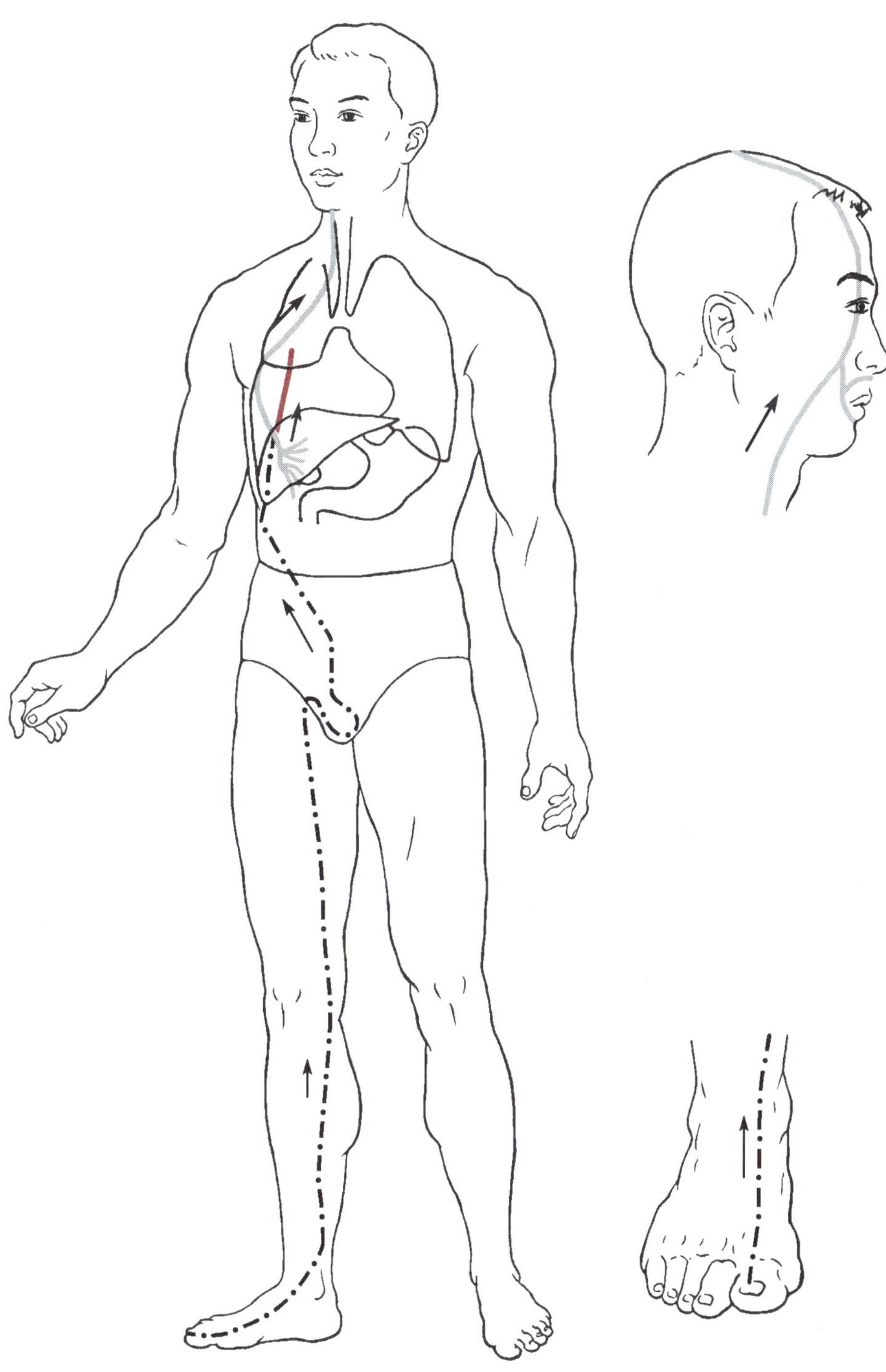

Leg *Jue Yin* Liver Channel

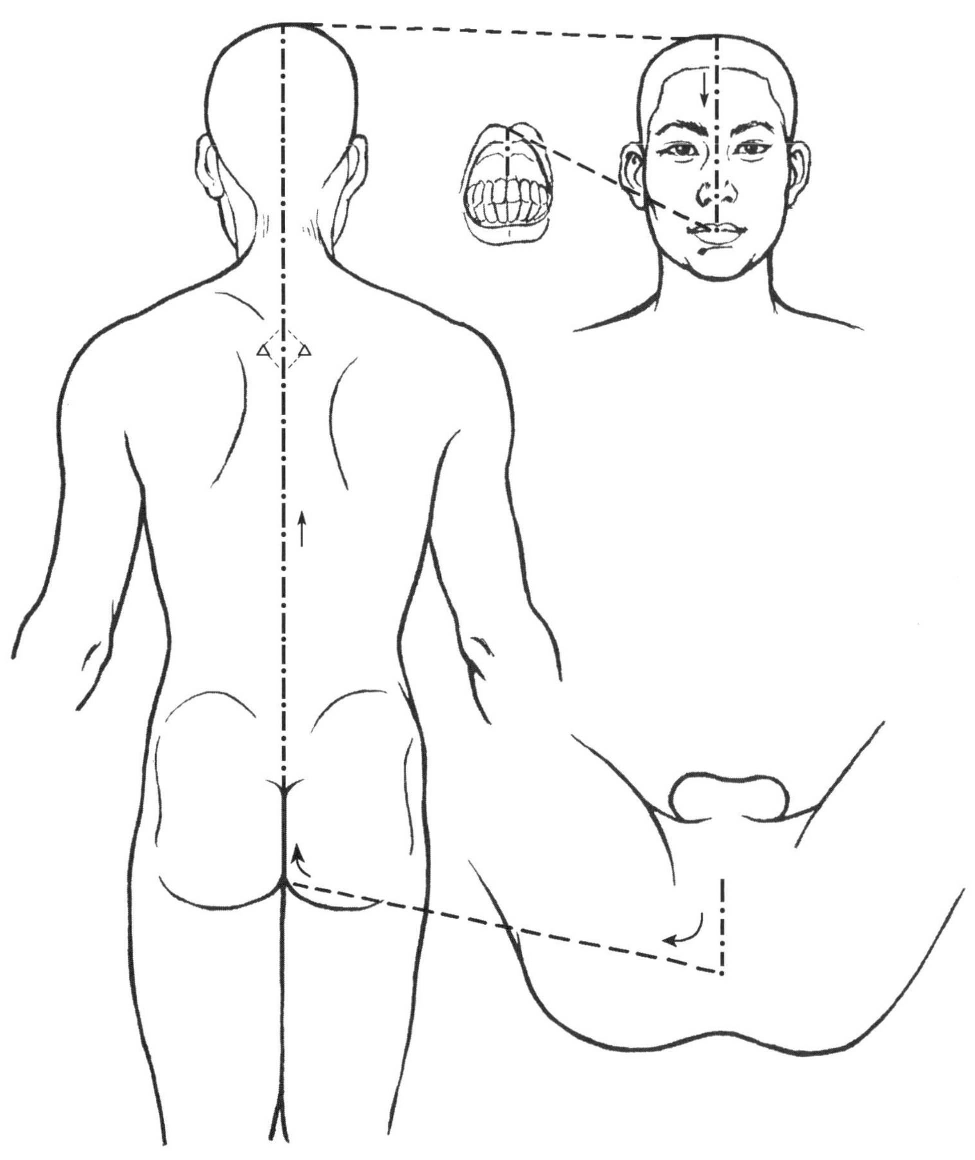

Governing Vessel

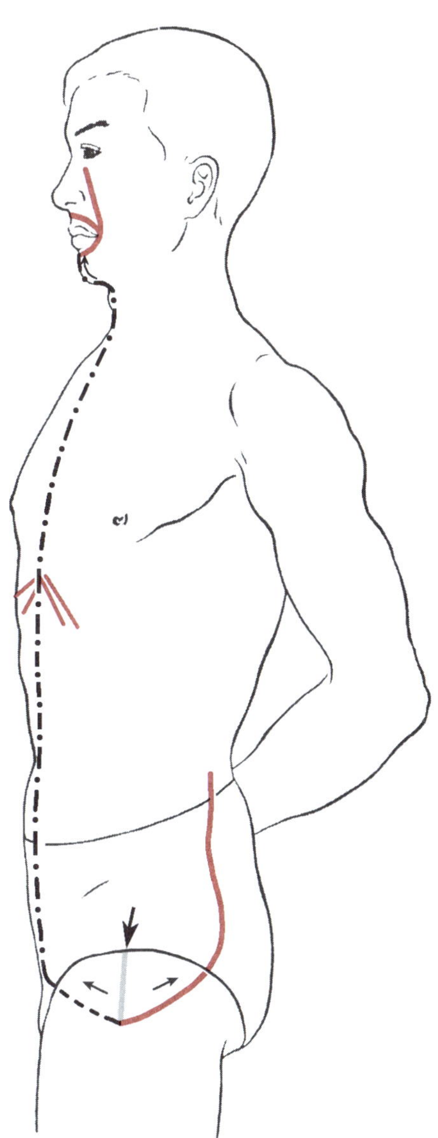

Conception Vessel

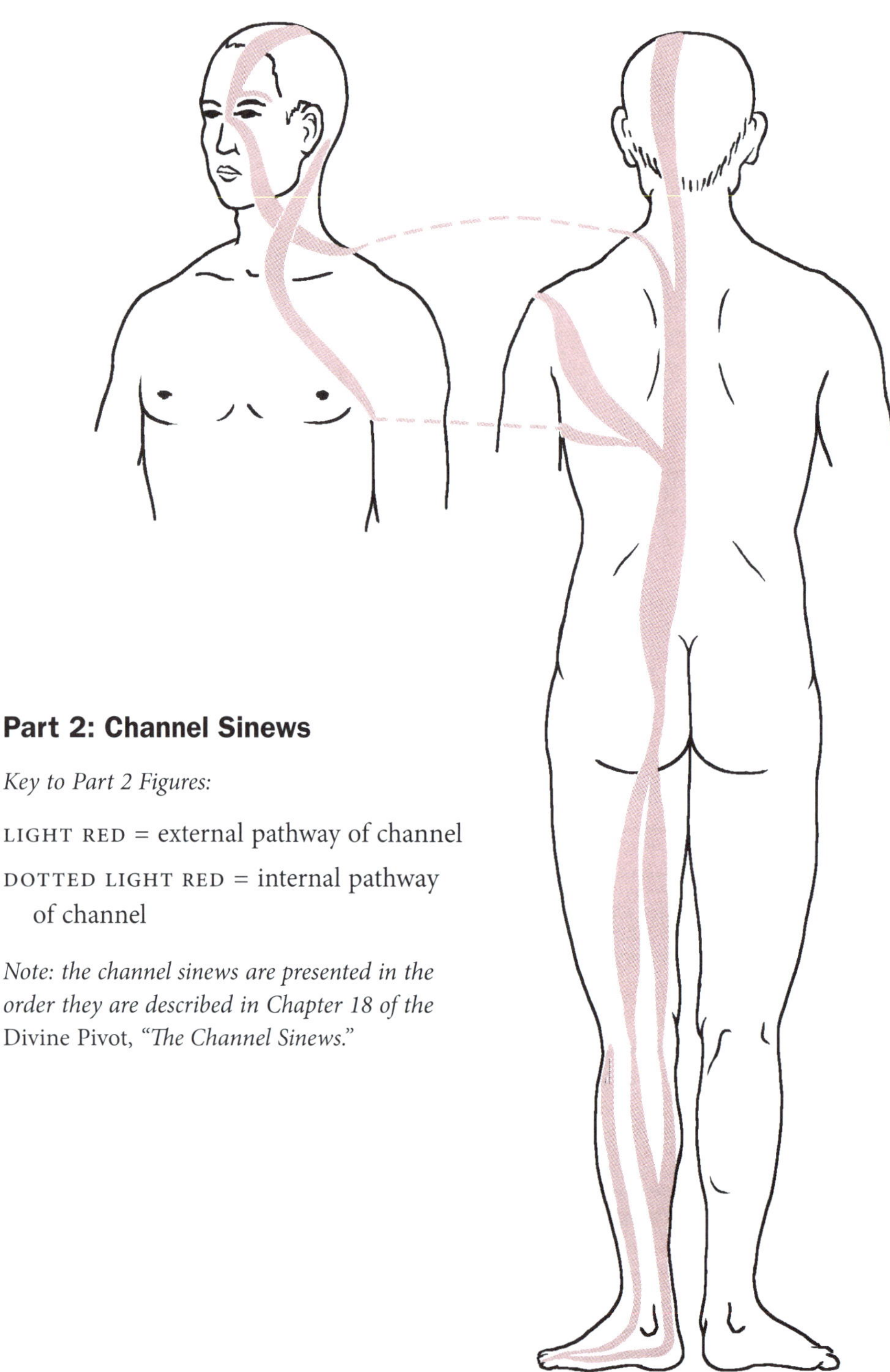

Part 2: Channel Sinews

Key to Part 2 Figures:

LIGHT RED = external pathway of channel

DOTTED LIGHT RED = internal pathway
   of channel

Note: the channel sinews are presented in the order they are described in Chapter 18 of the Divine Pivot, "The Channel Sinews."

Leg *Tai Yang* Channel Sinew

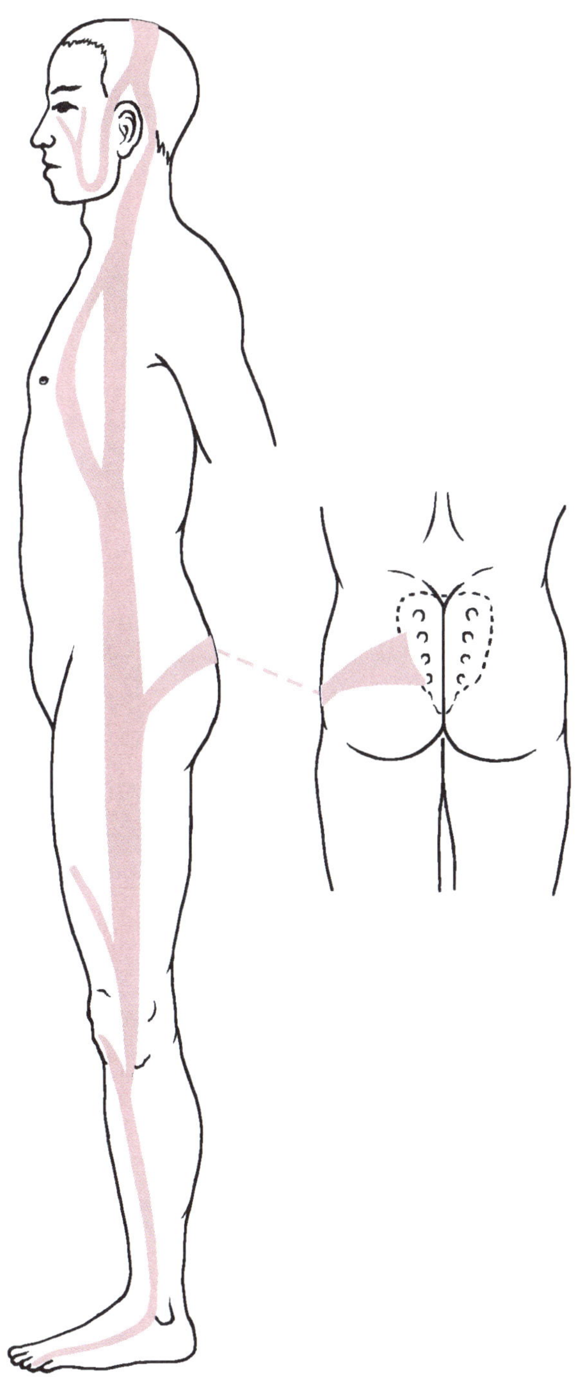

Leg *Shao Yang* Channel Sinew

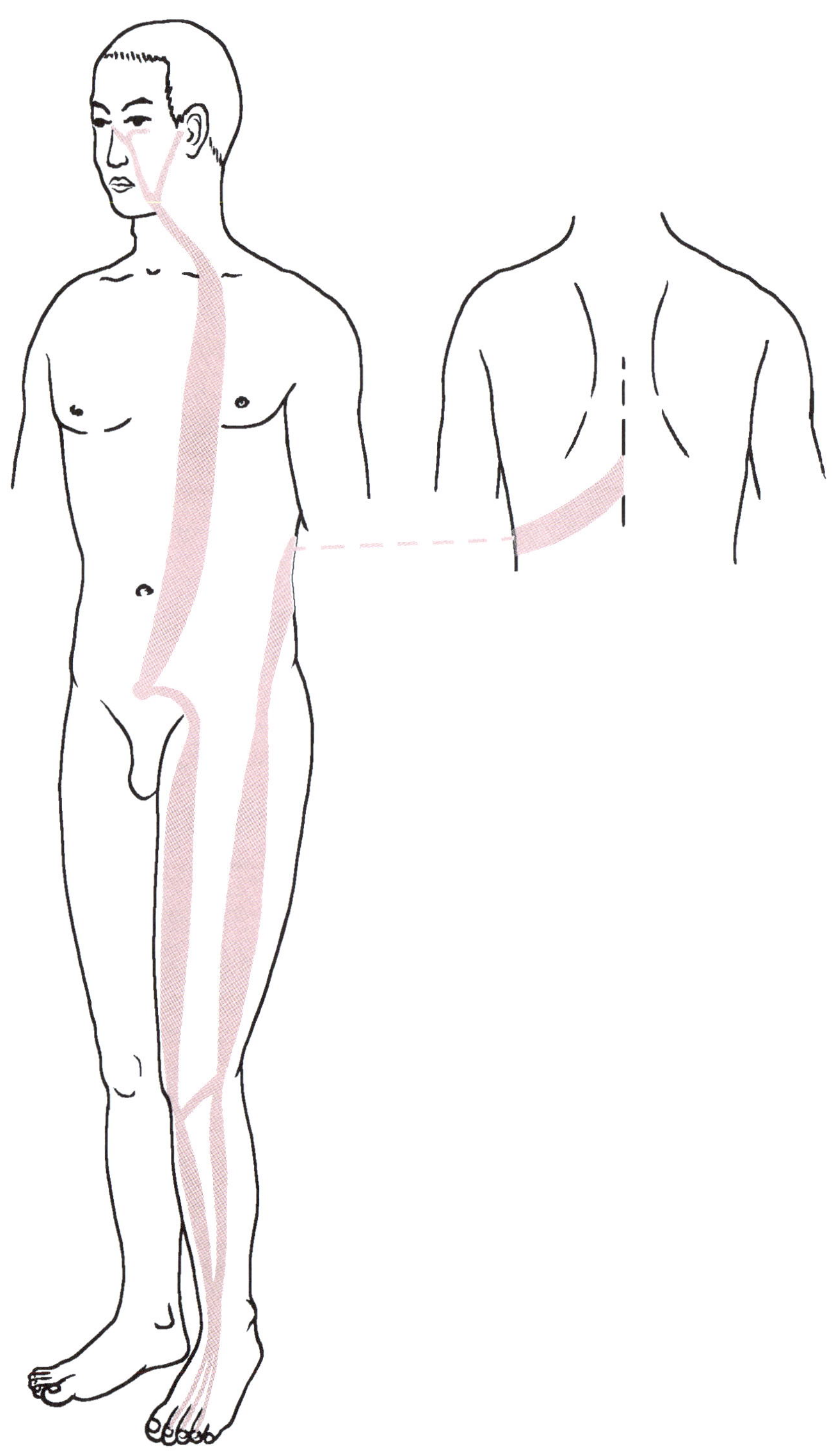

Leg *Yang Ming* Channel Sinew

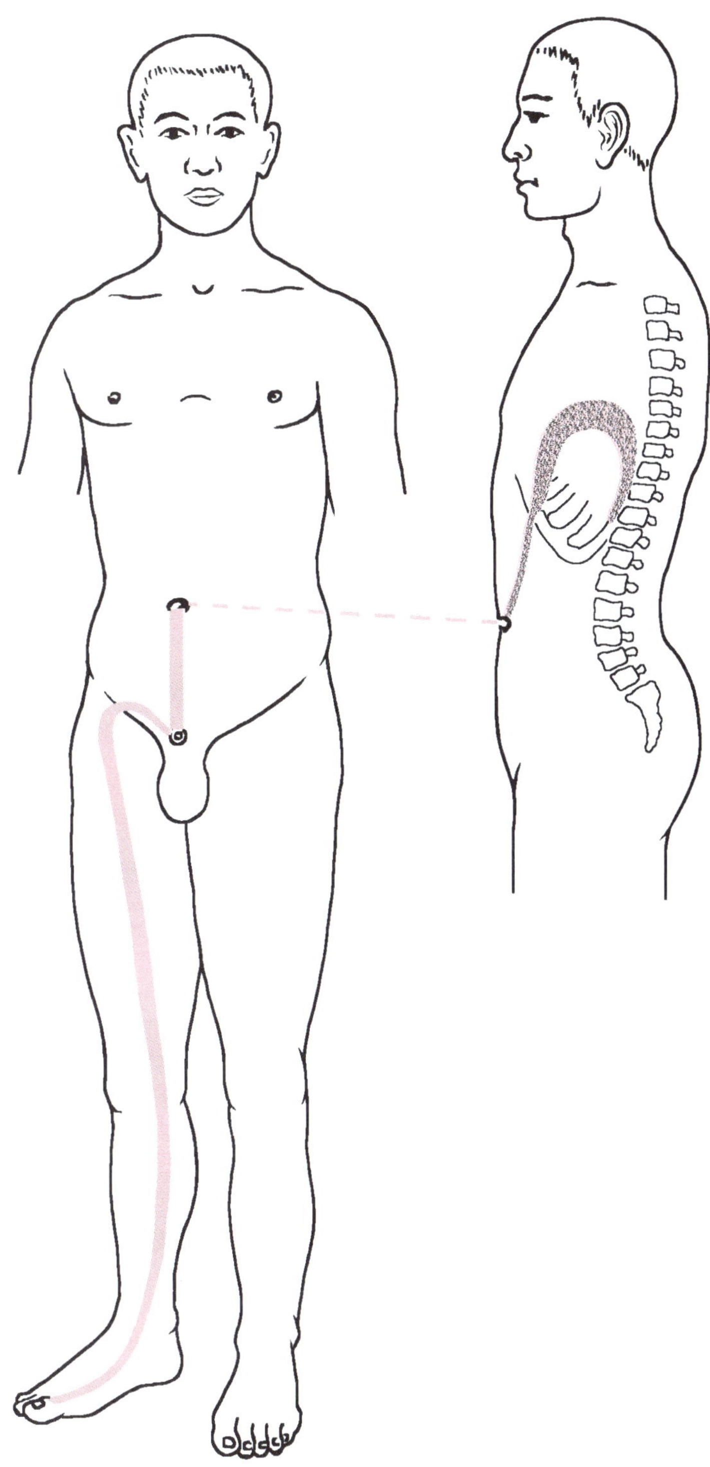

Leg *Tai Yin* Channel Sinew

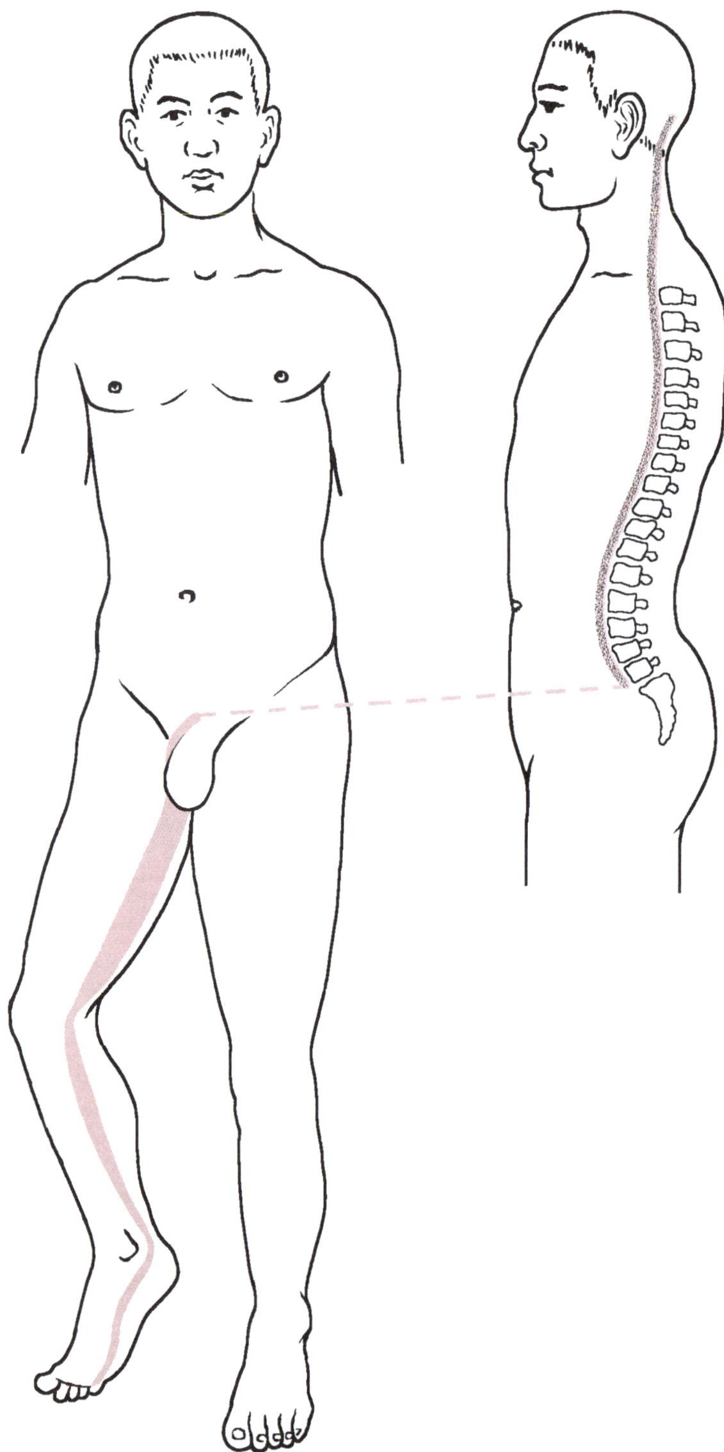

Leg *Shao Yin* Channel Sinew

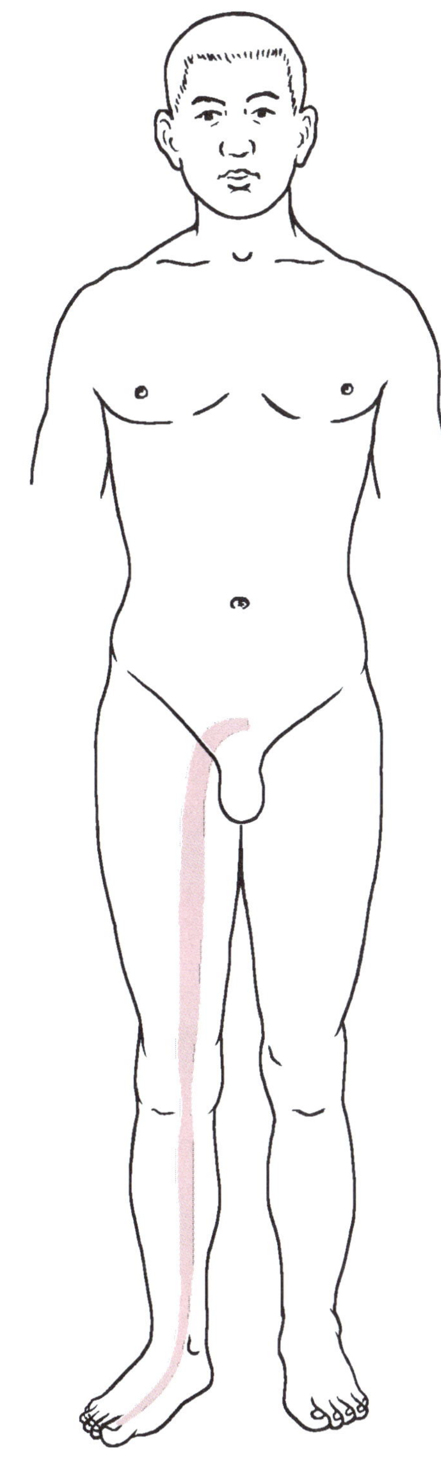

Leg *Jue Yin* Channel Sinew

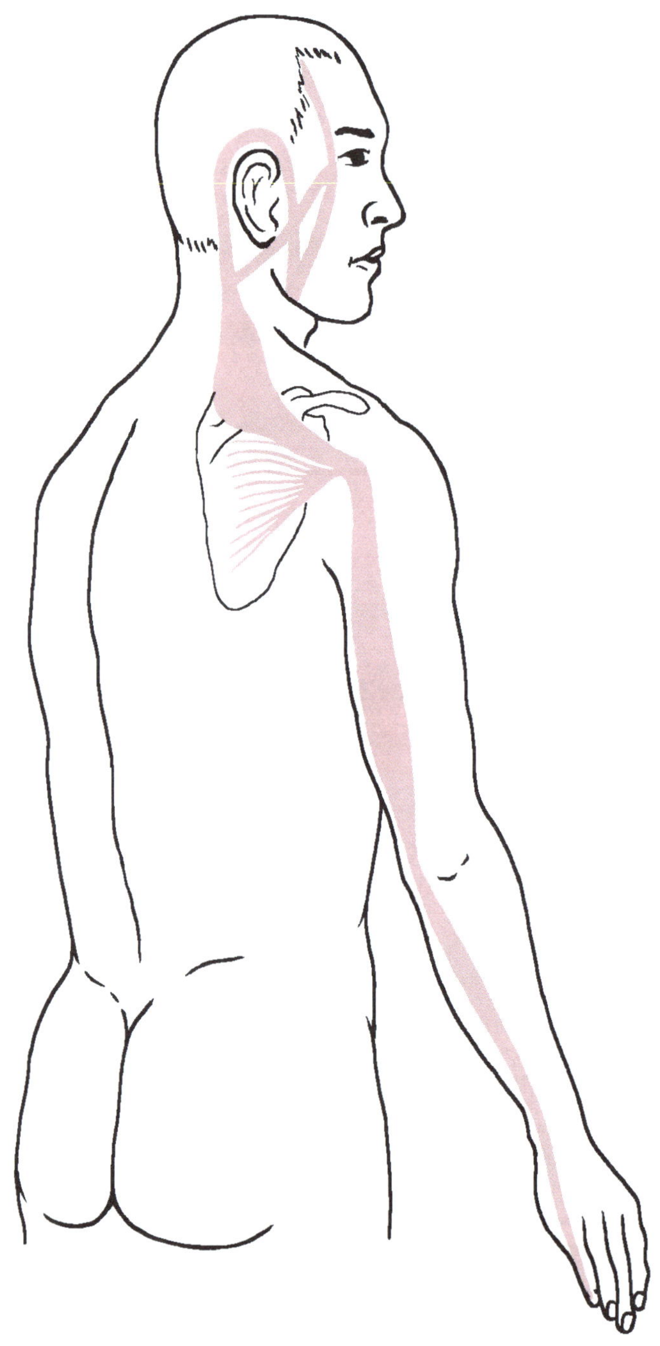

Arm *Tai Yang* Channel Sinew

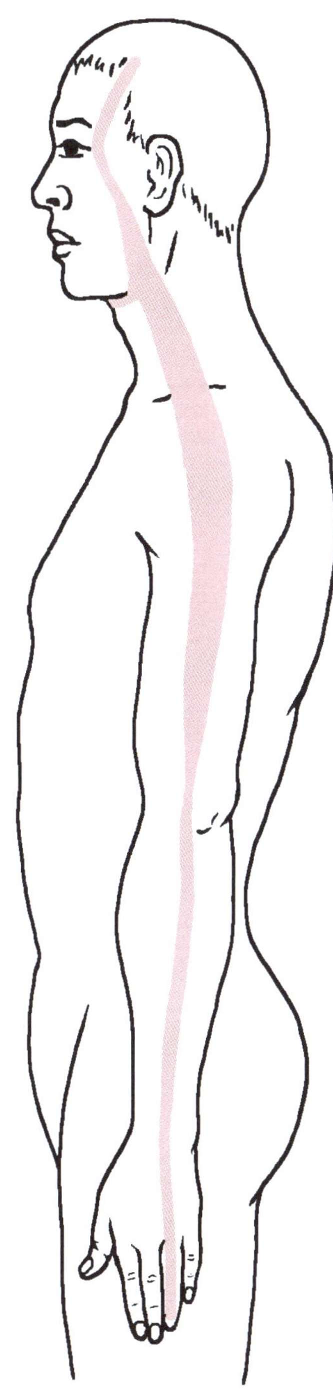

Arm *Shao Yang* Channel Sinew

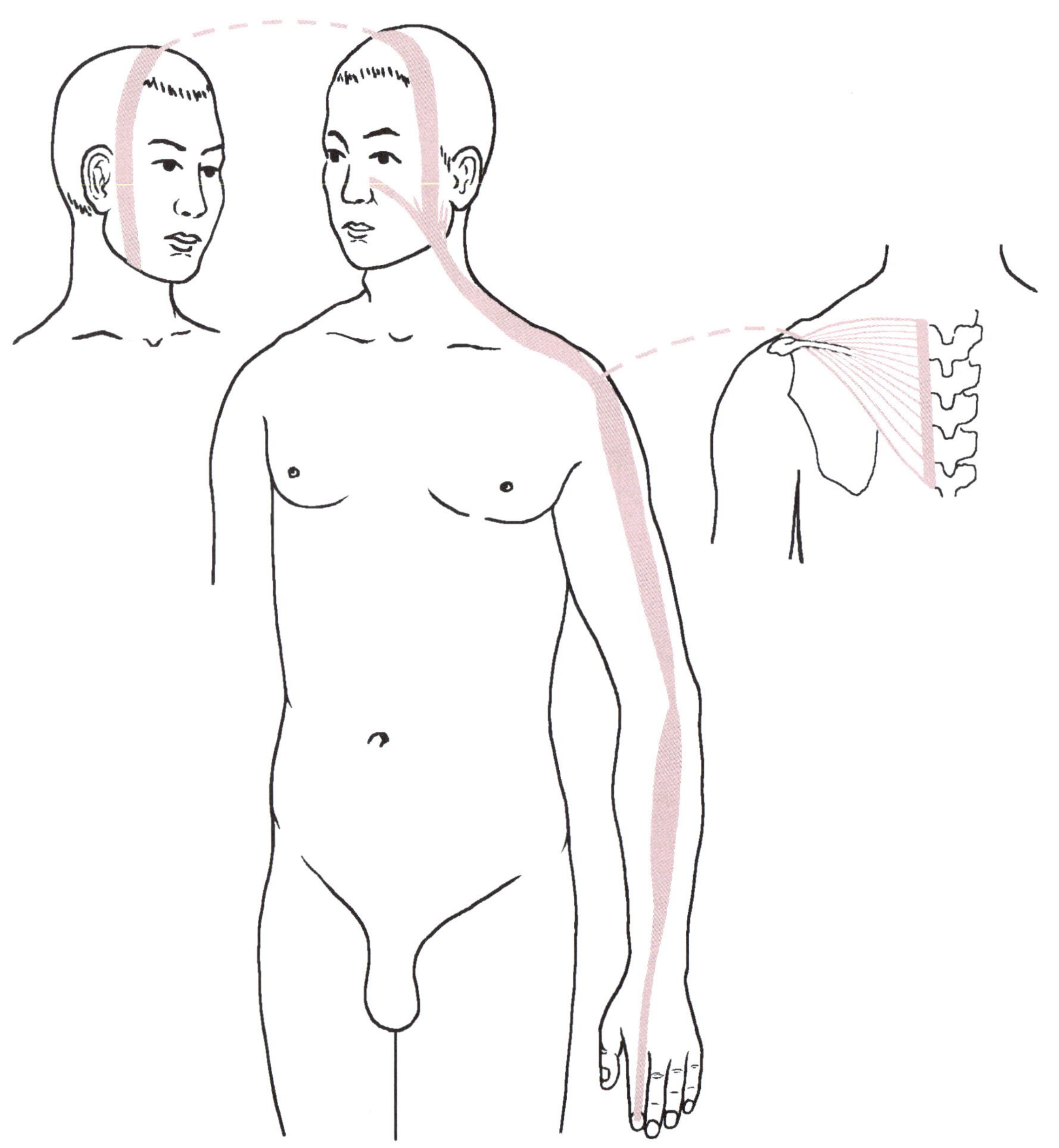

Arm *Yang Ming* Channel Sinew

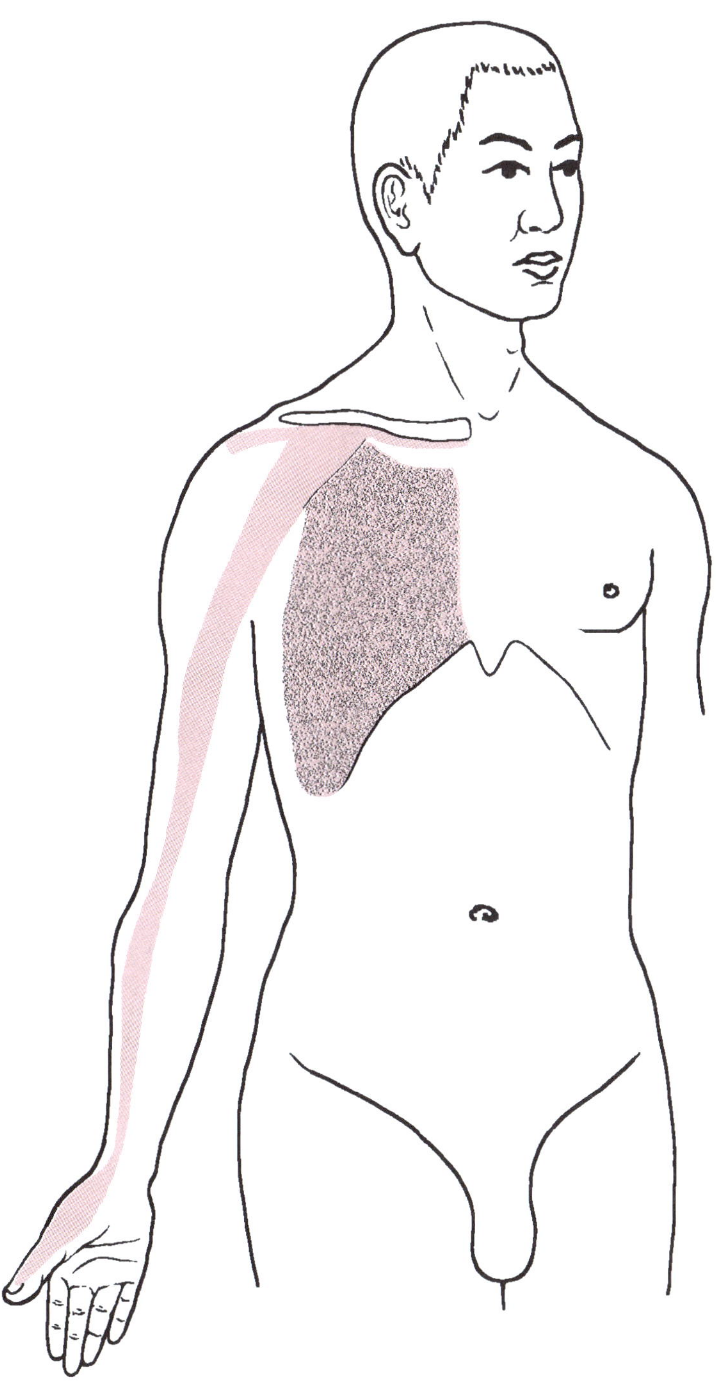

Arm *Tai Yin* Channel Sinew

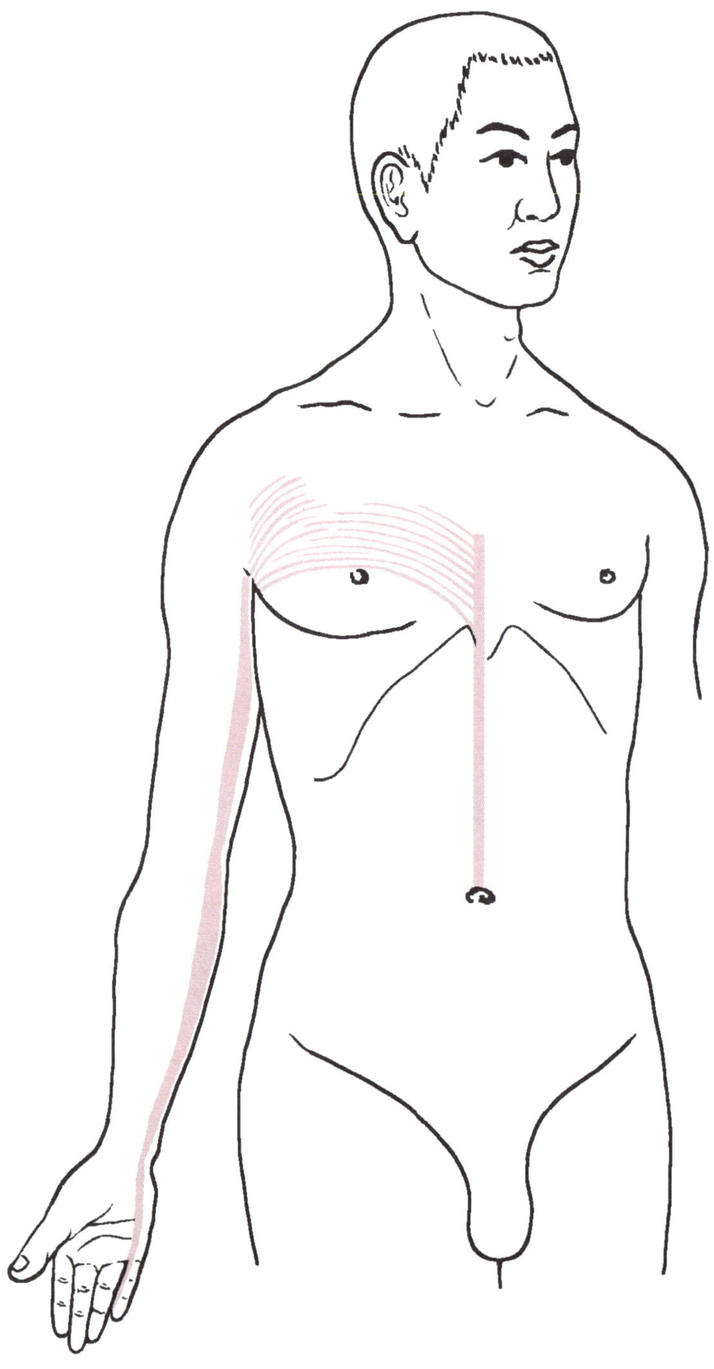

Arm *Shao Yin* Channel Sinew

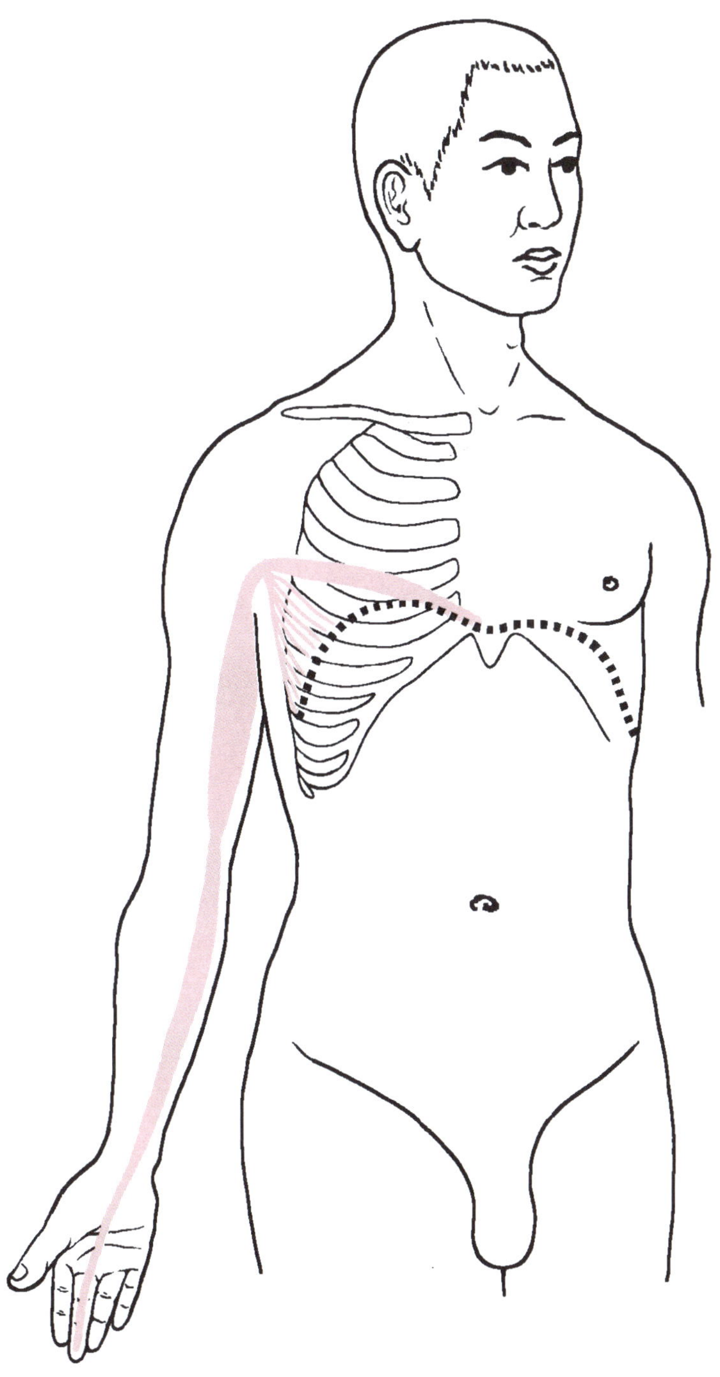

Arm *Jue Yin* Channel Sinew

NOTES

Preface

1. A. Chamfrault, *Traité de Médecine chinoise*. Angoulême: Ed. Coquemard, 1964. The translation of the *Inner Classic* has been superseded by that of A. Husson published in 1987 (*see* the Bibliography).

2. K. Schipper, *The Taoist Body*. Berkeley: University of California Press, 1994.

Ch. 1: Indispensable Preliminaries

1. This chapter is adapted from my book, *L'homme et ses symboles en M.T.C.* Paris: Albin Michel, 2002.

2. F. Jullien, *The Impossible Nude: Chinese Art and Western Aesthetics*. Chicago: University of Chicago Press, 2007, p. 34.

3. M. Bitbol, *De l'intérieur du monde: Pour une philosophie et une science des relations*. Paris: Flammarion, 2010.

4. Red Pine, *Lao tzu's Taoteching*. San Francisco: Mercury House, 1996, p. 4.

5. Institut Ricci, ed. 1976.

6. S. J. Wieger, *Caractères chinois: étymologie, graphies, lexique*. Taichung, Taiwan: Kuangchi Press, 1963, p. 485.

7. S. J. Wieger, *Caractères chinois: étymologie, graphies, lexique*. Taichung, Taiwan: Kuangchi Press, 1963, p. 285.

8. *Les grands traités du Huainanzi*, translated by C. Larre, I. Robinet and E. Rochat de la Vallée. Paris: Institut Ricci, Le Cerf, 1993, Ch. 7.

Ch. 2: Introductions

1. S. J. Wieger, *Caractères chinois: étymologie, graphies, lexique*. Taichung, Taiwan: Kuangchi Press, 1963. Note that only the most essential canonical books are called *jing*. Others are called *lun* 論, as in the *Discussion of Cold Damage (Shang han lun)*.

2. I. Robinet, *Méditation taoïste*. Paris: Albin Michel, 1995, p. 30.

3. S. J. Wieger, ibid.

4. Trinh Xuan Thuan, *Voyage au cœur de la lumière*. Paris: Découverte Gallimard, 2008.

5. S. J. Wieger, ibid.

Ch. 3: Pathophysiology and Therapy

1. Body, emotional, family, professional, social, etc.

2. The most common of these are aphthae, herpes, heartburn, foul-smelling diarrhea, malodorous urine, cystitis, pruriginous vaginal discharge, eczema, dermatomycosis.

3. See below the connecting points and exterior-interior (*biao-li*) pairs in the section "Primary Channels."

4. The heart *xin* 心 has two appellations in the classics: sovereign (君 *jun*) and master (主 *zhu*).

5. G. Soulié de Morant, *L'acupuncture chinoise*. Paris: Maloine, 1972.

6. Regarding the "desire to kill" found in disorders of the corporeal soul, this also appears as an indication for other Lung points. It seems as if the qi allotted to a person in order to "come out into life," and in order to incarnate under the control of corporeal soul, could not be fully accomplished and therefore turns against itself with its dedication to life or death, resulting in the desire to kill or to die. These symptoms can also be found in some other Lung points such as BL-13, BL-42, GV-12.

7. G. Guillaume, *Dictionnaire des points d'acupuncture*. Paris: Trédaniel—La Tisserande, 1995.

8. A symptom due to excess is aggravated by local pressure. When due to deficiency, it is improved by pressure.

9. I already mentioned this case history involving GV-5 briefly at the beginning of the book. Here it is described in more detail.

10. If there is a deficiency of qi (e.g., in the upper burner), the qi will not retain the blood that escapes. In case of an excess of qi (e.g., in the pelvis), the qi pushes the blood outside of its normal channels of circulation. These are two different mechanisms that may cause hemorrhages.

11. While the Kidneys, closely linked to the Stomach, are said to be the "root of production of the five organs."

Ch. 4: Maintenance of Life: Nutrition and Transmission

1. Gate of vitality and source qi are two Kidney functions that emerge at GV-4 and CV-4 respectively.

2. Note once again how a point is the conjunction of several functions that, clearly, are not unrelated.

3. It is "thoracic" and said to protect the Lung and Heart. "It controls the interior, not excretion." (*Classic of Difficulties,* No. 31)

4. "It controls excretion and not the interior." (*Classic of Difficulties,* No. 31) It is "pelvic" and protects the Liver and Kidneys.

5. A. Duron, C. Laville Mery, J. Borsarello. *Bioenergetique et médecine chinoise.* Moulins les Metz: Maisonneuve, 1973.

6. Nguyen Van Nghi, *Pathogénie et pathologie énergétique en Médecine chinoise.* Paris: Ed. N.V.N., 1971, p. 446.

7. Op cit.

8. To me the Heart envelope (心包 *xin bao*) can be seen as an agent of the Heart Master (心主 *xin zhu),* as it envelops and protects the Heart Master.

9. This "phlegm" may be material (sputum) or subtle: the latter is involved in some cases of epilepsy, ophthalmic migraines, mental disturbances, etc.

10. Gallbladder—gestational envelopes are of the order of *man.*

11. In Chinese medicine, no distinction is made between bone marrow and the spinal cord, as both are considered 髓 *sui.*

Ch. 5: Channels

1. We will see later that each main channel is divided into two primary channels, one upper, linked to the arm *(shou),* and one lower, linked to the leg *(zu).* They are known as arm *tai yang,* leg *tai yang,* arm *shao yang,* leg *shao yang,* arm *tai yin,* leg *tai yin,* etc.

2. To borrow the words used by Mrs. L. von Benedek, in a lecture. One of the functions of the Lung, associated with the autumn harvest, is to separate from the mother as the fruit separates from the tree.

3. From a seminar given in 1979.

4. I. Robinet, *Méditation taoiste.* Paris: Albin Michel, 1995.

5. These lists of symptoms come from 13 of *Divine Pivot,* as well as my studies with Nguyen Van Nghi and Chamfrault.

6. Nguyen Van Nghi, *Pathogénie et pathologie énergétique en Médecine chinoise.* Paris: Ed. N.V.N., 1971, Ch. 12.

7. Originating, in connection with the source, the origin of life: "When source qi condenses, it is life; when it disperses, it is death." The beginning of a creation (remember that we are recreated with each breath) is marked by the eruption of source qi, the source of life, at this crossroads. We can see how a disturbance in the Penetrating vessel could occur in all the first moments of intra-uterine life, when no authorization to live has been granted by the parents. It leads to great difficulty with emerging into life.

8. A portion of this comes from G. Soulié de Morant, *L' acupuncture chinoise*, Paris: Maloine, 1972, and the remainder from a lecture given in 1990 in Geneva by Dr. Mémé of Barcelona.

Ch. 6: Acupuncture Points

1. A. Chamfrault, *Traité de Médecine chinoise*. Angoulême: Ed. Coquemard, 1964.

2. G. Soulié de Morant, *L'acupuncture chinoise*. Paris: Maloine, 1972.

3. Op cit.

4. Because it controls the exit of *tai yang* qi, this point is of necessity located on a *tai yang* channel; since this exit occurs at the shoulder, it is a *tai yang* channel of the upper limb, arm *tai yang*, called the Small Intestine channel. Experience shows that the qi spreads out along the channel on which the exit point is located. So in a case of cervical-brachial pain linked with a failure of qi to exit at TB-15, there is an excess upstream, a deficiency downstream, and pain along the *shao yang* channels of the arm and leg, in the arm and neck.

5. See below for more about the channel sinews.

Ch. 7: Humans in the Cosmos: the Four Seasons and the Human Body

1. This paragraph takes up ideas expressed in my book *L'homme et ses symbols en MTC*. Paris: Albin Michel, 2002.

2. The quotations concerning the seasons come from *Basic Questions,* 2, translated by Husson (I), and from *Assaisonner les esprits*. Paris: Institut Ricci, 1983.

3. S. J. Wieger, *Caractères chinois: étymologie, graphies, lexique*. Taichung, Taiwan: Kuangchi Press, 1963.

4. There are various aspects to the Heart in Chinese medicine. The two main aspects are referred to schematically as the Heart Sovereign, at the center of the body, and the Heart Master (Pericardium), or Minister of the Heart, that by which the Heart commands, symbolically located in the south, in connection with fire. Naturally, these Heart functions emerge at different points. This corresponds to two different types of fire: central-sovereign fire for the Heart Sovereign, summer-minister fire for the Heart Master.

5. Marcel Granet, *La Pensée chinoise*. Paris: Albin Michel, 1968, p. 286.

6. A. Chamfrault, *Traité de Médecine chinoise*. Angoulême: Ed. Coquemard, 1964.

7. G. Soulié de Morant, *L' acupuncture chinoise*. Paris: Maloine, 1972.

8. Note the coincidence of function and location, in this case the junction between the abdomen and the thorax.

9. A. Chamfrault, ibid.

10. This is the reason why it is an important point of the Penetrating vessel (*see* the section on the extraordinary vessels). We should note in passing the way that several converging functions emerge in line with the same point, which often makes it difficult to find a clinical example that only corresponds to one of these functions.

11. This is from the *Great Compendium of Acupuncture and Moxibustion,* as quoted by Nguyen Van Nghi, *Pathogénie et pathologie énergétique en Médecine chinoise.* Marseille: Ed. N.V.N., 1971.

Ch. 8: Symbolic Language of Chinese Medicine

1. S. J. Wieger, *Caractères chinois: étymologie, graphies, lexique.* Taichung, Taiwan: Kuangchi Press, 1963.

2. "La Terre des Wuwing, cinq agents est Tu, 土 radical de Di."

3. Both of these definitions come from Institut Ricci, ed., *Dictionnaire français de la langue chinoise.* Paris: Institut Ricci-Kuangchi Press, 1976.

4. Lao Tseu, Tchoug Tseu, Lie Tseu, *Philosophes taoistes.* Paris: Gallimard, 1996.

5. The fact that I was old enough to be his father probably contributed to the result as well.

6. *Yuan Shen* is cited in reference to the brain.

7. The Heart is the sun of man. The Spleen corresponds to the earth (土 *tu)* of the five phases. Remember that this is a different word from the earth (地 *di)* in the heaven/earth pair and therefore of the Kidneys, in this case. The Heart and Spleen, central, heliocentric and geocentric, are respectively turned towards the one and the many. This dialogue between sun and earth is different from the heaven/earth relationship discussed above, between the Lung and Spleen.

8. These symbolic locations are obviously not anatomical. As stated in the *Classic of Difficulties,* No. 25, the Triple Burner "has a name but no form."

9. One representation of heaven is a roof with a central opening and two slopes that must be in harmony.

10. Which originates at CV-1, located between the anus and the genitals, on the fibrous central core of the perineum.

11. Here again it should be pointed out: the mechanisms placed under the symbolism of water or fire, etc.

12. Here the number does not reflect an arithmetic calculation: it is symbolic. The Chinese, who had practiced dissection, knew full well that there were two lungs and two kidneys.

13. I. Robinet, *Comprendre le Tao.* Paris: Albin Michel, 2002.

14. S. J. Wieger, ibid.

15. Lao Tseu, ibid.

Ch. 9: Diagnosis and Treatment

1. Jean-Marc Kespi, *L'homme et ses symboles en M.T.C.* Paris: Albin Michel, 2002.

2. Ms. Lisbeth von Benedek, psychoanalyst, during a lecture in 2002.

3. This passage draws from my book, *L'homme et ses symboles en M.T.C.,* ibid.

4. F. Cheng, *Empty and Full: The Language of Chinese Painting.* Boston: Shambala, 1994, pp. 39-40.

5. E. Klein. *Discours sur l'origine de l'univers.* Paris: Flammarion, 2010.

6. I will only discuss the salient aspects of the pulse and a few other findings here that may not be familiar to the reader. Otherwise I refer the reader to the standard works on pulse diagnosis.

Ch. 10: Summary: Ignore the Symptoms and Treat the Person

1. E. Klein, *Discours sur l'origine de l'univers.* Paris: Flammarion, 2010.

BIBLIOGRAPHY & REFERENCE

Medical and Other Chinese Classics

Huang Di Nei Jing Su Wen, A. Husson. Paris: Méridiens, 1987.

Les grands traités du Huainanzi, C. Larre, I. Robinet and E. Rochat de la Vallée. Paris: Institut Ricci, Le Cerf, 1993.

Ling-Shu: Bases de l'acupuncture traditionnelle chinoise, Ming Wong. Paris: Masson, 1997.

Lingshu, C. Milsky, G. Andres. Paris: Ed. de La Tisserande, 2010.

Nan-Ching (The Classic of Difficult Issues), P. Unschuld. Berkeley: University of California Press, 1986.

Philosophes taoïstes, tome 1 : Lao-Tseu, Tchouang-Tseu, Lie-Tseu, Etiemble. Paris: Gallimard, 1980.

Suwen: Les 11 premiers traités, C. Larre and E. Rochat de la Vallée. Moulins les Metz: Maisonneuve, 1993.

Tao Te King : Le livre de la Voie et de la Vertu, Lao Tseu, trans. by C. Larré. Paris: Desclée de Brouwer, 1995.

Zhenjiu jiayin jing Classique ordonné de l'acupuncture, trans. by C. Milsky and G. Andrès. Paris: Guy Trédaniel Éditeur, 2004.

Other References

Chamfrault, A., *Traité de Médecine chinoise.* Angoulême: Ed. Coquemard, 1964.

Cheng, F. *Vide et plein.* Paris: Seuil, 1979.

Granet, M. *La pensée chinoise.* Paris: Renaissance du livre (1934) and Albin Michel (1968).

Guillaume, G., *Dictionnaire des points d'acupuncture.* Paris: Trédaniel–La Tisserande, 1995.

Julien, F. *Procès ou création.* Paris: Seuil, 1989.

Kaltenmark, M. *Lao Tseu et le taoisme.* Paris: Seuil, 1976.

Kespi, J.M. *Acupuncture.* Moulins les Metz: Maisonneuve, 1982.

Robinet, I. *Méditation taoiste.* Paris: Albin Michel, 1995.

Schipper, K. *Le corps taoiste.* Paris: Fayard, 1982.

Soulié de Morant, G. *L'acupuncture chinoise.* Paris: Maloine, 1972.

Traité d'acupuncture de *l'IMTC de Shanghai,* trans. by C. Roustan. Paris: Masson, 1977.

Van Nghi, Nguyen, *Pathogénie et pathologie énergétique en Médecine chinoise.* Marseille: Ed. N.V.N., 1971.

Van Nghi, N., T. Dzung and C. Recours-Nguyen. *Art et pratique de l'acupuncture et de la moxibustion selon Zhen Jiu Da Cheng de Yang Chi Chou.* Marseille: Edition NVN, 1982.

Dictionaries

Institut Ricci, ed., *Dictionnaire français de la langue chinoise.* Paris: Institut Ricci-Kuangchi Press, 1976.

Wieger, S.J., *Caractères chinois : étymologie, graphies, lexique.* Taichung, Taiwan: Kuangchi Press, 1963.

POINT INDEX

Heart channel

(arm *shao yin*)

HT-1 51, 195, **213**

HT-2 113

HT-4 113, 122, 145, 197, **214**

HT-5 62, 65, 78, 99, 145, **214**

HT-6 133, 197, **214**

HT-7 38, 44, 79, 197, **214**

HT-9 79

Heart Master (Pericardium) channel

(arm *jue yin*)

HM-1 32, 49, 65, **227**

HM-2 132, 133, **227**

HM-3 **228**

HM-4 133, 199, **228**

HM-5 65, 197, **228**

HM-6 9, 10, 62, 65, 89, 99, 100, 152, **228**

HM-7 44, 62, 65, 87, **228**

HM-8 62, 65

HM-9 87, **228–229**

Kidney channel

(leg *shao yin*)

KI-1 70, **223**

KI-2 188, **224**

KI-3 29, 33, 62, 63, 101, 102, 115, 127, 177, 186, 188, **224**

KI-4 99, **224**

KI-5 62, 133, **224**

KI-6 89, 96, **224**

KI-7 58

KI-8 89, **224**

KI-9 10, 56, 89, 96, **224**

KI-11 26, 101, **225**

KI-12 26, **225**

KI-13 26, 124, **225**

KI-14 26, 124, **225**

KI-15 17, 18, 26, **225**

KI-16 55, 56, 57, **226**

KI-17 30, 62, 107, **226**

KI-18 17, 101, 102, **226**

KI-20 17, 19, 188, **226**

KI-21 28, 29, 30, **226**

KI-22 23, 24, 119, 122, 199, **226**

KI-23 17, 18, 54, 55, 169, **227**

KI-24 113

KI-25 22, **227**

KI-26 17, 18, 119, **227**

KI-27 24, 32, 33, 116, 119, 120, **227**

Large Intestine channel

(arm *yang ming*)

LI-4 117, **205**

LI-5 62, 63, 116

LI-6 62, 63, 64, 99, 103, 127, 162, **205**

LI-9 62, 63, 132, 133, **205**

LI-10 117, 178, **205**

LI-15 82, 85, 132, 133, **205–206**

LI-17 49, 50, 117, **206**

LI-18 117, 125, **206**

LI-19 125, 127, **206**

Liver channel

(leg *jue yin*)

LR-2 77, 78, **235**

LR-3 194, **235**

LR-4 136, **235–236**

LR-5 77, 79, 100, 148, **236**

LR-6 30, 40, 119, 133, 194, 197, **236**

LR-7 52, **236**

LR-9 73, **236**

LR-10 28, 29, 182, **236**

LR-11 xviii, xx, 24, 116, 132, 133, 136, 194, **236**

LR-13 62, 107, 119, 144, 146, **237**

LR-14 62, 144, 147, 149, 188, **237**

C

L

observing patient's, 185
   three powers, 165
Mother issues
   association with earth, 160
   earth and, 46
   and Governing vessel, 92
   tai yin and, 72
Mother-son rule, 79
Motion sickness, 29
Moxibustion, 190
Muscle cramps, case history, 29–30
Muscles, ethereal soul and, 52–53
Myths and rites (禮 *li*), xv
   and symbolic language, 157

N

Names, association with Governing vessel, 93
Nasal allergies, 32
Natural order, xv, 12, 200
Navel
   heaven and earth correspondences, 161
   tension under, 62–64
Neck
   tension and control needs, 196
   window-of-heaven points, 49
Needling
   asking permission, 185
   assisting organism recall through, 10
   duration, 190
   number of needles, 112
   painlessness in, 189
   treatment basics, 189–190
Neurasthenia, 55
Neuroendocrine systems, 9
Neurological disorders, phlegm and, 58
Neuropathy, case history, 106–107
Nighttime sweating, 150. *See also* Sweating
   case history, 48
   yin deficiency and, 47
Nonactive action (無為 *wu wei*), 183
North, five-phase correspondences, 143
Nothingness (無 *wu*), 183
Nurturing qi (*ying qi*), 46
Nutrition, 43, 171
   and *yang ming* channel, 74
Nutritive and protective qi, 182
Nutritive heat (肓 *huang*), 55
Nutritive heat transport, 56

O

Obsessive-compulsive disorder, xx
Old age, winter and, 143
Opening points, 9
   Girdle vessel, 105, 114
   Yang Linking vessel, 114
Openness, channels linked to, 108
Ophthalmic migraines, 47, 58
Opposite side, treating, 195
Organ drainage, points for, 17–19
Organ dysfunction, evocation through dreams, 186
Organ impairment, diagnosis, 14
Organ qi, 14
Organ symptoms, 14–15
Organic lesions, 181
   irreversible, xx–xxi
   reversible, xix
Organs, three powers symbology, 165–166
Orifices, communication through, 12
Original qi (*yuan qi*), 46
Original spirit (*yuan shen*), 67
Outlaw metaphor, 101
Overall qi disturbance, 47
Overall yin/yang stagnation, 47
Overeating, case history, 106
Overexcited speech, 39
Overflowing pulse, in summer, 187
Overwork, case history, 181

P

Pain
   accessibility to psyche, 201
   aggravated by fall, 197–198
   from barometric pressure changes, 51
   barrier points approach, 127
   blood-related, 46
   from deficiency of yin, 128
   from excess of yang, 128
   from excess of yin, 128
   fixed and stabbing, 54
   pulsatile, 46–47
   radiation to foot, 136
   right-sided case history, 113–114
   role in diagnosis, 128
   seeking non-local causes of, 193
   from stagnation, 69, 128

Q

Qi
  barrier points encouraging circulation of, 127
  in Chinese medicine, 3–4
  externalization of, 22–23
  failure to rise from Spleen/Kidneys, 34
  as mechanism, 3
  overall disturbance of, 47
  poor exit from trunk, 68
  as process, 3
  pulse diagnosis, 187
  rising from Kidneys, 172, 173
  symbolic correspondences, 168
  as Triple Burner product, 46–47
Qi barrier, 135
Qi blockage/obstruction, 4, 128, 135
  above, 101
  case history, 137–138
  in center, case history, 146
  unblocking point, 40
Qi breakdowns, 52–53
Qi circulation, Liver and, 14
Qi constraint, 52
  case history, 149–150
Qi counterflow. *See* Counterflow
Qi deficiencies
  and cold zones, 186
  in Lower Burner, 163
  points for, 14–17
Qi emergence, in spring, 140
Qi failure to descend, 57, 63, 176–177
  case history, 63
Qi failure to return, 154
Qi headaches, 46
  case history, 46–47
Qi meeting point, 119
Qi movements
  in autumn, 142, 152
  defect in ascending/descending, 31
  dreams of flying and, 32
  evocation through dreams, 186
  in organs, 31–35
  pulse signs, 188
  in summer, 142
  in winter, 142, 153
Qi obstruction
  as root of pathology, 9

by seven emotions, 180–181
Qi pathologies, 47–49
  overall qi disturbance, 47
  overall yin/yang deficiency, 47
  overall yin/yang stagnation, 47
  regional/local circulatory problems, 49
Qi phases, diaphragm points by, 62
Qi problems, points for, 15
Qi reserves, KI-3 pulse as indicator, 186
Qi storage, in winter, 142, 153
Qi vessels, 11

R

Radial artery pulse, 186
Rage, 41
  expression through Lung, 23
Rapid pulse, 187
Raw vegetables, 38, 39
Reactive elimination, 28
Reactivity, 77
Reality, particle *versus* vibrational aspects, 1
Recall, 180. *See also* Body memory
  assisting by needling, 10
  as function of acupuncture points, 112
Receiving fullness (承满 *cheng man*), 36
Regional disturbances, 112
  causing local problems, 193–195
  importance of context, 195–198
  understanding the person in, 199–200
Regulatory functions, of eight extraordinary vessels, 88, 89
Relationship breakups, 65, 149
Relationships, 8, 201
  Chinese medicine emphasis on, 200
  in Chinese thought, 1
  primacy of, 3
Relativity, 2
Renal colic, case history, 96
Resolve (志 *zhi*), 26
  case history, 27–28
  disorder of, 28
Resonances, 8
Respiratory allergies, case history, 17–18
Respiratory problems, case history, 163
Return the fire, 20
Reversible organic lesions, xix–xx
  acupuncture for, 16